Author
Paul Nicolazzo

Medical Editor
Andrew Ross, MD

Copy Editors
Kyle Branin
Ryan Conklin
Christine Jacobsen
Sarah Kaye
Katrina Michaelis
Joan Strobel
Susan Waters
John Winkley
Beth Wolff

Illustrations
Amanda Joubert
Paul Nicolazzo

Layout
Paul Nicolazzo

Cover Photo
Larry Goldie

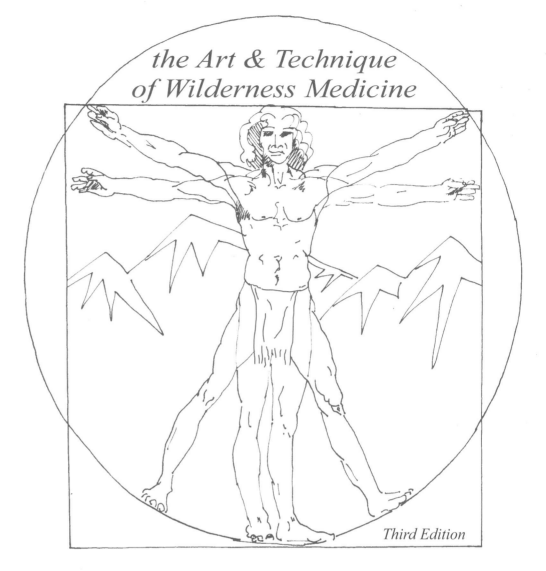

the Art & Technique of Wilderness Medicine

Third Edition

Publisher
the Wilderness Medicine Training Center Inc.
POB 11
Winthrop, WA 98862
URL: www.wildmedcenter.com
509.996.2502
office@wildmedcenter.com
© 2014 by Paul Nicolazzo
ISBN 978-0-9670228-6-4

CONTENTS

CONTENTS

CONTENTS

SECTION I

Introduction

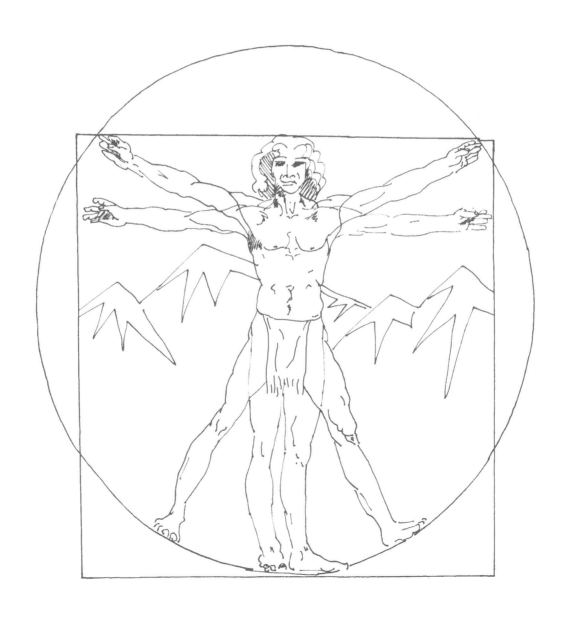

Introduction
General Information

Medicine is a blend of art and technique. Skills in both areas are acquired through rigorous training, practice, and insight. Your ability to use the information within these pages is directly related to your skill level. The techniques described and illustrated in the text require training, practice and experience in order to be effective; they are based on the practice guidelines published by the Wilderness Medical Society and position papers published by the National Association of EMS Physicians. Some of the recommended treatments should only be undertaken under the supervision of a licensed physician. You are encouraged to take an in-depth course in wilderness medicine, to solicit the advice of a licensed physician where necessary, and to remain current with developing information. Neither the author, editors, or publisher assume any liability for any injury, illness, or damage to persons or property arising from the use or misuse of the information contained in this text. For state-of-the-art courses in wilderness medicine, contact the Wilderness Medicine Training Center via their website at http://www.wildmedcenter.com.

The primary focus of this text is expedition medicine. That said, practitioners of rescue medicine and those working in remote clinics will find much of the information contained herein useful. While the three practices are related, there are also critical differences between them: Expedition medicine relies on prevention, early assessment, prompt field treatment and safe, yet often rapid, evacuation. Rescue medicine depends on effective communication and dispatch procedures, rapid deployment, assessment, field treatment and evacuation. Rescue teams tend to bring advanced care and equipment to the scene and are generally able to provide transport shortly after their arrival. In contrast, resources available to expeditions are limited and emergency evacuation, if possible, is often delayed. Harsh environments, difficult terrain, limited space and often severe weight restrictions prevent transportation and use of most standard pre-hospital equipment and medications. Hence, expedition medics and trip leaders require a deeper knowledge of the body's structure and function to effectively prevent, assess and treat the injuries and illnesses they encounter in the field. While healthcare providers at remote field clinics *may* have access to more sophisticated equipment and drugs, they may also be short-staffed, resource shy, and benefit from the improvisation techniques described in the text.

How to Use This Book

This textbook was written for advanced courses in wilderness medicine taught by the Wilderness Medicine Training Center and was designed to integrate smoothly with our course material. With a focus on understanding anatomy, physiology and pathophysiology, and with the inclusion of clear full-color diagrams and photographs of difficult-to-visualize problems, it is the most complete and easily understood lay textbook available. The Wilderness Medicine Training Center's waterproof, tear-proof, and pocket-sized field manual, *the Wilderness Medicine Handbook*, provides a useful summary of key information found in this text and can be purchased online at http://www.wildmed-center.com/store.html.

Major topics covered in the text are listed in the Contents. Specific problems can be located using the Problem and Treatment Index in Section XIII at the end of the book. Section II discusses legal issues surrounding wilderness medicine, according to United States law; if you work within the United States, read this section. Section III is devoted to normal anatomy and physiology: The better you understand how your body is "supposed" to work, the better equipped you will be to respond when it doesn't. Section IV is devoted to understanding our patient assessment system and Section V describes basic life support. Sections VI through IX are the specific problem-based sections. The first three problem-based sections correspond to one of the three mechanisms of injury or illness (MOI): Traumatic Injuries, Environmental Injuries and Illnesses, and Medical Illnesses; the fourth section is devoted to Infectious Diseases. Section X discusses basic pharmacological principles and includes drug and herb tables for many of the problems listed in the text. Section XI discusses expedition first aid kits in a unique and practical way. Section XII summarizes common medical abbreviations and symbols and Section XIII contains the Problem and Treatment Index.

About the Author

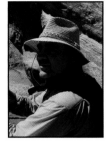 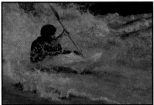

Paul Nicolazzo

Paul Nicolazzo is a widely respected professional in the outdoor field with over thirty-five years experience leading trips, training staff, and designing and managing outdoor programs. An EMT for 38 years, he has worked for a number of ski patrols and technical rescue teams across the country. He has been teaching wilderness medicine since 1987 and is the Director and President of the Wilderness Medicine Training Center, Inc. An articulate and sought-after speaker, Paul presents annually at national outdoor education and recreation conferences. His professional writing includes *the Art & Technique of Wilderness Medicine*, *Case Studies in Wilderness Medicine*, *the Wilderness Medicine Handbook*, *Effective Outdoor Program Design & Management*, *the Site Management Handbook*, numerous articles, and a weekly blog on the WMTC website. He has extensive technical and field expertise in general mountaineering, ski mountaineering, rock climbing, canyoneering, and all inland whitewater and expedition paddle and rowing sports. He has a number of kayak, canoe, and ski first descents coupled with a few remote climbing first ascents in his skills résumé. Paul plays outside with his son whenever possible and continues to teach medical and risk-management courses at the WMTC classroom in Mazama, WA and elsewhere.

Note from the Author

In this text I've tried to be selective and yet include most everything about wilderness medicine that I've found helpful over the years as a student, world traveler, expedition member, trip leader, outdoor program supervisor, and wilderness medicine instructor. The balance between just enough and way too much anatomy, physiology, pathophysiology and even problems seems to me impossible to strike. There is a lot of information here. For those of you who find the depth of anatomy and physiology on the "way too much" side of things, simply skip those parts. For those who find it's not enough, I suggest taking an anatomy and physiology course from a nursing or medical school; and if you are a visual learner, one with a cadaver lab. For those who want to know general concepts, focus on those. For those who want more, consider advanced training as a herbalist, paramedic, nurse, physician assistant, physician (naturopathic, osteopathic, allopathic, oriental, etc.). Seriously.

Please keep in mind that both the art and technique of wilderness medicine are constantly changing. As evolving research expands our understanding of how the human body works, as new drugs, treatments, and technologies are developed, these changes will refine what we carry and how we respond. Fortunately, I keep learning. Unfortunately, this book won't reflect all the new stuff...until the next edition. Remember to double check all the information here with reliable sources for updates; this is especially important when it comes to drugs and their uses. It's taken me a lifetime to learn this much; I hope it takes you far less.

About the Medical Editor

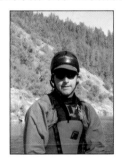

Drew Ross M.D.

Drew is a paddler, skier, climber, and mountaineer. He graduated from Lewis and Clark College where he was active in their outing club. After spending several years as an itinerant guide and Outward Bound instructor, he began teaching courses for the Wilderness Medicine Training Center Inc. Teaching wilderness medicine sparked a dormant gene—his father is a pathologist—and nine years later he graduated with honors from Oregon Health & Science University in Portland to pursue a career in medicine. Drew's unique résumé—college outdoor club leader, Outward Bound instructor, professional guide, wilderness medicine instructor, and physician—makes him well suited to edit a text on wilderness and expedition medicine.

SECTION II

Medical Legal Considerations in Wilderness Medicine

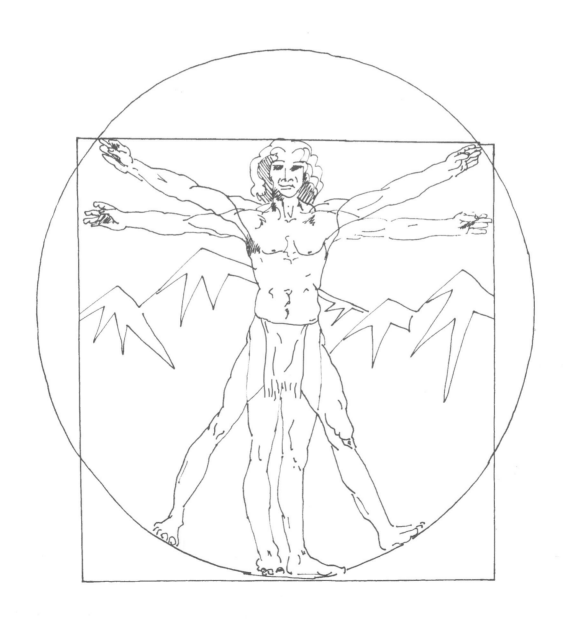

Medical Legal Considerations in Wilderness Medicine

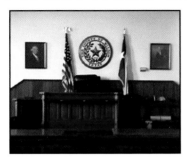

Wilderness medicine is a relatively new form of medicine that emerged with the increase in wilderness travel (and subsequent injuries) in the mid 1980s. Wilderness Medicine is defined as the skills necessary to prevent, assess and treat injuries or illness in a prolonged pre-hospital setting. Since assessment and treatment often occur in severe environments with minimal facilities available, practitioners require a broader range of knowledge and skills than those offered by standard urban medical courses. The United States legal system is complex. The following paragraphs outline some of the legal concepts you should be aware of whether you are a guide, outdoor instructor, Search and Rescue (SAR) team member, or simply part of the general public.

Substantive versus Procedural Law

Conceptually our legal system is divided into substantive and procedural law. Substantive law dictates the rules people should follow within a given society, essentially how they should act. Procedural law dictates how a person is treated after they break a law, essentially the procedure that is followed.

Criminal versus Civil Law

The legal system is also divided into criminal and civil law. Criminal law prohibits specific acts (theft, murder, assault, etc.) and sets a range of punishments for violations. The intent is for the severity of the punishment (imprisonment, fine, etc.) to match the severity of the crime. A violation of criminal law requires that the government bring charges against the defendant and prove guilt beyond a reasonable doubt. Law enforcement is a branch of criminal pro-

cedural law. Instead of prohibiting specific acts, civil law dictates what a "reasonable" person's conduct should be in a given situation. Violations of civil law are not punished but the violators may be required to provide compensation for damages. Any given act may violate criminal law, civil law, or both, depending on the act and circumstances; however, a person cannot be judged in violation of civil law if there is a criminal law prohibiting the act. Contract law and tort law are two subdivisions of civil law that relate to wilderness medicine practitioners.

Contract Law

Contract law is the area of civil law that deals with agreements between people and/or organizations. Contracts may be expressed or implied, written or oral. A person may bring a civil suit against a person or organization if they think a contract has been breached or broken.

Tort Law

Social responsibility dictates that people within a given society have a duty to act reasonably towards one another. Tort law is the area of civil law that deals with injury or damage to people and property as a result of a person's "unreasonable" actions. Injured persons are entitled to compensation for the damages caused by the defendant's unreasonable conduct. The standard for what is considered "reasonable" is usually set by the defendant's profession and called the "standard of practice."

Standards of Practice

There are two standards of practice commonly applied to cases involving wilderness medicine. One pertains to sponsoring organizations (outfitters, schools, etc.) and the other to individual caregivers. An organization or individual who fails to meet their standards of practice may be in violation of criminal law, civil law, or both. Organizations are held to the industry standards of their profession as defined by committees within their respective industry and/or by the state where the organization operates. Industry standards usually dictate the minimum level of training, certification, and/or licensure required for the organization's staff. They may also include requirements or recommendations for expedition equipment. In general, an organization sponsoring a trip into a remote area is responsible for providing adequate medical care until the patient has entered the local health care system. The Wilderness Medical Society (WMS), a nonprofit physician and professional organization, reviews, endorses, and publishes practice guidelines for wilderness medicine. While the WMS does not offer certifications in wilderness medicine, they do hold annual conferences in wilderness medicine that are approved for continuing medical education credit for physicians, nurses, and EMTs. Similar conferences are also held by other national organizations. The National Association of Emergency Room Physicians (NAEMSP) has published a series of position papers that address advanced skills performed in a wilderness environment. Care rendered by wilderness medicine providers is likely to be held to the practice guidelines established by the WMS and the position papers published by the NAEMSP. Training, certification, and standing orders/protocols should be in alignment with both industry and medical standards of practice and should be reviewed regularly.

Duty to Act

Duty to act (in this case to provide reasonable medical care) is defined by law. How you should act is defined by your profession's standard of practice (as described above), your training, certification, the protocols set by your medical advisor, and state and federal laws. In most cases wilderness medicine providers have been sued for a failure to act rather than for their actions. You have a duty to act if:

- You have a prior relationship with the person.
- The person is under your direct care.
- The person is a participant in an activity you have been hired to instruct or supervise.
- You have entered into a contractual agreement to provide medical services.

If you are a guide or trip leader, you have a duty to provide medical care to trip participants under your direct care.

Good Samaritan Laws

To encourage trained people to act in emergencies when they do not have a duty to act, most states have enacted "Good Samaritan" laws that protect physicians and health care providers against simple negligence. They do not protect against gross or willful negligence. In order to be protected by Good Samaritan laws, the aid must be unscheduled and

unplanned and it must be provided at or near the scene where the illness or injury occurred. The provider must act without compensation and outside of their normal scope of employment. They must also have consent from and not abandon their patient(s). In emergencies, consent is usually implied. Implied consent may be indicated by a patient's lack of resistance prior to and during treatment. It may also be indicated by the situation. Patients with a normal mental status have the right to refuse treatment. Once aid has begun, medical providers are under a legal obligation to see that it continues until the patient is no longer in danger. Based on their training, a medical provider is also expected to anticipate and plan for common problems that may arise en route to definitive care. Abandonment occurs when a patient's care is terminated prematurely and they suffer subsequent harm as a result of the lack of treatment. Leaving a patient to go for help is NOT considered abandonment.

Increasing Your Legal Umbrella

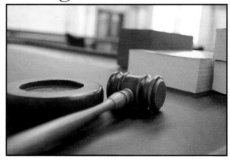

The law requires only what a reasonable patient would require in similar circumstances and protects medical providers who act according to their training and in the best interests of their patient. For a defendant's action(s) to be labeled unreasonable and the plaintiff to prevail in a civil suit, the plaintiff must prove four things:

- That the defendant had a duty to act;
- That the defendant did not adhere to the standard of practice of their profession (negligence);
- That the plaintiff suffered a loss or injury; and
- That the plaintiff's loss or injury was caused by the defendant's negligence.

If a court finds against a defendant, the defendant may be required to pay damages consistent with the plaintiff's injury or loss as determined by

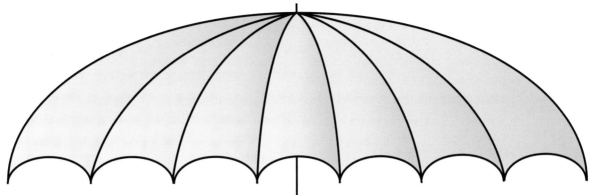

Increasing Your Legal Umbrella

Institutional

- Meet or exceed Industry standards.
- Use Participant Release and Assumption of Risk forms.
- Have an active medical control physician who provides oversight and protocols.
- Have your staff trained and certified by a nationally accepted provider according to WMS and NAEMSP Practice Guidelines.
- Ensure field and follow-up documentation using SOAP format.
- Ensure emergency field communication.
- Have an Emergency Action Plan.
- Follow state and federal laws.

Individual

- Keep your certification current.
- Maintain your skills.
- Accurately document what happened, the patient's signs and symptoms, your assessment, and your treatment/evacuation plan using the SOAP format.
- Follow your organization's protocols.
- Follow state and federal laws.

the judge and/or jury. Given the above information, there are a number of things organizations and individuals can do to increase the size of their legal umbrella (amount of legal protection) before an illness or injury occurs.

Institutions

While it may not be feasible to enact all the recommendations on this list, the more you can do, the greater your legal protection. Needless to say, make sure you have adequate liability insurance. Consider rescue and evacuation insurance, especially for third world countries.

- The sponsoring organization should be aware of and meet or exceed the industry standards for their profession.
- Have all participants sign a release form giving advance permission for the sponsoring organization's staff to render appropriate aid in the event of

injury or illness. If prescription drugs are to be carried and used, participants and their personal physicians should grant permission for their use as per the organization's protocols or provide alternative field treatments and protocols for the individual in question. The form should also acknowledge that the participant is aware of, accepts, and releases the sponsoring organization and its staff from the risks associated with the activity. The release form is a contractual agreement and should be drawn up by an attorney licensed in the state where the business is registered or licensed.

- The sponsoring organization should employ a physician advisor that is aware of the WMS and NAEMSP standards and acts in an active advisory capacity. In the absence of direct on-line control via radio or cell phone, the medical advisor should issue written "standing orders" or "protocols" appropriate to the staff's certification and the activities and environmental conditions likely to be encountered during the sponsoring organization's trips.

- Staff should be trained and certified by an organization that teaches according to the WMS practice guidelines, the Wilderness First Aid & Wilderness First Responder Scope of Practice documents, and the NAEMSP position papers.

- Staff should document their patient care in a standardized SOAP format that includes: time, dates, a description of the mechanism of injury, environmental conditions, a detailed patient history, the staff's assessment, treatment and evacuation plans, and changes in the patient's condition while still under their care. If it isn't written down, it is difficult, and often impossible, to prove. Judges and juries generally place greater weight on field notes written during the incident than on notes recorded after the patient has passed from the staff's care. It is also important for staff to document a patient's refusal of treatment. Many SAR organizations, ambulance squads, ski patrols, etc. require a patient to sign a contractual document releasing them of all liability from damages resulting from a refusal of treatment. Such a document is usually signed in the presence of a witness who in turn signs as well.

- If the geographic area and finances permit, organizations should carry cell or satellite phones for emergency communication and have an assigned on-call person, preferably a physician familiar with the program, available at all times.

- Have an Emergency Action Plan (EAP) with detailed procedures and contact information (names, phone numbers, addresses and directions to health care facilities, location of pre-placed evacuation vehicles, etc.).

- Have a licensed attorney work with your physician advisor to assure that the organization is aware of and compliant with all state and federal laws.

Individuals

If you are going to work professionally in the outdoors, you should keep current with all recommendations on this list. That said, outdoor work is both seasonal and transient making keeping track of state and federal laws extremely difficult; do the best that you can.

- It is important to keep your certifications current. You have invested a lot of time, energy, and money into your certifications and training. Maintain them.

- Most wilderness medicine providers certify you based on an evaluation of your skills during a training course and do NOT warrant that you will be able to perform at that level during an actual emergency. It's up to you to maintain and improve your skills. This may mean taking a refresher course before your actual certification expires, retaking your original course, or seeking work within the outdoor medical field where you will gain experience, such as ski patrol, bike patrol, local Search and Rescue teams, etc.

- Make sure you are familiar with your organization's rules for documentation. Carry your own Patient SOAP note if your organization does not provide one. Alternately, get permission to use the one you prefer. Always keep a copy of your own field notes; they are a legal document and go a long way to verifying your thoughts and actions at the time of the incident.

- Make sure you understand and follow your organization's protocols. Consider carrying an approved medical field manual.

- Make sure you understand and follow state and federal laws. Be aware that laws often vary from state to state and may change at any time.

8 *Medical Legal Considerations*

SECTION III

General Concepts in Human Anatomy & Physiology

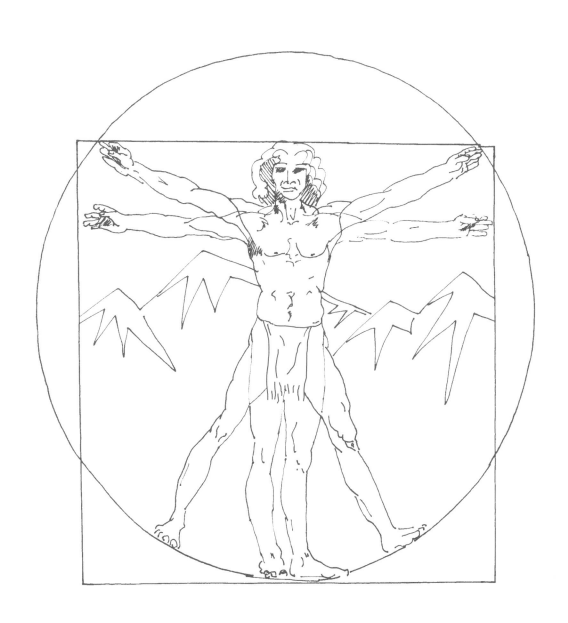

General Concepts in Human Anatomy & Physiology

Introduction

Human anatomy is the study of the physical parts of the human body and their relationship to each other; human physiology is the study of their functions. The collective goal for each of the body's systems is to maintain a balance between the body and its environment. Biologically, this balancing act is known as homeostasis. Built into each complex body system are numerous compensating mechanisms that work to correct problems before they become critical. If any problem overwhelms the body's compensatory mechanisms, outside intervention is necessary to tilt the balance in favor of healing.

Problem
Compensatory Mechanisms

Homeostasis

Levels of Organization

The human body contains many parts, both small and large; all are interdependent, and damage to one part affects the entire system. At the chemical level, atoms make up molecules. The shape of each molecule determines its function. Molecules can be organic or inorganic and combine to form the individual parts of a cell (organelles). As such, a change in body chemistry may alter cell function. Cells are the smallest living components of the human body; they behave like tiny organisms and act independently to maintain homeostasis with the body's internal environment. Similar cells working together form tissue. Tissue function, like cellular function, is specialized. Multiple types of tissue work together to form organs, while multiple organs work together to form organ systems. Organ systems work together to make up the body. Each level of organization has its own specific, and somewhat restricted, set of functions.

In general, gross functions are carried out by individual organs and organ systems. Structurally, fluids and gases are transported between organs and systems via tubes. Blood, for example, travels throughout the body in the tubes of the circulatory system. Oxygen enters and carbon dioxide leaves the body through air tubes, as part of the respiratory system. Digestive, excretory, and reproductive systems all rely on tubes for transporting both fluids and solids. Control and integration are provided by the brain, as its messages are conducted throughout the body via nerves. *In its simplest form, the major components of the human body are organs, tubes, and nerves.*

Water, Fluid Spaces, & Stuff Sacks

All living cells are in contact with body fluids, and all body fluids contain water. As such, water accounts for approximately 65% of the body's total weight and is arguably its most important compound. The majority of the body's chemical reactions take place in water. Water is an excellent solvent capable of dissolving numerous chemical compounds. Water is also an essential reactant in and by-product of cellular metabolism. It is both an input in chemical reactions that break down specific compounds in the cell, as well as a by-product of cellular reactions that build the specialized compounds required for life. The chemical reactions necessary to maintain life occur within a narrow temperature range. Since water has an enormous capacity for holding and transferring heat, it plays a key role in regulating body temperature. Water retains its liquid form throughout a broad range of temperatures. This property, combined with the small size of its molecules, enables it to pass freely through most body membranes and effectively transport molecular compounds , such as nutrients, wastes, and toxins, throughout the body.

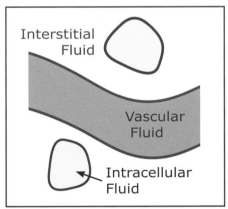

There are three basic types of fluid and fluid spaces within the human body: vascular, tissue, and cellular. Vascular spaces contain blood, plasma, and lymph; tissue spaces are filled with interstitial

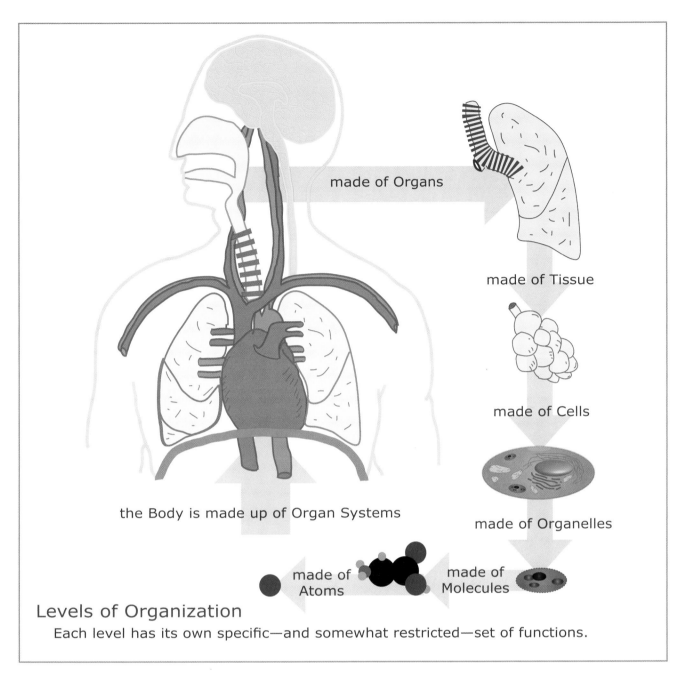

made of Organs

made of Tissue

made of Cells

made of Organelles

the Body is made up of Organ Systems

made of Atoms

made of Molecules

Levels of Organization
Each level has its own specific—and somewhat restricted—set of functions.

fluid; and, cells contain intracellular fluid. Solutes and structures contained in each of the three fluid matrices are slightly different and help to define the density and characteristics of each. Blood, plasma, and lymph have the consistency of vegetable juice, interstitial fluid is syrupy, while intracellular fluid is gel-like. Extracellular fluid (vascular and extracellular fluid) contains high levels of sodium (Na^+) and chloride (Cl^-) ions, while intracellular fluid contains high levels of potassium (K^+) and protein (A^-) ions. Any significant change in the volume or chemical composition of the fluids in any of the spaces will affect overall body chemistry and homeostasis.

Each of the body's components—cells, tissues,

organs, body cavities—and the body collectively and individually, is surrounded by a membrane. Structural proteins attach each component to one another. Essentially, everything in the body is in "stuff sacks" and "on-belay." Membranes serve to separate, contain, and protect. Increases in membrane permeability encourage fluid or gas movement across the membrane in accordance with the pressure and concentration gradients.

Swelling indicates structural damage and is caused by one of two mechanisms: bleeding or edema. Bleeding occurs when blood vessels are broken. Blood leaks from the damaged vessels into the local tissue spaces until the pressure is equalized

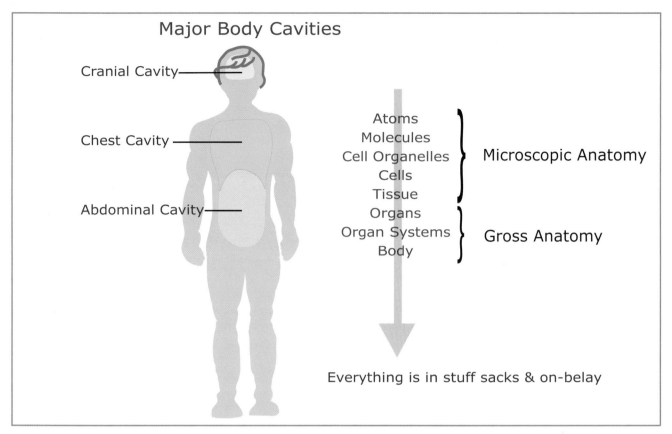

Major Body Cavities

Cranial Cavity

Chest Cavity

Abdominal Cavity

Atoms
Molecules
Cell Organelles } Microscopic Anatomy
Cells
Tissue
Organs
Organ Systems } Gross Anatomy
Body

Everything is in stuff sacks & on-belay

and is referred to as a hematoma or bruise. Edema occurs when plasma (not blood cells) leaks into tissue spaces due to an increase in vascular permeability. Numerous mechanisms, each discussed in depth later in the text, may lead to increased vascular permeability and subsequent edema: altitude, a weak heart, poor muscle tone, inflammatory response, etc. If the structures of the body are viewed as cells, tissue, organs, and organ systems, where fluids and gases are transported through tubes, the concept of "stuff sacks" has clinical significance. If a rupture or leak occurs in any tube or stuff sack, the leak is contained within the next largest stuff sack. *This idea is perhaps the single most important concept in understanding the pathophysiology of most traumatic injuries (Section VI).*

Basic Chemistry

Atoms are the smallest components of matter and can chemically bond to one another to create molecules. Chemical reactions between molecules alter the shape and properties of matter while leaving the atoms essentially unaffected. Atoms are comprised of neutrons, protons, and electrons. Neutrons and protons make up the nucleus, or core, of the atom. Electrons orbit around the nucleus in a

prescribed cloud or shell. Each electron shell holds a fixed number of electrons. If the outermost shell is full, the atom will NOT react with other atoms. ONLY atoms with space in their outermost electron shell are available to participate in chemical reactions. Atoms bond to one another by sharing electrons with another atom, accepting electrons from another atom, or donating electrons to another atom. Once their outermost electron shell is full, they are unavailable for further reactions.

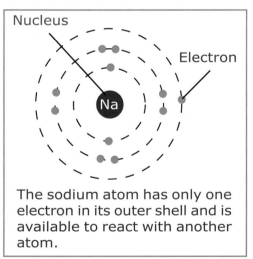

The sodium atom has only one electron in its outer shell and is available to react with another atom.

Energy is stored in chemical bonds. Cells break the chemical bonds in food to release energy. They

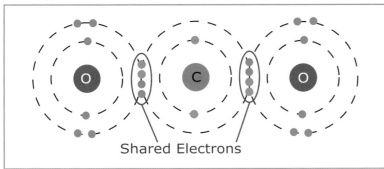

Covalent Bond

In carbon dioxide (CO_2), the electrons are equally shared and the atoms remain electrically neutral.

Shared Electrons

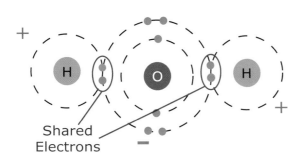

Polar Covalent Bond

In water (H_2O), the electrons are NOT shared equally and spend more time orbiting the oxygen atom than the hydrogen atoms. As a result, the oxygen atom becomes slightly negatively charged and both hydrogen atoms become slightly positively charged.

Shared Electrons

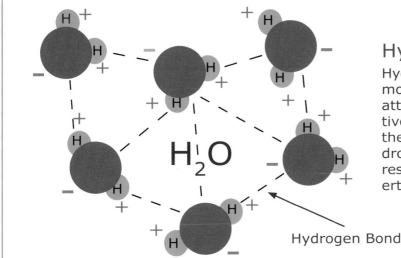

H_2O

Hydrogen Bond

Hydrogen Bonds

Hydrogen bonds form between water molecules because of the electrical attraction between the weak negative charge of the oxygen atom and the weak positive charge of the hydrogen atom. This hydrogen bond is responsible for the evaporative properties and surface tension of water.

capture and use the energy to construct many of the molecules necessary to create and maintain life. Excess energy is released as heat.

There are three types of chemical bonds: covalent bonds, hydrogen bonds, and ionic bonds (refer to the above diagram). When atoms share electrons, they form covalent bonds. Covalent bonds are the strongest of the three types of atomic bonds and therefore store the most energy; the more electrons shared, the stronger the bond. Covalent bonds are formed and broken in the process of cellular metabolism. Metabolism provides cells with the energy required to grow and to maintain homeostasis.

Most atoms in covalent bonds remain electrical-ly neutral because the electrons are shared equally. In some cases, water is one example, unequal sharing of the electrons results in slight electrical charges within the molecule known as a polar covalent bond. The weak charges are not strong enough to create separate new molecules. However, they can alter the shape of a given molecule and are sufficient to pull other charged molecules together. When hydrogen forms polar covalent bonds with oxygen, the hydrogen bonds that form between water molecules are responsible for the unique surface tension of water and its rather slow evaporative properties.

Protons have a positive electrical charge, electrons have a negative electrical charge, and neutrons have no charge. Atoms are electrically neutral as long as the number of protons equals the number of electrons. Atoms or molecules become electrically charged when they give up or receive electrons. Atoms or molecules with an electrical charge are called ions. An ionic bond is formed when one atom donates one or more electrons to another. The atom donating the electron becomes positively charged while the atom receiving the electron becomes negatively charged. The two atoms remain next to each other after the electron transfer because the opposing electrical charges attract one another. Ionic compounds break into their individual ions when dissolved in water. The slight electrical charges within each water molecule, a result of the polar covalent bonds that form the molecule, keep them apart as long as they remain in solution.

Mineral Salts & Electrolytes

Mineral salts are inorganic ionic compounds, excluding acids and bases, that disassociate in water to release their respective ions. They are naturally occurring elements and work with enzymes to maintain homeostasis. During digestion, they are coated with a protein molecule (chelated) to aid in their absorption. Large amounts of fiber eaten along with mineral salts inhibit the chelating process and restrict mineral absorption.

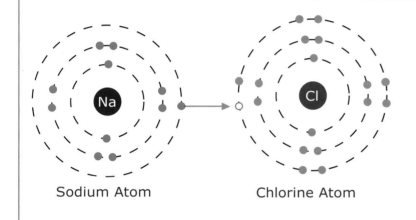

Sodium Atom   Chlorine Atom

Ionic Bond

The sodium atom donates an electron to the chloride atom leaving the outer electron shells of both atoms full.

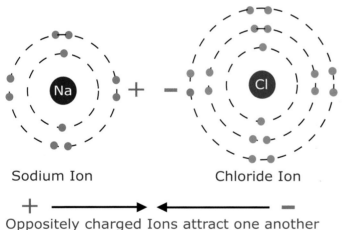

Sodium Ion   Chloride Ion

+ ⟶ ⟵ −
Oppositely charged Ions attract one another

After donating an electron, the sodium atom has a positive charge because it has one more proton than electrons. After receiving an electron, the chloride atom has one more electron than proton giving it a negative charge and becoming the chloride ion.

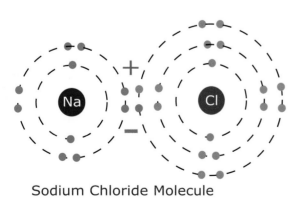

Sodium Chloride Molecule

Opposite charges attract creating the sodium chloride molecule. The molecule disassociates when dissolved in water. The weak negative charges in the oxygen atoms of water are attracted to the positive charges in the sodium ion and the weak positive charges in the hydrogen atoms of water are attracted to the negatively charged chloride ion. The difference in electrical charges keeps the ions apart as long as they remain in solution.

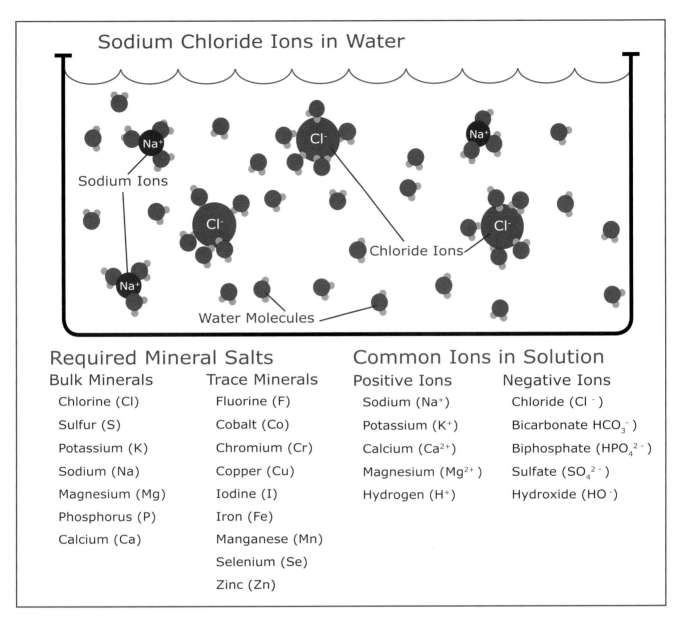

Sodium Chloride Ions in Water

Sodium Ions

Chloride Ions

Water Molecules

Required Mineral Salts

Bulk Minerals
Chlorine (Cl)

Sulfur (S)

Potassium (K)

Sodium (Na)

Magnesium (Mg)

Phosphorus (P)

Calcium (Ca)

Trace Minerals
Fluorine (F)

Cobalt (Co)

Chromium (Cr)

Copper (Cu)

Iodine (I)

Iron (Fe)

Manganese (Mn)

Selenium (Se)

Zinc (Zn)

Common Ions in Solution

Positive Ions
Sodium (Na^+)

Potassium (K^+)

Calcium (Ca^{2+})

Magnesium (Mg^{2+})

Hydrogen (H^+)

Negative Ions
Chloride (Cl^-)

Bicarbonate HCO_3^-)

Biphosphate (HPO_4^{2-})

Sulfate (SO_4^{2-})

Hydroxide (HO^-)

Ions capable of carrying an electrical charge when in solution are called electrolytes. All mineral salts are electrolytes. Changes in the concentration of electrolytes in the extra and intracellular fluids will disrupt all body functions and, if severe, lead to death. While calcium and phosphate ions are stored in bone, most mineral salts are excreted in urine and require frequent replacement. Many diseases may be traced to a lack of specific minerals and the adverse-effects reversed if detected early. Sodium is the primary electrolyte in the extra cellular fluid, while potassium is the primary electrolyte in the intracellular fluid. Both are crucial materials for maintaining water balance within the body and hence, neurological function. Together with glucose, which is required for electrolyte absorption, sodium and potassium are the major components in all oral rehydration salt (ORS) preparations used to treat dehydration. (Dehydration and ORS preparations are discussed in more detail in Section VII, Environmental Injuries and Illnesses.)

Acids, Bases, & pH

Hydrogen has only one electron in its electron shell and regularly donates it to other atoms creating an EXTREMELY reactive positive ion with one proton. *Acids are compounds that break down in solution to release hydrogen ions, while bases bind with hydrogen ions and remove them from solution.*

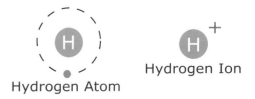

Hydrogen Atom

Hydrogen Ion

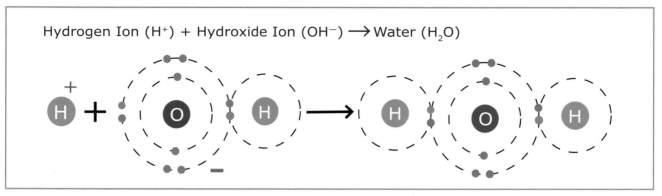

Hydrogen Ion (H⁺) + Hydroxide Ion (OH⁻) ⟶ Water (H₂O)

Many common bases dissociate in solution to form a hydroxide ion (OH^-); hydroxide ions readily combine with hydrogen ions (H^+) to form water ($OH^- + H^+ \longrightarrow H_2O$).

pH is an abbreviation that stands for "potential of Hydrogen." The pH of a solution is measured by a logarithmic scale designed so that the large values of the hydrogen ions present in a given solution correspond to small values in the scale. The scale varies from 0 to 14. The lower the number, the greater the concentration of hydrogen ions present in the solution. Each change in pH value represents a tenfold change in the concentration of hydrogen ions. Therefore, small changes in pH reflect huge changes in the number of ions present. The pH of water is 7 and the number of hydrogen ions in solution equals the number of hydroxide ions. Solutions having pH lower than 7 are acidic and those having pH above 7 are considered basic. ***An excess of hydrogen ions (acid) can upset the stability of cell membranes, break chemical bonds, and change the structure of proteins.*** Normal blood pH varies between 7.35 and 7.45; variation of 0.5 pH units outside this normal range can be fatal.

In order for the body to remain in balance the concentration of hydrogen ions in the body fluids (pH) must be carefully regulated. There are three processes responsible for balancing pH in the human body: chemical buffering, respiration, and renal (kidney) filtration.

Hydrogen Ions   Hydroxide Ions

pH Regulatory Processes
1) Chemical Buffering
2) Respiration (rate of)
3) Renal Filtration

Carbon Dioxide (CO_2), a byproduct of cellular metabolism, combines with water to produce carbonic acid, which promptly dissociates in solution to release a hydrogen ion and a bicarbonate ion ($H_2O + CO_2 \longleftrightarrow H_2CO_3 \longleftrightarrow H^+ + HCO_3^-$); excess CO_2 in the blood produces more hydrogen ions and lowers blood pH (the blood becomes acidic). Buffering compounds in the blood, tissues, and cells chemically stabilize pH by removing or replacing hydrogen ions. This buys time for the lungs and kidneys to reestablish normal body chemistry. The lungs respond to

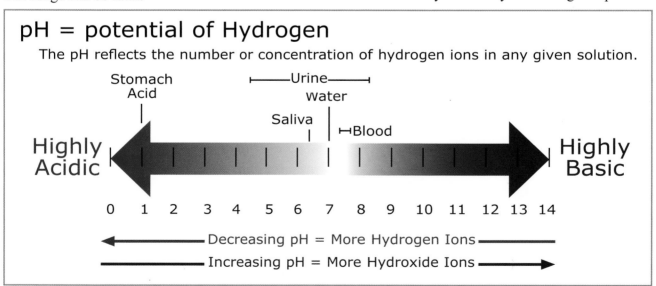

pH = potential of Hydrogen

The pH reflects the number or concentration of hydrogen ions in any given solution.

Stomach Acid · Urine · water · Saliva · Blood

Highly Acidic — Highly Basic

0 1 2 3 4 5 6 7 8 9 10 11 12 13 14

Decreasing pH = More Hydrogen Ions

Increasing pH = More Hydroxide Ions

decreasing pH levels by increasing respirations and exhaling CO_2, essentially removing the excess acid. A prolonged increase in respiration rate, for instance, as experienced at high altitude or by a medical condition, blows off too much acid and raises blood pH. The kidneys respond to pH changes in both directions by either excreting hydrogen or bicarbonate ions as needed and by producing either acidic or basic urine respectively. Problematic changes in pH are either metabolic or respiratory in nature and treated by correcting the underlying cause.

Organic Compounds

The numerous organic compounds in the body fall into six major classes: carbohydrates, lipids, proteins, nucleic acids, high-energy compounds (ATP), and vitamins; all contain carbon and hydrogen atoms, and most contain oxygen.

Carbohydrates

Carbohydrates are the body's primary energy source. Simple sugars, including glucose, are relatively small molecules whose covalent bonds are quickly broken to provide energy. Two simple sugars combine to form disaccharides. Large complex carbohydrate molecules called polysaccharides, starches are one example, are either plant or animal based and do not dissolve in water. Animal starch (glycogen) is composed of a large chain of glucose molecules and is stored in liver and muscle cells. Stored glycogen is broken down into glucose when energy demands are high. Excess sugar is stored as fat.

Lipids

Lipids are fats, waxes, or oils; most are insoluble in water and require special transport proteins to carry them in the blood. There are four basic types of lipids: fatty acids, fats, steroids, and phospholipids. Each has a slightly different molecular shape specific to its individual function. Fatty acids provide an alternate energy source to carbohydrates and are subdivided into saturated and unsaturated fatty acids. Fatty acids, stored in triglyceride chains, are the building blocks of fat molecules. Saturated fats tend to come from animal sources and are solid at room temperature, while unsaturated fats are usually plant-based and liquid at room temperature. A diet high in saturated fats increases the risk of arteriosclerosis and related circulatory system problems. In addition to providing an emergency energy source, fats also offer subcutaneous insulation and organ protection. Steroids, such as cholesterol, and phospholipids are the primary components of cell membranes. Their water insolubility helps maintain the integrity of the cell and the specific concentrations of the extracellular and intracellular fluids. Cholesterol is also required to manufacture many of the body's messenger hormones.

Proteins

Proteins make up the largest group of organic compounds in the human body. They are composed of long chains of amino acids and are responsible for most of the physical structure of the body and its numerous components. The number and order of the amino acids in a protein determine its shape and function. Minor changes in the concentration of ions, temperature, and pH in the surrounding environment can cause proteins to denature—irreversibly break down. Denaturation ultimately leads to death as tissues, organs, and organs systems fail.

Nucleic Acids

Nucleic acids—DNA and RNA—store and process all the genetic information responsible for our individual characteristics. Both DNA and RNA are composed of nucleotide chains. Both work together to direct the synthesis of proteins in the body. As such, they directly control cellular metabolism.

High Energy Compounds

As previously discussed, cells break the covalent bonds in food to release energy. Much of the released energy is captured by creating high energy phosphate bonds; the remainder emerges as heat. Cells add a phosphate group to adenosine diphosphate (ADP) creating adenosine triphosphate (ATP). The reaction is completely reversible. When cells need energy, the bond is broken under controlled conditions within the cell, leaving the ADP and phosphate group intact for future storage: ATP $\longleftrightarrow$ ADP + phosphate group + energy.

Vitamins

Vitamins are organic nutrients related to lipids and carbohydrates; they work with enzymes to facilitate chemical reactions and maintain homeostasis. Vitamins B and K are produced by bacteria in the intestinal tract; vitamin D is manufactured by skin cells when exposed to sunlight; beta-carotene is converted into vitamin A by the body; and the B com-

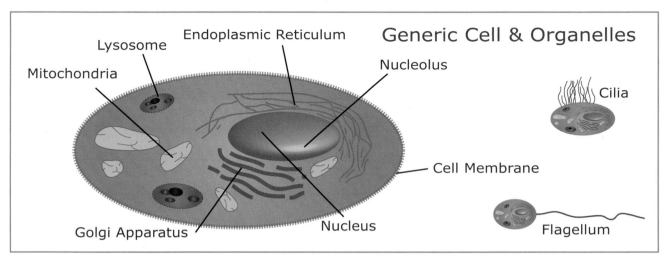

Generic Cell & Organelles

Lysosome · Endoplasmic Reticulum · Nucleolus · Mitochondria · Cilia · Cell Membrane · Golgi Apparatus · Nucleus · Flagellum

plex vitamins, along with vitamin C, are absorbed through the intestinal tract from outside sources. Vitamins are broken down into two major categories: fat soluble and water soluble. Fat-soluble vitamins: A, D, E and K, bind to and are transported with lipids. While fat-soluble vitamins may be stored for long periods of time within muscle tissue and specialized liver cells, water-soluble vitamins must be replaced frequently. Most water-soluble vitamins, such as B complex and C, are excreted by the body within four days. Numerous diseases may be traced to a lack of specific vitamins. Often the disease process may be reversed with early assessment and treatment using the appropriate supplements.

Required Vitamins	
Fat Soluble	**Water Soluble**
Vitamin A	Vitamin C
Vitamin D	All B Vitamins
Vitamin E	
Vitamin K	

Cell Structure & Physiology

Cells are the smallest form of life and, as the basic building blocks for the human body, they are responsible for creating tissues, organs, and organ systems. While there are numerous types of cells within the body, all respond to internal and external stimuli in order to maintain homeostasis. The shape of a cell reflects its function. Each cell is surrounded by a lipid membrane (stuff sack) that separates the contents of the cell from the extracellular fluid and contains the cell's organelle (refer to the above diagram). Each organelle has its own stuff sack and

is held in place by structural proteins. Additional proteins are embedded in the cell membrane and act as receptors, channels, enzymes, molecular carriers, anchors, or identifiers. Individual organelles are responsible for specific functions within each cell: mitochondria process glucose and store energy as ATP. The endoplasmic reticulum synthesizes and stores proteins, carbohydrates, and lipids. Lysosomes are responsible for digestion, defense, and recycling. Golgi apparatus package secretions and enzymes in small vesicles and maintain the cell membrane. The nucleus controls metabolism, reproduction and protein synthesis. Some cells produce hair-like extensions of their cellular membrane to increase their surface area and speed absorption (microvilli), to move liquids across their surface (cilia), or to move through tissue and body fluids (flagella).

In order to perform efficiently, all cells require a constant supply of nutrients and the steady elimination of waste products. Both nutrients and wastes are transported to and from the cells via the circulatory system. They are either suspended within the blood or lymph as solutes or bound to carrier cells. They must be able to freely pass through the semipermeable membranes of the capillaries and cells. Passage generally depends on a combination of their molecular size, shape, electrical charge and lipid solubility. It is through the extracellular fluid that the cells either absorb nutrients or dispose of wastes. Movement of both nutrients and wastes across the cell membranes takes place by filtration, diffusion, active transport or vesicular transport (refer to the diagrams on the following page). Filtration happens when particles are forced through the cell membrane by hydrostatic pressure. Diffusion occurs when solutes move across

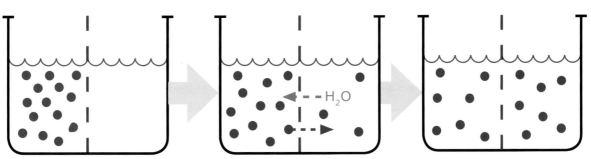

Diffusion
In a freely permeable membrane, solutes and water diffuse through the membrane until they are equally distributed on both sides.

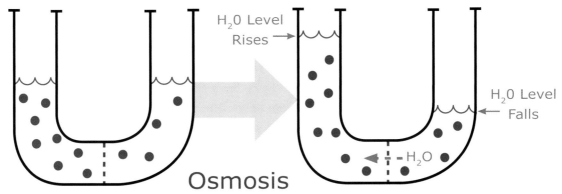

H₂0 Level Rises →

← H₂0 Level Falls

Osmosis
In a semi-permeable membrane, where the solutes are too large to pass through the membrane, water moves across the membrane to dilute the solutes until the concentrations are equal or until an opposing pressure halts the process.

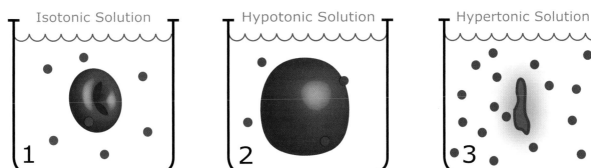

Isotonic Solution

Hypotonic Solution

Hypertonic Solution

Water moves towards the highest concentration of solute via osmosis. 1. Solutes are equal inside cell and in solution (isotonic solution). 2. A higher concentration of solute is inside of the cell than in the solution (hypotonic solution). 3. A lower concentration of solute is inside of the cell than in the solution (hypertonic solution).

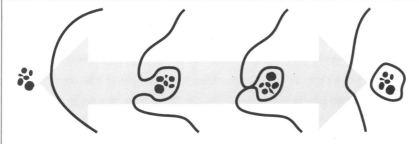

Vesicular Transport
In order to import material into the cell, the cell membrane extends to surround extracellular fluid and the material, and then fuses, to form a vesicle. The reverse happens to export cellular products and/or debris.

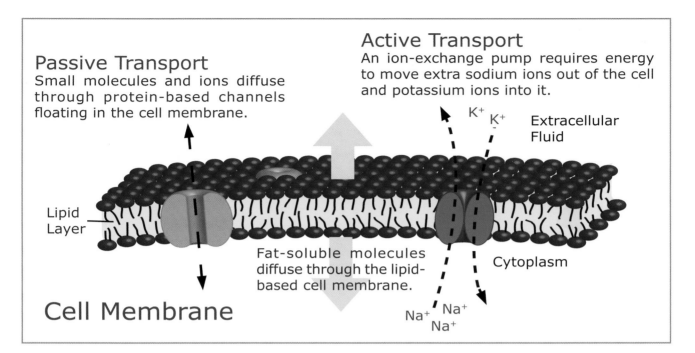

a membrane from an area of higher concentration to an area of lower concentration. Carbon dioxide and oxygen are transported across cell membranes by diffusion. Glucose is also transported across the cell membrane by diffusion; however, its entry is facilitated by the presence of the hormone, insulin. Osmosis is a form of diffusion, wherein water, not a solute, diffuses through a semipermeable membrane to equalize the concentration on each side of the membrane. A working knowledge of osmosis is necessary to prevent, assess, and treat heat-related illnesses.

Active transport occurs when a cell uses energy, that is, converts ATP into ADP, to move solutes across its membrane, often against the concentration gradient. Sodium, potassium, other ions, and proteins are often carried into and out of cells by active transport (shown in the diagram above).

In vesicular transport, nutrients, products, waste, or pathogens are packaged in extensions of the cell membrane for transport into or out of the cell.

As stated previously, all cells require oxygen and glucose in order to survive. Cells break down glucose to produce chemical energy, primarily in the form of ATP, and heat: $C_6H_{12}O_6 + 6O_2 \longrightarrow 6CO_2 + 6H_2O + ATP$. The energy is used by the cell to carry out its functions. A cell deprived of oxygen and glucose will eventually die. Carbon dioxide is a waste product of cellular metabolism. It is picked up by the blood and eliminated through the lungs. Other cellular waste must be transported to the kidneys

for removal. If waste products build to toxic levels, cellular function will decrease and the cell will die. *In order for the transportation of both nutrients and wastes to be effective, fluid levels within the human body must remain within tight parameters. Cellular function will significantly decrease or stop if fluids fall below acceptable levels.*

Body Systems
The Circulatory System

The function of the circulatory system is twofold: it picks up nutrients from the proper organs and delivers them to all the cells of the body; and, of equal importance, it picks up cellular wastes and delivers them to the proper organs for removal. Medically, this transportation process is known as perfusion. Without perfusion, cellular function decreases or ceases altogether as the affected cells are denied access to the nutrients they need to support life or as toxic wastes begin to poison them. Both nutrients and waste are carried by the blood through an interconnected series of tubes to all the cells of the body. The blood is forced through the tubes by a powerful muscular pump. The circulatory system may be structurally divided into three major components: the heart or pump; the vessels or tubes; and the entire fluid volume of the body: blood, plasma, intracellular fluid, and lymph. A problem that disrupts the function of any one of the components of the circulatory system will affect the function of the entire system, and subsequently the entire body. Severe problems with the circulatory system usually lead to a systemic decrease in cellular perfusion (shock) and death. See page 22 for a diagram of the circulatory system.

The Heart

The heart is a single organ comprised of two pumps, known as ventricles, and two receiving chambers, known as atria. The larger of the two pumps, the left ventricle, pumps blood to the body while the smaller pump, the right ventricle, pumps blood to the lungs. Oxygen-poor blood returning from the body is collected in the larger of the two receiving chambers, the right atrium, and oxygen-rich blood returning from the lungs is collected in the smaller chamber, the left atrium. Each chamber is separated by independent valves, and the timing of these valves, as well as the contraction of each ventricle, is critical to functional circulation. The characteristic "lub-dub" sounds associated with a heartbeat are the opening and closing of the four paired valves that regulate blood flow between the atria and ventricles and its exit from the heart. The heart contains specialized cardiac nerves that are responsible for generating and coordinating the electrical impulses necessary for efficient pumping. The rate and strength of cardiac contractions is dependent upon both the specialized cardiac nerves and signals from the autonomic nervous system. Cardiac perfusion is accomplished via the coronary arteries and veins.

The Vessels

The blood and lymphatic vessels create a system of tubes that carry fluids to and from all the cells of the body. Arteries are muscular blood vessels that carry blood away from the heart and are responsible for the pickup and delivery of nutrients—vitamins, minerals, amino acids, glucose, etc.—from the gastrointestinal system and liver, and oxygen from the lungs. They also deliver cellular waste to the kidneys for elimination. Because they are under increased pressure due to their proximity to the heart, arteries have thicker and more muscular walls than either veins or lymph vessels. Veins and lymphatic vessels return blood and lymph, which is similar to plasma, back to the heart. They are also responsible for delivering carbon dioxide to the lungs for oxygen exchange. All vascular muscles are under the control of the autonomic nervous system and capable of vasoconstriction or vasodilation when properly stimulated.

Upon leaving the heart, arteries continually divide and subdivide until they form an interwoven web of microscopic tubes called capillaries. Capillaries form the link between the circulatory system and the cells of the body and are found within all body tissues. Nutrients suspended in blood plasma move through the thin permeable walls of the capillaries to bathe and nourish individual cells. Waste products are released into the extracellular fluid, picked up by the capillaries and lymph vessels, and eventually removed from the blood by the kidneys. Small sphincters surround the entrance to each capillary and dilate or contract in response to autonomic nervous system commands to control the amount of blood entering each capillary.

Blood leaving the capillaries returns to the heart via veins. Movement of venous blood towards the heart is driven by the muscular contraction of the surrounding striated muscle groups, especially those in the legs, by "squeezing" the blood back to the heart. Since the blood pressure is lower on the venous side, the veins contain one-way valves to aid the return of deoxygenated blood to the heart and to prevent it from pooling in the extremities.

Lymph vessels also pick up extracellular fluid and wastes and pass it through lymph nodes, where most of the white blood cells (WBC) in the body are located, before returning it to general circulation via the central veins. WBCs are an integral part of the body's defenses and leave the lymph nodes to fight systemic infections. Fluid moves through the lymphatic vessels in the same manner as venous blood returns to the heart—through contractions of the surrounding muscle groups. Of the blood leaving the capillaries, about one fifth is picked up by the lymph vessels; the remainder is reabsorbed at the venous end of the capillaries. Lymph nodes become enlarged during an infection, when the flow of WBCs *into* the node exceeds the rate of outflow.

Blood, Plasma, and Fluids

Blood is made up of approximately equal proportions of blood cells, including platelets, and plasma. Under normal circumstances, the overwhelming majority of blood cells are red blood cells

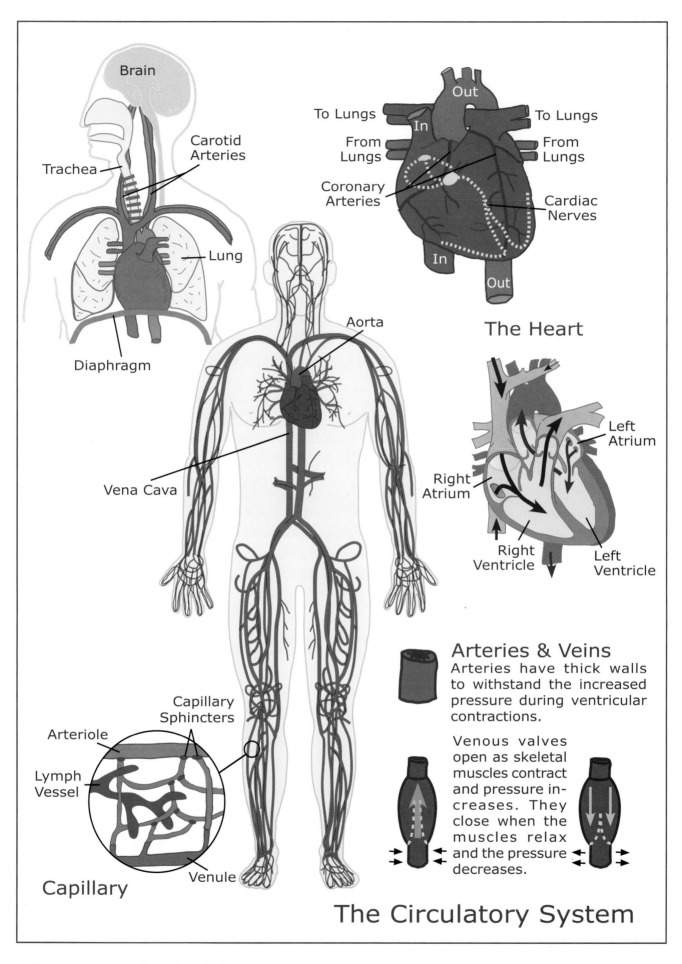

Brain

Carotid Arteries

Trachea

Lung

Diaphragm

To Lungs

In

Out

To Lungs

From Lungs

From Lungs

Coronary Arteries

Cardiac Nerves

In

Out

The Heart

Aorta

Vena Cava

Left Atrium

Right Atrium

Right Ventricle

Left Ventricle

Capillary Sphincters

Arteriole

Lymph Vessel

Venule

Capillary

Arteries & Veins

Arteries have thick walls to withstand the increased pressure during ventricular contractions.

Venous valves open as skeletal muscles contract and pressure increases. They close when the muscles relax and the pressure decreases.

The Circulatory System

(RBCs) responsible for binding with and carrying oxygen to all the tissues of the body. The spleen is responsible for recycling old RBCs while new red blood cells are formed by stem cells within bone marrow. Unless an infection is present, relatively few white blood cells (WBCs) are present in general circulation. Platelets are also present in small numbers and are responsible for clotting. Plasma is a water-based, nutrient-rich solution containing the salts, sugars, proteins, vitamins, and minerals required by the body's cells for normal functioning. Because of their large size, blood cells remain within the capillary network, while the vital nutrients held within the plasma are able to pass through the semipermeable walls of the capillaries to nourish individual cells. Lymph is similar to plasma in that it does not contain blood cells. Each type of fluid contains a slightly different combination of nutrients and waste products, and each fluid has a unique electrical charge depending upon the needs of the local tissue. Sodium is the predominant ion in the extracellular fluid, while potassium dominates the intracellular fluid or cytoplasm. Because sodium and potassium ions are small enough to pass through the channel proteins in the cell membrane,

they freely diffuse into and out of the cytoplasm. In order to maintain the correct ion concentration levels, cells utilize a protein-based ion-exchange pump to move each ion against the concentration gradient. The respective concentrations of sodium and potassium in the extracellular and intracellular fluid are particularly important because, as illustrated earlier, water follows salt, diffusing in or out of the cell, according to the concentration gradient.

Shock

Shock is the major life-threatening problem of the circulatory system. It is medically defined as a loss of systemic perfusion. There are three basic types of shock: heart shock (cardiogenic shock), volume shock (hypovolemic shock), and vascular shock (septic shock, anaphylactic shock and spinal shock). Each is directly related to a failure in one of the major components of the circulatory system. All forms of shock, regardless of the mechanism, may lead to death.

Failure of the pump (heart shock) may be caused by a variety of mechanisms, all resulting in a drop in perfusion pressure and arrest. Medical mechanisms involving the heart usually disrupt the heart's intrinsic electrical system by blocking

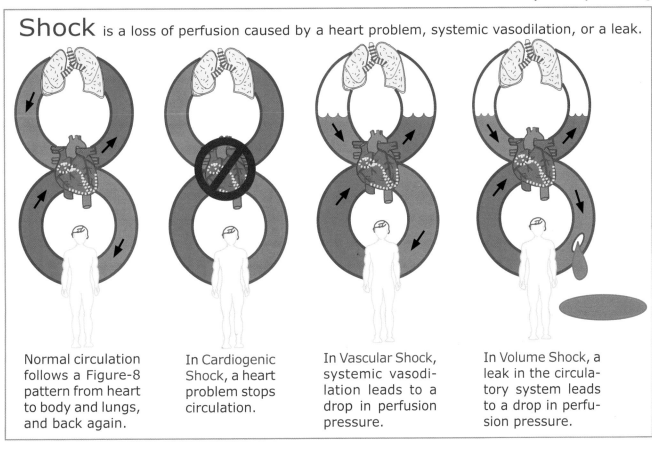

Shock is a loss of perfusion caused by a heart problem, systemic vasodilation, or a leak.

Normal circulation follows a Figure-8 pattern from heart to body and lungs, and back again.

In Cardiogenic Shock, a heart problem stops circulation.

In Vascular Shock, systemic vasodilation leads to a drop in perfusion pressure.

In Volume Shock, a leak in the circulatory system leads to a drop in perfusion pressure.

one or more of the coronary arteries and depriving cardiac cells of oxygen and nutrients (heart attack). In addition, infection may damage the heart muscle or any of its various components. Trauma can directly impair the heart's electrical system or injure the organ itself. Environmental mechanisms, such as lightning, may disrupt the electrical system directly, while drowning affects the heart indirectly by damaging the respiratory system and depriving the heart of oxygen.

A break in any vessel causes an immediate fluid loss at the site of the break. If the vessel is an artery, the amount of fluid loss is increased because of the arterial pressure. Fluid loss may also be caused by an increase in the permeability of the walls in the capillary beds (inflammatory response). Any loss of red blood cells causes an immediate decrease in the oxygen carrying capacity of the blood. A loss of water (dehydration) causes an immediate decrease in the efficiency of the circulatory system's delivery system. Both cause a decrease in cellular function, as the delivery of nutrients and the removal of wastes slow. Large amounts of fluid loss (blood, plasma, water), regardless of the cause, will cause a systemic loss of perfusion (volume shock).

Problems with the vessels that affect the entire circulatory system tend to be those that cause systemic vasodilation (anaphylaxis, spinal shock, and septic shock). All may lead to a loss of perfusion pressure (vascular shock).

The Respiratory System

The function of the respiratory system is to supply the blood with oxygen and to remove carbon dioxide. (See page 26 for a diagram of the respiratory system.) The removal of carbon dioxide helps to balance blood pH. When the amount of carbon dioxide in the blood becomes too high, or the oxygen level too low, chemical receptors in the brainstem signal the diaphragm and intercostal muscles to contract and begin inhalation. The muscular contractions enlarge the intrathoracic space, expand the lungs, and cause a negative pressure to develop internally. In a process similar to that of an expanding bellows, air is pulled into the body through the mouth or nose by the negative pressure. It passes through a series of smaller and smaller tubes (tra-

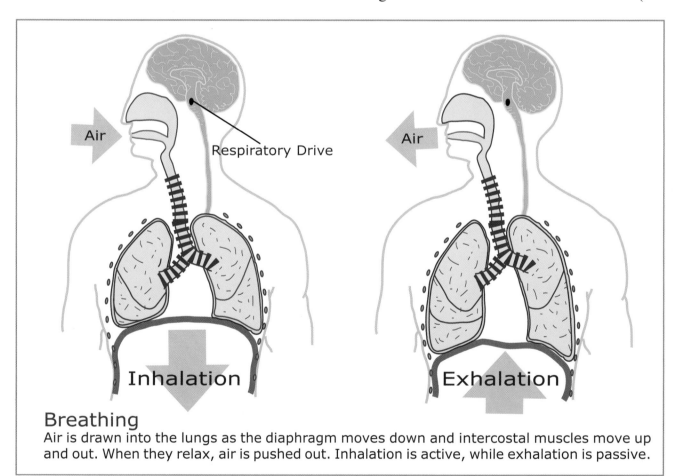

Breathing
Air is drawn into the lungs as the diaphragm moves down and intercostal muscles move up and out. When they relax, air is pushed out. Inhalation is active, while exhalation is passive.

24 Anatomy & Physiology

chea, bronchi, bronchioles) until it fills microscopic air sacs (alveoli) and the pressure is equalized. The alveoli are enveloped by capillary beds; it is through the thin walls of the alveoli and the adjacent capillaries that the gas exchange takes place. While inhalation is an active process, expiration is passive. During expiration, the muscles relax, intrathoracic pressure increases, and air is expelled. Normal respirations are smooth, easy, and quiet.

For diagnostic purposes, the respiratory system may be structurally divided into five major components: the respiratory drive located in the brainstem; the upper airway; the lower airway; the air sacs or alveoli; and the musculoskeletal structure consisting of the chest wall, diaphragm, and pleura (the stuff sacks surrounding each lung). Any problem that disrupts the function of any of the components will affect the function of the entire system and subsequently the entire body. Problems with the respiratory system decrease or stop the gas exchange, causing systemic cellular hypoxia (lack of oxygen) and often death.

The Respiratory Drive

All cells require oxygen to produce energy and do work; carbon dioxide and water are waste products of the metabolic process. An increased demand for work from individual organs, increases the oxygen requirement of their cells. Chemical receptors located in the brainstem monitor blood pH, carbon dioxide, and oxygen levels. When the blood pH falls too low (becomes more acidic) due to increasing levels of carbon dioxide or the oxygen levels fall too low, the chemical receptors stimulate the diaphragm and intercostal muscles to contract. This begins a breathing cycle. The respiratory drive regulates the rate and depth of the body's respirations to facilitate oxygenation and assist the kidneys with balancing blood pH. It is the interface between the nervous system and the respiratory system.

The Upper Airway

The upper airway consists of the nasal and oral pharynges. Both are hollow tubes surrounded by soft tissues that intersect at the back of the throat; both are capable of carrying air. Air entering the nose is filtered before entering the lungs, while air entering the mouth may contain particulate matter. Food is prevented from entering the main air tube,

called the trachea, by the contraction of a muscular flap, called the epiglottis. During swallowing, the epiglottis lowers, directing food or liquids into the esophagus. Large contaminants or foreign bodies are removed from the upper airway by sneezing and coughing. Directly below the epiglottis is the larynx or voice box. The upper airway ends at the larynx.

The Lower Airway

The lower airway is a series of air tubes that begin with the trachea. Immediately below the larynx, the trachea divides into bronchi, then subdivides into secondary bronchi, then again into tertiary bronchi, and then finally into bronchioles, before terminating in the alveoli. The walls of the larger tubes, the trachea and bronchi, are supported by cartilage and are lined with smooth muscle and ciliated mucosa; cilia are small hair-like fibers that help remove tiny particulate matter from the bronchi. The smaller bronchioles consist almost entirely of smooth muscle and are covered by a mucous membrane. Within the lower airway, large particulate matter is removed by coughing while smaller particles are trapped by the mucous layer and expelled by ciliary action. An extensive lymphatic network within the lining of all the tubes is responsible for the removal of microscopic particles and organisms. The lower airway ends at the alveoli.

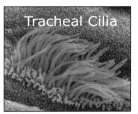
Tracheal Cilia

The Alveoli

The alveoli are microscopic air sacs or chambers completely enveloped by a capillary network. In structure, each air sac resembles a grape clustered with other grapes. It is through the alveolar walls that oxygen is exchanged for carbon dioxide. The alveoli are the interface between the respiratory system and the circulatory system. Both systems must be functioning to ensure the oxygenation of cells.

The circulatory system is responsible for transporting oxygen and carbon dioxide between the alveoli and cells. Once oxygen has diffused through the thin alveolar and capillary walls, it is quickly dissolved in the plasma. Because plasma can only hold a small amount of gas in solution, most of the oxygen binds with hemoglobin molecules in the red blood cells for transportation. Upon reaching its destination, the oxygen is released into the plasma, passes

The Respiratory System

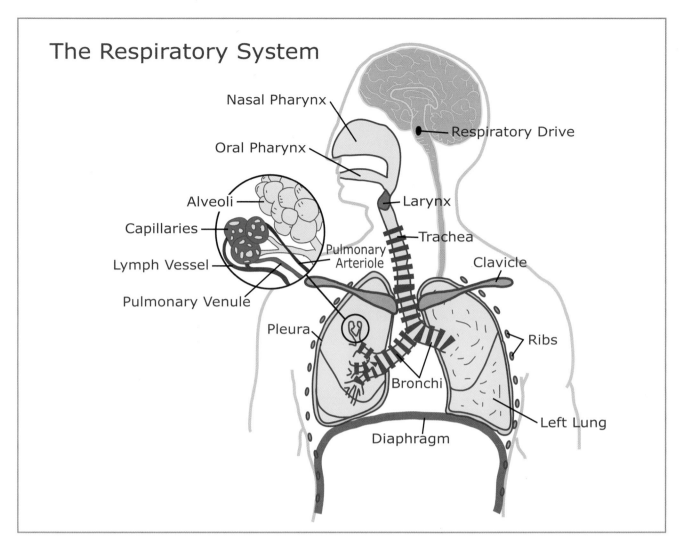

Labels in figure:
- Nasal Pharynx
- Oral Pharynx
- Alveoli
- Capillaries
- Lymph Vessel
- Pulmonary Venule
- Pleura
- Pulmonary Arteriole
- Respiratory Drive
- Larynx
- Trachea
- Clavicle
- Ribs
- Bronchi
- Left Lung
- Diaphragm

through the capillary walls into the tissue, and then diffuses into the cells where it is used to produce energy. Simultaneously, carbon dioxide diffuses from the cells into the adjacent capillaries. Carbon dioxide is carried by the blood in three ways: a small amount remains dissolved in the plasma as a solute; approximately one third combines with hydrogen ions and is carried in the red blood cells as carbonic acid; and, the remainder, over half, is carried in the plasma as a bicarbonate ion. Once in the lungs, the carbonic acid breaks down into water and carbon dioxide, diffuses into the alveoli, and is exhaled. The breakdown of carbonic acid and the elimination of the resulting water and carbon dioxide decreases the acidity of the blood (increases blood pH). Prolonged rapid respirations (hyperventilation) may lead to respiratory alkalosis if too much carbon dioxide is lost.

The Musculoskeletal Structure

The musculoskeletal structure of the respiratory system includes the sternum, ribs, and thoracic vertebrae; the diaphragm and intercostal muscles; and, the lungs and their pleura. The bone and cartilage of the sternum, ribs, and thoracic vertebrae provide support, while the intercostal muscles allow for movement. Together, these components form the chest wall. As the intercostal muscles contract, the ribs pivot along the spine and lift anteriorly, causing the chest to expand both externally and internally. The diaphragm is a large muscle that separates the chest cavity from the abdominal cavity. When stimulated, it contracts downward pushing the abdominal organs out of the way to internally expand the chest cavity. Movement of the diaphragm can be seen as an expansion in the upper abdominal quadrants (aka: belly breathing). The interior of the chest wall, or thoracic cavity, and diaphragm are lined with a smooth resilient membrane, known as the parietal pleura. The lungs are enclosed by a second membrane, the visceral pleura, that lies against the parietal pleura separated

Respiratory Distress ...or Arrest

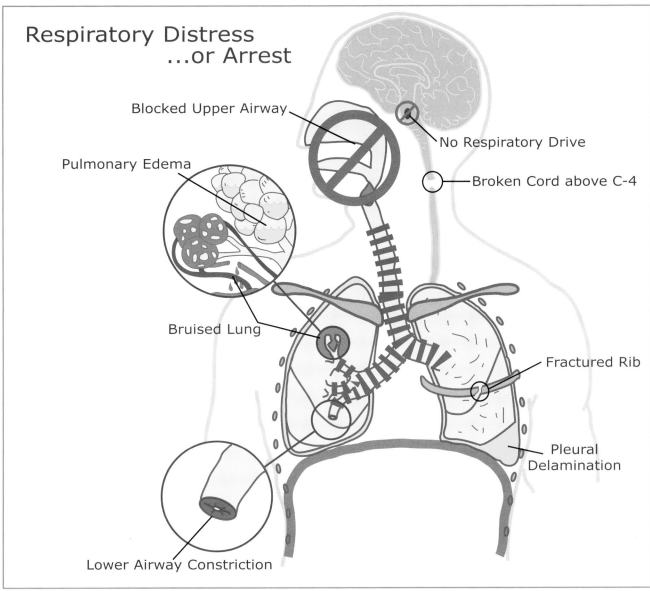

Blocked Upper Airway

Pulmonary Edema

No Respiratory Drive

Broken Cord above C-4

Bruised Lung

Fractured Rib

Pleural Delamination

Lower Airway Constriction

only by a lubricating fluid. The parietal and visceral pleuras separate the lungs from the middle section of the thoracic cavity (mediastinum) that contains the heart. The lungs contain the lower airway, the alveoli and the blood vessels that are responsible for the delivery of oxygen and the removal of carbon dioxide. In their most basic form, the lungs are a series of air tubes and sacs tied to a second series of tubes containing blood and surrounded by a stuff sack. It is the integrity of the individual pleura and the surface tension of the fluid between them that permits the lungs to expand with the contraction of the chest and the diaphragm.

Respiratory Distress & Arrest

The major problems of the respiratory system are a complete or partial failure of the system's ability to supply the blood with oxygen and remove carbon dioxide. Partial failure of any of the system's components may cause respiratory distress, while complete failure will cause respiratory arrest and potentially death.

The respiratory drive may be damaged by head trauma, toxins, lack of oxygen (hypoxia), electricity, stroke, altitude, etc. Serious damage leads to a decrease in the patient's level of consciousness and a decreased respiratory rate that is rapidly followed by respiratory arrest. Problems in the upper airway are usually related to a complete or partial blockage. Blockage may occur from foreign objects (usually food or gum), localized swelling, fluids (typically blood or vomitus), or simply poor positioning of an unresponsive patient. Lower airway problems are usually related to the constriction of the smooth muscular lining of the respiratory tree due to a bronchial spasm and/or swelling. Common causes range from asthma to anaphylaxis to smoke inhalation. If the alveoli fill with fluid, as occurs with congestive heart failure, pneumonia, high-altitude pulmonary edema, and after near drowning or smoke inhalation, the gas exchange cannot take place. If the integrity of the chest wall or diaphragm is broken during trauma, air or blood can leak into the pleural space and prevent one or both lungs from inflating. These types of injuries are medically referred to as hemothorax, pneumothorax, hemopneumothorax, or tension pneumothorax depending on whether blood, air, or both are responsible for the collapse of the patient's lung and whether one lung is so badly damaged that the leaking air and/or blood puts pressure on the patient's opposing lung and heart; the latter quickly leads to death if not promptly treated. An abrupt pressure change through trauma or an improper ascent with SCUBA may rupture multiple alveoli and cause a similar phenomenon.

The Nervous System

The nervous system works with the endocrine system to maintain homeostasis by generating and sending the electrochemical signals that provide control and integration for most body functions. (See page 33 for a diagram of the nervous system).

There are two types of cells within the nervous system: nerve cells, or neurons, and neuroglia. Neurons are responsible for generating and carrying the electrochemical signals that control the body; neuroglia are specialized cells that support neurons. Structurally, the nervous system is divided into the central nervous system (CNS) and the peripheral nervous system (PNS). The CNS is further subdivided into the brain and spinal cord. The cells of the CNS are delicate and well protected by tough stuff sacks, circulating cerebrospinal fluid (CSF), and bone; damage to these cells is permanent. The nerves of the peripheral nervous system are far stronger and require less protection; they tend to

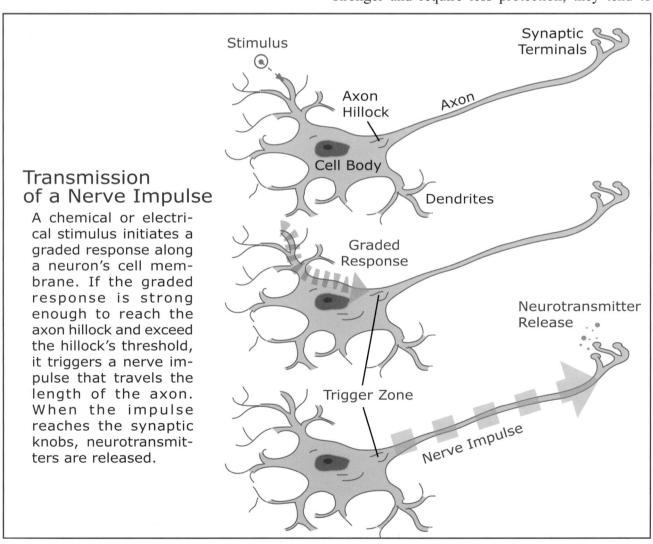

Transmission of a Nerve Impulse

A chemical or electrical stimulus initiates a graded response along a neuron's cell membrane. If the graded response is strong enough to reach the axon hillock and exceed the hillock's threshold, it triggers a nerve impulse that travels the length of the axon. When the impulse reaches the synaptic knobs, neurotransmitters are released.

Stimulus

Axon Hillock

Axon

Cell Body

Synaptic Terminals

Dendrites

Graded Response

Neurotransmitter Release

Trigger Zone

Nerve Impulse

follow the medial aspect of the long bones as they travel through the extremities. Peripheral nerves are capable of regeneration.

On a functional level, the nervous system is divided into two divisions: the voluntary (somatic) nervous system and the involuntary (autonomic) nervous system. The voluntary division of the nervous system contains both sensory and motor nerves. Sensory nerves carry input to the spinal cord and brain, while motor nerves carry messages from them. Through its nerves, the somatic nervous system controls conscious functions, primarily striated muscle contractions. The autonomic division of the nervous system maintains or restores homeostasis by regulating smooth muscle contractions and the glandular secretion of hormones. Most autonomic functions are beyond conscious control.

The autonomic division of the nervous system is subdivided into the sympathetic and the parasympathetic systems. The sympathetic system stimulates effectors (cells or organs) while the parasympathetic system inhibits them. Both systems continually transmit impulses to the same effector and act in an antagonistic manner, with the stronger impulse assuming control. Under normal conditions, the sympathetic system is responsible for waking us up and the parasympathetic system is responsible for sleep and digestion.

Neurons and Nerve Impulses

Neurons have three distinct parts—a cell body, a dendrite, and an axon—each with a specific purpose. The cell body houses the nucleus and, as is true for all cells, is responsible for maintaining the neuron's homeostasis. Dendrites receive a stimulus from the extracellular environment, from a neural receptor, or from another neuron and send a local or graded impulse to the cell body and axon. If the graded signal is strong enough to overcome the stimulus threshold at the start of an axon (axon hillock), it initiates an electrical impulse that continues along the axon to its terminus where it communicates with another neural cell, a muscle cell, or other effector via specialized chemicals called neurotransmitters. (Refer to the diagram on the previous page.) Graded signals occur in all cells in response to environmental stimuli and trigger changes in cell function. They are a local phenomenon and the signal travels only a short distance before dissipating; graded signals do NOT affect the entire cell membrane. Motor neurons control cells by releasing neurotransmitters near the cell that stimulate a graded response. In highly excitable neurons or

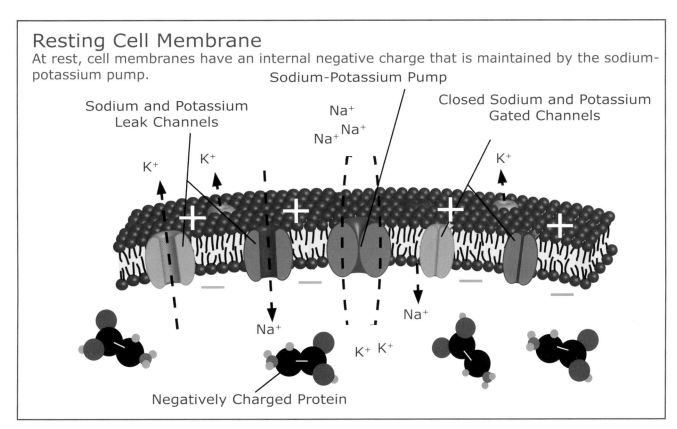

Resting Cell Membrane
At rest, cell membranes have an internal negative charge that is maintained by the sodium-potassium pump.

Sodium-Potassium Pump

Sodium and Potassium Leak Channels

Closed Sodium and Potassium Gated Channels

Na^+
Na^+
Na^+ Na^+

K^+ K^+

K^+

Na^+

Na^+

K^+ K^+

Negatively Charged Protein

muscle cells, a strong graded signal can initiate an electrical impulse that is capable of traveling long distances and affect the entire cell membrane. The motor and sensory neurons of the extremities are several feet long in an adult. These nerve impulses originate from one of three points: a sensory receptor, the spinal cord via a reflex arc, or the brain.

Nervous system signals are electrochemical in nature and directly related to the concentration of electrolytes in the extracellular and intracellular fluids. The intracellular fluid contains more potassium (K^+) and protein (A^-) ions, while the extracellular fluid has more sodium (Na^+) and chloride (Cl^-) ions. There are two types of protein channels in a neuron's cell membrane: leak channels that are always open and gated channels that open only in response to a stimulus. Ions move down the concentration gradient and continually diffuse through specific leak channels in the cell membrane. Because there are more potassium leak channels than sodium leak channels, potassium diffuses out of the cell faster than sodium leaks into the cell. The lipid structure of the cell's membrane acts as a layer of insulation permitting opposing electrical charges to exist simultaneously on either side of the membrane. The net movement of the sodium and potassium ions through the cell membrane, in combination with the negatively charged protein ions that are too big to pass through the membrane channels, leaves the inside of the membrane with a slight negative charge. The sodium-potassium pump acts to maintain the concentration gradient across the cell membrane by exchanging two potassium ions for three sodium ions. Without the sodium-potassium pump, the ion concentration would eventually equalize and neural communication as we know it would not exist.

In addition to moving down the concentration gradient, ions also move along electrical gradients from positive to negative and vice versa. Electrical and chemical stimuli change the permeability of the cell membrane by opening gated ion channels. If sodium gates are opened, sodium ions flow through the channel and the negatively charged interior cell membrane becomes positive at that point. Nearby negative ions move inward towards the positively charged region and the positive ions move outward; the ion movement along the interior of the cell membrane creates an electrical current that eventually dissipates (graded signal) or, if strong enough, stimulates a nerve impulse in the axon. Typically, nerve impulses are generated at the axon hillock and flow like a wave to its other end. It is clinically important to note that a change in the ion (electrolyte) concentration on either side of a cell membrane or a change in the permeability of the cell membrane is capable of generating a signal. (Refer to the diagram on the following page.)

Neuroglia

There are four types of neuroglia in the central nervous system: astrocytes,

Ion Movement & Current

When chemicals or electricity stimulate the receptor site on a gated sodium channel, the channel opens and positively charged sodium ions flow into the cell, depolarizing the cell membrane at that point. When the cell membrane depolarizes, positive ions flow outward from the point of depolarization, creating a electrical current along the inside of the cell membrane towards the synaptic knob at the terminus of the axon.

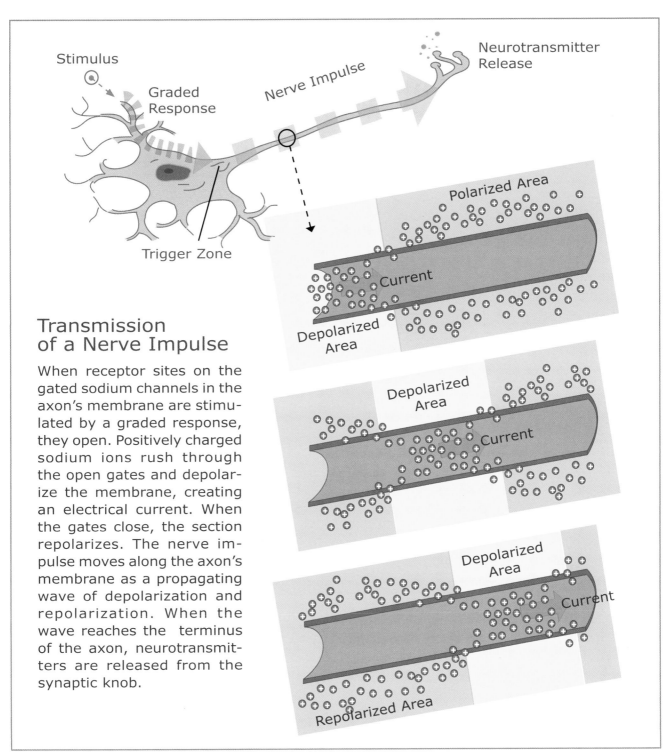

Stimulus

Graded
Response

Nerve Impulse

Neurotransmitter
Release

Trigger Zone

Polarized Area

Current

Depolarized
Area

Depolarized
Area

Current

Depolarized
Area

Current

Repolarized Area

Transmission of a Nerve Impulse

When receptor sites on the gated sodium channels in the axon's membrane are stimulated by a graded response, they open. Positively charged sodium ions rush through the open gates and depolarize the membrane, creating an electrical current. When the gates close, the section repolarizes. The nerve impulse moves along the axon's membrane as a propagating wave of depolarization and repolarization. When the wave reaches the terminus of the axon, neurotransmitters are released from the synaptic knob.

microglia, ependymal cells, and oligodendrocytes; and two in the peripheral nervous system: satellite cells and Schwann cells. Astrocytes are star-shaped cells that make up roughly half of the mass of the brain. In addition to providing the basic structure of the brain, their projections surround almost all of the brain's capillary network and help to create an impermeable blood-brain barrier to many circulating compounds and even the cells of the immune system. In general, only fat-soluble compounds and water can cross the blood-brain barrier freely; water-soluble compounds, including ions, require the assistance of specific carrier cells in order to diffuse into the interstitial tissue. The blood-brain barrier is necessary to maintain the stability of the fluid environment surrounding the brain. In this way, the normal changes in the blood's fluid matrix from general metabolism will not negatively impact

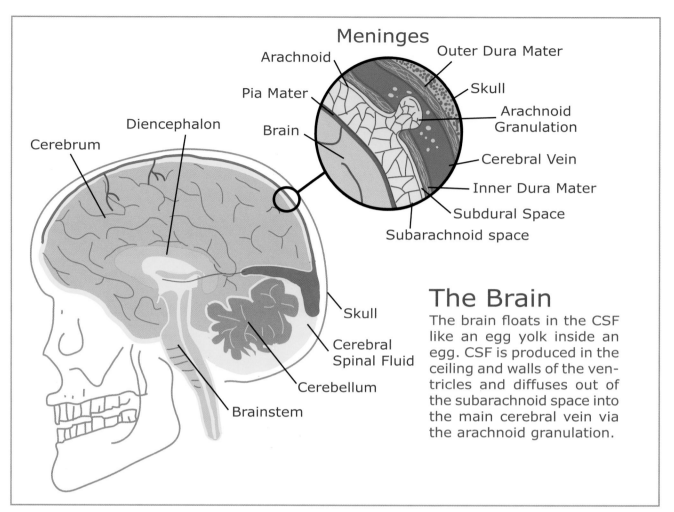

Meninges

Arachnoid
Pia Mater
Brain
Outer Dura Mater
Skull
Arachnoid Granulation
Cerebral Vein
Inner Dura Mater
Subdural Space
Subarachnoid space

Cerebrum
Diencephalon

Skull
Cerebral Spinal Fluid
Cerebellum
Brainstem

The Brain

The brain floats in the CSF like an egg yolk inside an egg. CSF is produced in the ceiling and walls of the ventricles and diffuses out of the subarachnoid space into the main cerebral vein via the arachnoid granulation.

brain function, as metabolic waste, many proteins, drugs, and toxins are denied entry. Only the parts of the brainstem that require chemical input from the body's organs via the blood are exempt. Microglia are responsible for maintaining the health of neurons. They are essentially the brain's private defense system and are necessary because the blood-brain barrier denies the brain access to cells of the immune system. Ependymal cells line the tissue spaces and canals filled with cerebrospinal fluid (CSF) and have cilia to assist CSF circulation. While they separate CSF from the brain's interstitial fluid, they remain extremely permeable to ensure rapid diffusion of nutrients from the CSF into the brain tissue. Oligodendrocytes (CNS) and Schwann cells (PNS) wrap fatty extensions of their cell membranes, called myelin sheaths, around axons to insulate and increase the speed of neural transmissions. Schwann cells also assist with regenerating damaged peripheral nerves. Satellite cells surround and strengthen groups of cell bodies or ganglia in the PNS. This strengthens them which makes them

stronger and more resistant to physical damage.

The Central Nervous System

The brain is the primary source of the signals necessary to control bodily functions. Its texture closely resembles spongy cottage cheese. While the brain comprises only three percent of the body's total weight, because of its high metabolism, it uses 25% of the body's oxygen and 20% of its sugar. Higher functions, such as sensory awareness, thought and personality, reside in the brain's outer layers known as the cerebrum, while the more basic autonomic functions, such as cardiac, vasomotor, and respiratory centers, lie within the central region of the brain, in the diencephalon and the brainstem. The diencephalon is hollow and filled with CSF; its sides form the thalamus and its bottom the hypothalamus. The thalamus is responsible for processing sensory information, while the hypothalamus connects to the pituitary gland and contains centers for emotions, autonomic function, and hormone production. The brainstem consists of the pons, midbrain, and medulla oblongata. The brainstem contains numerous

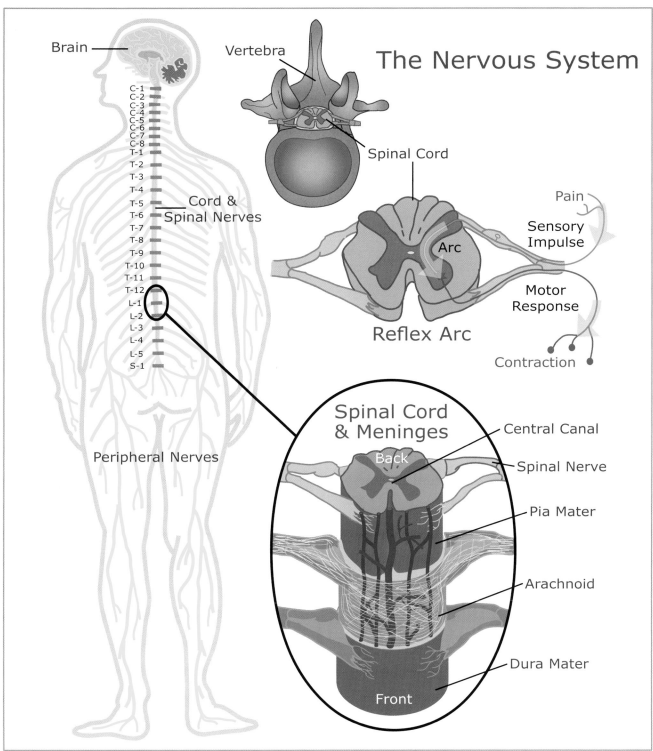

The Nervous System

Brain

Vertebra

C-1
C-2
C-3
C-4
C-5
C-6
C-7
C-8
T-1
T-2
T-3
T-4
T-5
T-6
T-7
T-8
T-9
T-10
T-11
T-12
L-1
L-2
L-3
L-4
L-5
S-1

Cord & Spinal Nerves

Spinal Cord

Pain

Sensory Impulse

Arc

Motor Response

Reflex Arc

Contraction

Peripheral Nerves

Spinal Cord & Meninges

Back

Central Canal

Spinal Nerve

Pia Mater

Arachnoid

Dura Mater

Front

reflex centers, such as hearing, smell, pupil responses, coughing, sneezing, swallowing, and vomiting. The cerebellum lies adjacent to but outside the cerebrum and controls muscular coordination. Groups of specialized nerves carry signals from the brainstem throughout the brain, permitting it to function as a gestalt. The spinal cord is an extension of the brainstem. In both appearance and texture, the spinal cord resembles strands of "al dente" spaghetti. Both the

brain and cord contain white and gray matter. Gray matter is primarily composed of cell bodies, while the white matter is made up of axons.

While its primary function is communication, the cord also contains reflex centers which respond directly to pain. When pain receptors in the skin, joint capsules, bone membranes and in the tissue surrounding blood vessels are stimulated, a signal is sent to the brain via sensory nerves and the spinal cord. On the way, sharp or abrupt pain is routed *across* the spinal cord through a reflex arc causing an immediate muscle contraction away from the source of the pain *before* the pain message actually reaches the brain and consciousness.

Both the brain and spinal cord are surrounded by three stuff sacks, called meninges, and bone. The skull protects the brain much like the shell of an egg protects its yolk and the spine protects the cord. The leather-like outermost meningeal layer, the dura mater, is fused to the lining of the skull and is very tough. Between the two layers of the dura, lies a thin space containing plasma and blood vessels. The innermost layer of the dura extends into the cerebrum and anchors the brain to the skull, further supporting its fragile tissue. A second narrow space below the dura, the subdural space, is filled with lymphatic fluid that serves to lubricate the dura and the second meningeal layer, the arachnoid. Beneath the arachnoid membrane is the subarachnoid space. The subarachnoid space is a hollow elastic layer made of collagen fibers and filled with CSF. The third meningeal layer, the pia, is attached directly to the brain and is highly vascular; it is also extremely delicate.

Both the brain and spinal cord are hollow. The brain contains four interconnected chambers or ventricles: two lateral chambers, one in each of the cerebral hemispheres, a central chamber in the diencephalon, and a fourth in the pons. The cord has a hollow canal running down its center. Each ventricle, the central canal of the cord, and the subarachnoid space contain cerebrospinal fluid (CSF). While the primary purpose of CSF is support and protection—the brain essentially floats in CSF like an egg yolk inside an egg—it also transports nutrients, chemical messengers and waste products. A specialized capillary network, called the choroid plexus, in each ventricle actively filters plasma and selected nutrients from the blood to produce CSF. Once produced, CSF freely circulates until it diffuses through small projections of the arachnoid membrane, the arachnoid granulations, into the superior sagittal sinus and the cerebral veins where it joins general circulation.

The Peripheral Nervous System

The nerves of the PNS resemble strong elastic cords and are primarily responsible for both sensory and motor communication. Sensory nerves carry messages, including pain, pressure, heat, cold, taste,

sight, smell, and sound, back to the brain for processing. Conversely, motor nerves carry the brain's commands to specific muscle groups for action. Extreme stimulation of a sensory nerve causes the signal to arc across the spinal cord and send a preemptive message to local muscles to contract *before* the signal reaches the brain. In this manner, many injuries are avoided. In general, peripheral nerves follow the same routes through the body as do the major arteries and veins forming a neurovascular bundle. In the extremities, the neurovascular bundle follows the medial aspect of each limb, through the joints, to its terminus in the hands or feet. In this way, skeletal bones offer some protection from minor trauma.

Spinal nerves branch from the cord at each vertebra and form the interface of the CNS with the PNS. Spinal nerves are mixed nerves capable of transmitting both sensory and motor messages. It is important to understand that each spinal nerve root enervates a specific region of the body, such as the skin, muscles, organs, etc. The sensory nerves serving the skin have been mapped as shown in the diagram on the following page; each zone, or dermatome, overlaps slightly. Only C-1 lacks sensory fibers to the skin; instead, the face is served by the three branches of the trigeminal nerve, one of the twelve cranial nerves that connect directly to the brain. Knowledge of a few of the spinal nerves, their pathways, and their functions can assist in the field assessment of trauma patients with a suspected spine injury. Clinically useful motor functions and their nerve roots are: wrist and finger extension and finger abduction/adduction C-7 and C-8, big toe/foot dorsiflexion L-5, and foot plantar flexion S-1 and S-2. Clinically useful sensory functions and their nerve roots are: top of the foot L-4 and L-5, and hands (front and back) C-6, C-7 and C-8. Refer to Section VI, Traumatic Injuries, for the spine assessment (ruling-out) guidelines.

CNS Problems

The cells of the central nervous system are extremely delicate and require a constant supply of nutrients, via blood and CSF, and a stable internal environment to function normally. Changes in oxygen concentration, available sugar, temperature, electrical impulses, body chemistry, and pressure may adversely affect the brain and alter the patient's level of consciousness. Significant changes often result in death.

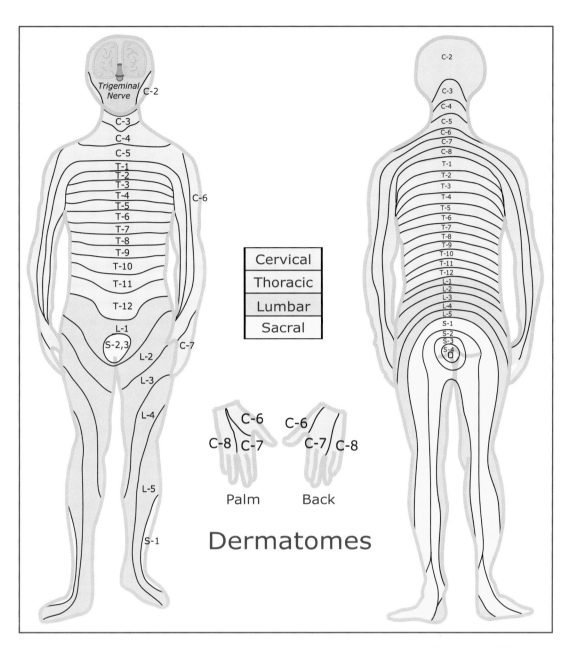

Dermatomes

Increased Intracranial Pressure (ICP)

An immediate life-threatening problem involving the brain is increased intracranial pressure. When brain cells become injured or die, the attendant cellular debris initiates the inflammatory process. If the damage is severe, localized swelling occurs within 24 hours of the insult. The swelling may occur quickly if caused by an arterial rupture, or more slowly, if due to a venous leak or inflammation. In the closed compartment of the skull, swelling means increased pressure. If the pressure builds to a point where it reduces perfusion to adjacent tissue, a negative spiral develops as the newly affected tissue dies. This results in additional swelling, a greater loss of perfusion, increased edema, and increasingly more pressure. If the cycle is not interrupted, the patient may die. Common causes of increased ICP are high altitude, suffocation, head trauma, and stroke.

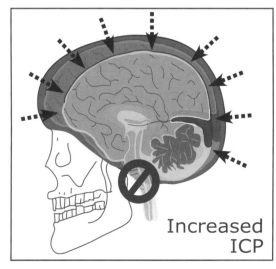

Increased ICP

Nerve Problems

Two mechanisms damage nerve fibers: pressure and cutting. Pressure on any nerve may interrupt its signals and cause numbness, pain and decreased function. Pressure applied for long periods of time may cause permanent nerve damage. The pressure may be *internally* caused by tissue damage and subsequent swelling from an injury or *externally* caused by poorly adjusted shoulder straps of a backpack or a splint that is too tight. The cutting of a nerve will effectively stop any communication beyond that point. Damage to the spinal cord is permanent, while peripheral nerves often regenerate or heal.

Autonomic Stress Response (ASR)

The autonomic nervous system responds to stress by stimulating either its sympathetic or its parasympathetic division. If the sympathetic nervous system is engaged, the body prepares for "fight or flight": pupils dilate to increase vision; pulse, respiration and blood pressure rates rise to meet an intense physical demand; awareness, often seen as anxiety, increases; sweating increases, while vasoconstriction leaves the skin pale, cool and moist; and endorphins are released to block pain. *A patient experiencing a sympathetic ASR cannot give accurate information about their injuries. In most cases, the patient is unaware of any physical problems and may not exhibit abnormal signs or symptoms upon examination. Their vital sign pattern may mimic or mask volume shock.*

If the parasympathetic nervous system is stimulated, the patient becomes nauseated, dizzy, and may faint. Blood pools centrally around their digestive tract and their pulse, respiratory and blood pressure rates fall. Their skin is pale and cool. Upon awakening, the patient is often confused. *A parasympathetic ASR may mimic the signs and symptoms of a concussion and make accurate assessment of a traumatic head injury difficult.*

ASR, regardless of the type of response, is not life threatening. Given the removal of the stressful incident, time, and reassurance, its signs and symptoms will disappear. The danger lies not in the ASR, but in the possibility that a serious problem will go unrecognized and untreated because of a lack of physical signs and symptoms in the patient. *Assume that all patients involved in a stressful in-*

Major Endocrine Organs & Effect

Hypothalamus	links nerves and hormones; sends regulatory hormones to pituitary gland
Pituitary Gland	controls other endocrine glands
Pineal Gland	controls body rhythms (wake/sleep cycles)
Thyroid Gland	controls rate of metabolism; can store its hormones
Parathyroid Glands	helps to regulate blood calcium levels
Thymus Gland	controls development of the immune system T-cells
Adrenal Gland	regulates metabolism of glucose, sodium and potassium; controls fluid balance
Pancreas	produces insulin and glucagon to respectively lower and raise blood glucose levels
Ovaries	produces female sex hormones
Testes	produces male sex hormones

Organs Containing Endocrine Glands & Effect

Heart	helps regulate fluid balance by controlling blood volume and pressure
Stomach	controls the release of digestive enzymes
Small Intestine	controls the release of digestive enzymes
Kidney	stimulates the production of red blood cells
Skin	produces vitamin D to stimulate the absorption of dietary calcium from the small intestine

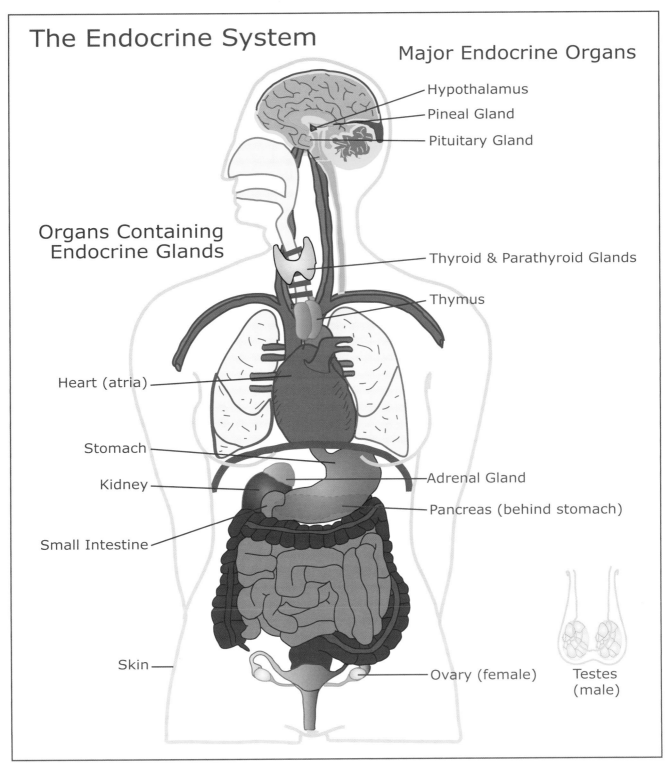

The Endocrine System

Major Endocrine Organs

- Hypothalamus
- Pineal Gland
- Pituitary Gland
- Thyroid & Parathyroid Glands
- Thymus
- Adrenal Gland
- Pancreas (behind stomach)
- Ovary (female)
- Testes (male)

Organs Containing Endocrine Glands

- Heart (atria)
- Stomach
- Kidney
- Small Intestine
- Skin

cident, especially major trauma, have ASR. Treat all patients under these situations as if they have the worst possible injuries indicated by the mechanism of injury or illness (MOI).

The Endocrine System

The endocrine system works with the autonomic nervous system to maintain homeostasis. Once stimulated by nerve impulses, its ductless glands release hormones directly into the circulating blood. In contrast to the short, quick nerve impulses generated by the nervous system, body responses to hormones are both slower and longer lasting. Hormones regulate metabolism, fluid and electrolyte balance, blood pressure, blood sugar levels, digestion, growth and repair of tissue, and stress responses. Damage to any of the glands of the endocrine system can usually be

The Digestive System

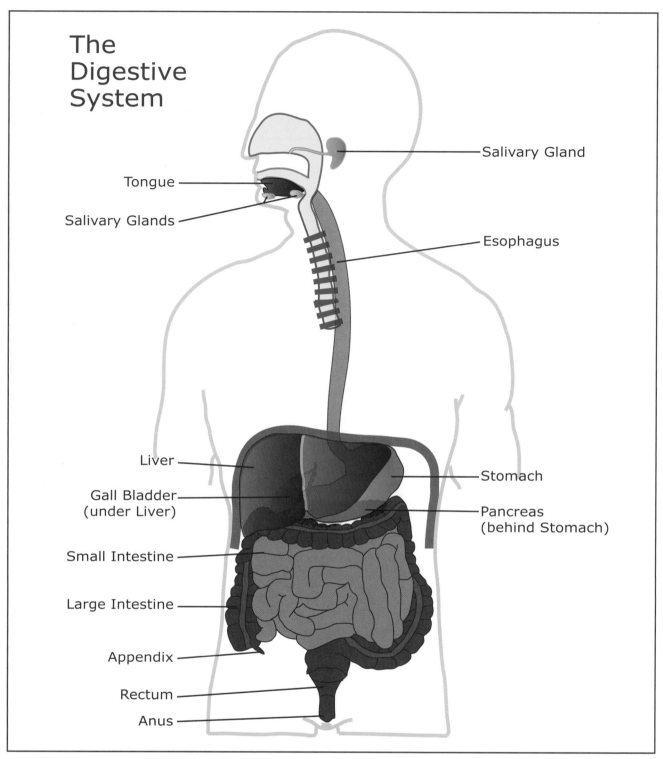

Salivary Gland

Tongue

Salivary Glands

Esophagus

Liver

Stomach

Gall Bladder
(under Liver)

Pancreas
(behind Stomach)

Small Intestine

Large Intestine

Appendix

Rectum

Anus

attributed a medical mechanism and generally has serious consequences.

The Digestive System

The digestive system is a series of interconnected hollow organs, connecting tubes, and solid organs. Many of the hollow organs are muscular tubes themselves and collectively form a "main" digestive tube. This main tube begins with the mouth and continues down to include the pharynx, esophagus, stomach, and small intestine. From the end of the small intestine, it continues past the appendix into the large intestine and rectum before ending at the anus. This central tube is connected to the liver, gall bladder, and pancreas through the portal vein, bile duct, and pancreatic duct respectively.

The digestive system mechanically and chemically breaks down food, absorbs nutrients and water, and eliminates unusable material. Mechanical breakdown is accomplished initially by chewing and then through the coordinated muscular contractions of the stomach and small intestine. The chemical breakdown of food requires the presence of specific enzymes that are released as food travels through the digestive system. Enzymes chemically break down food into amino acids, simple sugars and fats. These simple substances are then prepared for absorption. The process begins when saliva is released in the mouth and the enzymes contained in the saliva digest starch. In the stomach, gastric juices containing hydrochloric acid are released to initiate protein digestion. Food leaves the stomach as a thick liquid and enters the first part of the small intestine (duodenum), where the gallbladder releases bile and the pancreas releases pancreatic juice. Bile emulsifies fats, while the pancreatic juices continue to break down proteins, fats, and starches. In addition to secreting digestive enzymes, the pancreas secretes insulin and glucagon. Insulin and glucagon are hormones that act to balance blood sugar levels. Insulin lowers blood sugar levels by increasing glucose (sugar) transport into cells, while glucagon acts to increase blood sugar by stimulating the liver to release glucose. The primary purpose of the small intestine is absorption. Nutrients pass directly through the intestinal mucosa into the bloodstream and are immediately transported to the liver for filtering before entering general circulation. In addition to acting as a filter, the liver functions as a storage chamber for glucose and vitamins. Food passes from the small intestine through a valve into a pouch-like structure, called the cecum then past the appendix and into the large intestine. The appendix is a finger-like structure that protrudes from the cecum. It serves as a reservoir for healthy gut bacteria to repopulate the gut after severe diarrheal infections. The large intestine removes water and solidifies fecal matter. Once formed, fecal matter is eliminated through the anus.

While the digestive organs are susceptible to disease, most problems with the digestive system are associated with the structure and function of its tubes. These tubes can become blocked, kinked, cut, ruptured, irritated by toxins, or infected.

The Urinary System

The urinary system is a collection of tubes and solid filter organs. It removes waste products from the blood and eliminates them from the body. A mucous membrane lines the urinary tubes in both men and women. The kidneys are the organs primarily responsible for waste removal. They lie in the rear of the abdominal cavity separated from the other abdominal organs by a strong membrane, called the parietal peritoneum, and are somewhat protected by the floating ribs. In addition to blood filtration, the kidneys balance pH, fluids, and electrolytes in the blood. As the kidneys remove waste from the blood, urine is formed and carried via tubes (ureters) to the bladder where it is collected prior to elimination. Urine is eliminated from the bladder through another tube, the urethra. In women, the urethra is quite short and emerges as a small opening in the anterior vagina. In men, it travels a significantly longer route through the penis.

Normal urine is clear or pale yellow in color. Cloudy urine usually indicates bleeding or infection. High doses of B vitamins will produce a dark yellow or orange-colored urine. The pH of urine is usually acidic, but it may become basic with a predominantly vegetable diet. A high-protein diet increases its acidity. Normal urine does not contain sugar.

While the kidneys can be injured through trauma or by infection, the most common problems with the urinary system are associated with the blockage of its tubes from kidney stones in both sexes, bacterial infections in women, and sexually-transmitted diseases in men.

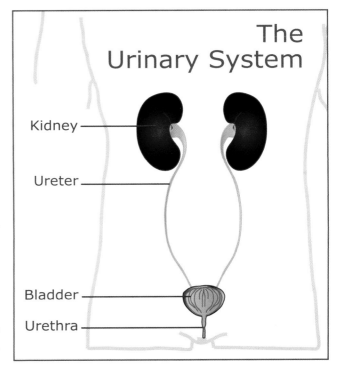

The Urinary System

Kidney

Ureter

Bladder

Urethra

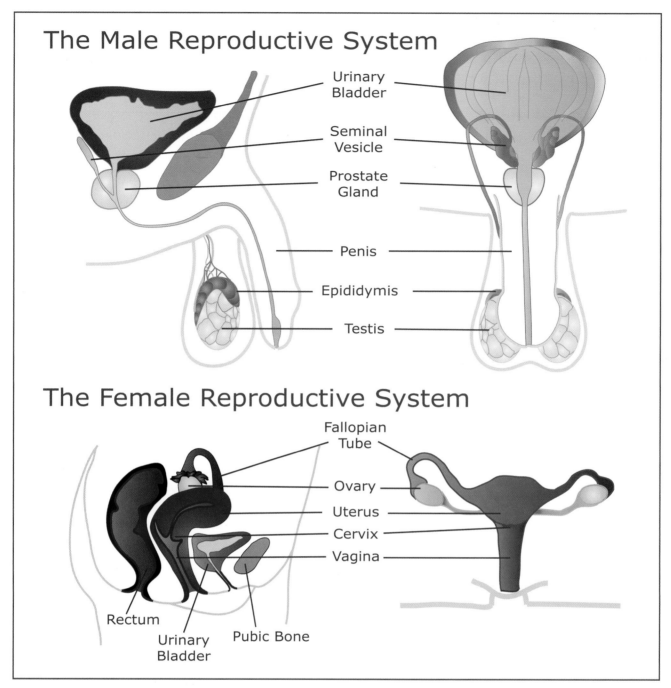

The Male Reproductive System

- Urinary Bladder
- Seminal Vesicle
- Prostate Gland
- Penis
- Epididymis
- Testis

The Female Reproductive System

- Fallopian Tube
- Ovary
- Uterus
- Cervix
- Vagina
- Rectum
- Urinary Bladder
- Pubic Bone

The Reproductive System

The reproductive system is a series of interconnecting tubes and sex glands. The function of the system in both men and women is reproduction of the species and the secretion of hormones necessary to develop and maintain secondary sex characteristics.

In men, the sex glands or testes are carried outside of the body in the scrotum with tubes connecting to the urethra. The prostate gland aids in semen production, lies below the urinary bladder, and surrounds the urethra, while the epididymis, the coiled tubes where sperm mature, lie above and behind each testis.

In women, the sex glands are internal (ovaries) with tubes leading to the pear-shaped uterus. The uterus is where the fertilized egg attaches and the fetus develops. The cervix is a muscular opening that separates the uterus from the vagina; its function is to preserve its sterility. A relatively short, muscular tube (vagina) leads from the cervix to the outside. Under normal conditions the mucous lining of the vagina contains a balanced mix of yeast and bacteria.

While both sexes may suffer from sexually transmitted diseases, yeast and bacterial infections are primarily female problems. Women may also suffer from problems arising during pregnancy and delivery. Men can suffer from a twisting of the blood vessels and spermatic cords leading to the testes (testicular torsion), an infection or enlargement of the prostate gland, or an infection of the epididymis.

The Integumentary System

The skin is the ultimate body stuff sack. It varies greatly in thickness, offering both physical protection from minor traumatic injury and denying access to potentially dangerous microorganisms. The outer layer of skin, the epidermis, is extremely tough and contains melanin, while the more sensitive underlying layer, the dermis, contains both blood vessels and nerve endings. Melanin offers protection from prolonged exposure to sunlight. Blood vessels within the dermis aid in thermoregulation as they contract to conserve heat or dilate to release it. Medically, skin color is not related to pigmentation, but to its perfusion status; hence, normal skin color is considered pink regardless of race. Sensory nerves in the dermis transmit environmental messages to the brain. Glands, also within the dermis, excrete water, electrolytes, and oils. Connective tissue (superficial fascia) lies directly underneath the dermis and ties it to underlying structures. A subcutaneous fat layer separates the layers of the skin from underlying muscle.

A number of mechanisms may cause damage to the skin. Any break in the integrity of the stuff sack may expose underlying structures to injury. Trauma may cut or abrade the skin, causing bleeding, tenderness, and pain. Extreme cold or heat may freeze or burn it. Infection may destroy cells locally and then move systemically.

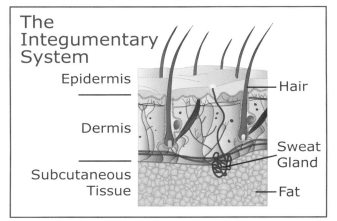

The Integumentary System
Epidermis
Dermis
Subcutaneous Tissue
Hair
Sweat Gland
Fat

The Musculoskeletal System

The musculoskeletal system is made up of bones, joints, cartilage, ligaments, tendons, and muscle. It provides the basis for support and movement. All components of the system require both perfusion and communication to develop, function, and heal. Arteries, veins, and nerves combine in the extremities to form neurovascular bundles that travel medially beside the long bones of the body to carry nerve impulses and blood to the hands and feet.

Bones form the rigid structure of the system and are highly vascular. They provide support and protection, are reservoirs for calcium and other minerals, and blood cells are formed in the bone marrow. Bones are surrounded by a highly vascular and innervated stuff sack, the periosteum, that contains special bone-forming cells known as osteoblasts. These bone cells, together with others called osteoclasts, regulate the density and strength of each bone. Continued stress on bones by walking, running, exercising, etc. causes an increase in both density and strength. Conversely, a decrease in stress-producing exercise causes a decrease in bone strength and density.

Joints hold bones together and permit movement. There are three basic types of joints in the human body: fibrous, cartilaginous, and synovial. Fibrous joints are formed when fibrous tissue securely binds the surfaces of the bones so tightly that no movement is possible (e.g.: skull sutures, teeth, radius/ulna, tibia/fibula). Cartilaginous joints have a limited amount of movement and are created when cartilage binds the bones together (e.g.: sternum to ribs, symphysis pubis). Synovial joints are very mobile and extremely complex; they make up the majority of the joints in the body (e.g.: elbow, knee, ankle, spine, etc.). In synovial joints the articulating bone ends are covered with cartilage and the entire joint is encased with a sleeve-like extension of the periosteum (bone stuff sack) that forms the joint capsule. Each capsule is lined with a slippery membrane that both contains and secretes a lubricating fluid. Ligaments are strong bands of fibrous tissue that complete the joint structure by firmly tying the bone ends together. Ligaments, like door hinges, help define the movement of synovial joints.

Muscle tissue comprises about half of the total weight of the body, is highly vascular, provides additional glucose storage, and produces most of the heat generated by the body. Muscles and tendons work together to create movement. Tendons are fibrous bands of tissue that connect muscle to bone. While tendons

The Musculoskeletal System

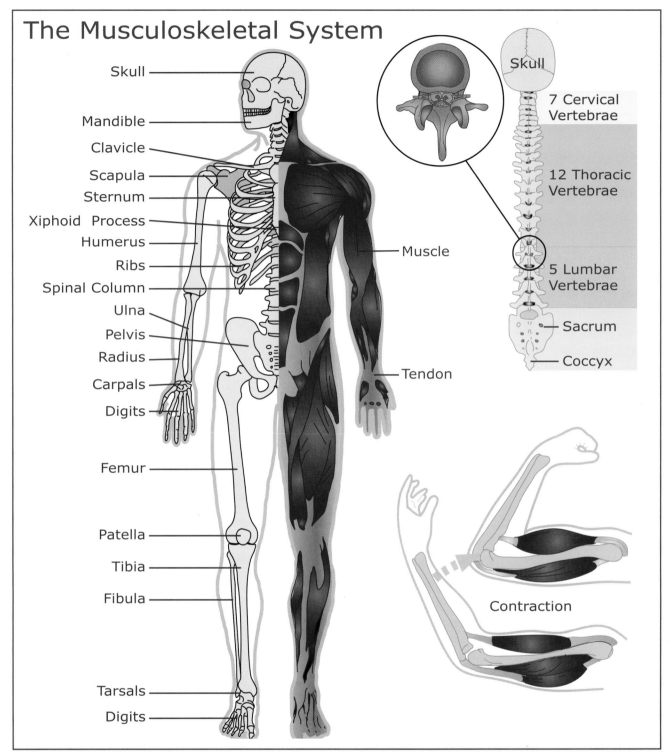

Skull

Mandible

Clavicle

Scapula

Sternum

Xiphoid Process

Humerus

Ribs

Spinal Column

Ulna

Pelvis

Radius

Carpals

Digits

Femur

Patella

Tibia

Fibula

Tarsals

Digits

Muscle

Tendon

Skull

7 Cervical Vertebrae

12 Thoracic Vertebrae

5 Lumbar Vertebrae

Sacrum

Coccyx

Contraction

do not cause movement, they must be intact for movement to occur. When stimulated, muscle fibers contract and pull on the tendon. The tendon transfers the energy of the muscles to the bone, creating movement. Since muscles can only contract and relax, they must work in pairs through opposition to produce movement in two or more directions. ***While both bone and muscle are highly vascular, tendons, ligaments, and cartilage have decreasingly less perfusion.***

Problems with the musculoskeletal system are usually those associated with traumatic injury and classified as stable or unstable. Significant musculoskeletal damage may indicate life-threatening internal injury.

Body Defenses

The body has three levels to its defense system: the skin and mucous membranes, nonspecific chemical and cellular responses, and the immune system. Each level is closely linked to the others and often responds in concert. Understanding the basic physiology of each level of the body's defenses provides a platform for successful prevention and intervention.

Nonspecific Body Defenses

As long as the skin and mucous membranes remain intact, they provide a mechanical barrier to pathogens and toxins. Skin and mucous membrane secretions are antimicrobial and help to protect against infection.

The second line of defense is also nonspecific and relies on chemical and cellular responses. Phagocytes, a type of white blood cell, engulf and destroy pathogens that penetrate the skin and/or mucous membranes. Natural killer cells directly attack and destroy infected and cancerous cells before the immune system is fully mobilized. The inflammatory response isolates the damage, assists in the destruction of invading pathogens, and begins the repair process. Antimicrobial proteins, complement and interferon, are present at all times in the blood and plasma. Complement binds to the cell membrane of invading microorganisms and causes them to explode or lyse. Interferon enters virus-infected cells and interferes with the virus's ability to replicate. Phagocytes actively engaged in fighting invading microorganisms secrete chemicals, called pyrogens, that stimulate the brain to raise the body's temperature. Low and moderate fevers ($\leq 102°$ F) increase general metabolism, raise the effectiveness of all the body's defenses, and speed repair processes; they also tend to suppress reproduction of most pathogens. High fevers are dangerous because too much heat breaks down (denatures) proteins and inactivates the enzymes required for normal body processes.

The Inflammatory Response

When cells are damaged or destroyed by any MOI, a chemical "alarm" is sounded, which activates the immune system and a complex healing process known as the inflammatory response. Numerous chemicals such as histamine, kinins, prostaglandins, complement, and lymphokines, are released locally by the injured cells, mast cells, nerve endings, platelets, and white blood cells (WBC). Together, the chemicals act to increase the permeability of the local capillary network and to encourage

healing. Clotting proteins build a fine net designed to wall off the damaged area and keep microorganisms out of healthy tissue. At the same time, specialized white blood cells, called phagocytes, move across the capillary walls and into the damaged tissue. Once there, the phagocytes begin cleaning up the cellular debris and actively devouring any bacteria or toxins present. The area remains "inflamed" until most of the damage has been repaired.

Vasodilation, a component of the inflammatory response, increases the local capillary pressure and forces plasma to move across the vessel walls into the extracellular space. Plasma continues to accumulate in the extracellular space until the pressure is equalized. The extra fluid (edema) helps to dilute any harmful substances and brings in the extra oxygen, nutrients, and clotting proteins necessary for repair. The clotting proteins form a gel-like fibrin mesh that act as an internal protective barrier and prevent the spread of pathogens to other areas. The mesh also acts as a framework for permanent repair.

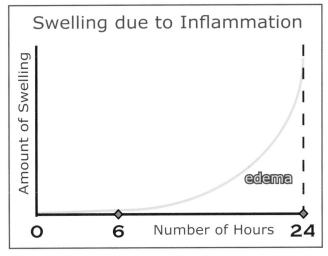

Local pain, redness, heat, and swelling are signs and symptoms of a healthy inflammatory response. The influx of fluid (edema) causes pain as local nerve endings are stimulated. Pain also results from the presence of toxins, a sudden decrease in nutrients and the sensitizing effects of prostaglandins and kinins. Non-steroidal anti-inflammatory drugs (NSAIDs) relieve pain by inhibiting prostaglandin synthesis. In addition to causing pain, prostaglandins decrease collagen production and slow surface healing. While this is helpful for deep wounds that are likely to become infected because it aids in drainage, it is not necessary for superficial wounds. The vasodilation causes redness and increased heat as more blood enters the damaged tissue. Another sign of increased permeability and vasodilation is localized swelling; the edema (and therefore the swelling) is confined to the stuff sack that surrounds the leaky tissue (e.g.: muscle facia, organ membranes, skin, etc.) Generally the greater the tissue damage, the greater the swelling. In the majority of trauma cases, clinically significant swelling due to the inflammatory response reaches its peak within 24 hours. Swelling primarily due to bleeding is much more rapid and usually occurs within six hours of a traumatic event.

Specific Body Defenses: Immunity

Unlike the first two defensive layers, the immune system is specific and has a memory. The cells of the immune system distinguish "self" from "non-self" (antigens) by recognizing specific "self molecules", called MCH proteins, on the surface of the body's cells. There are two types of immune responses: cellular (or cell-mediated) and humoral. Both responses occur at about the same time and both increase the inflammatory response. ***The cellular immune response is designed to attack invaders inside infected cells by chemically destroying the cell. The humoral immune response neutralizes invaders outside the cell and marks them for destruction by phagocytes.***

Both processes begin when a new antigen is engulfed and digested by one of several phagocytes, such as dendritic cells, macrophages, activated B-cells, etc. Once digestion is complete, the cell presents part of the antigen on its surface and travels through the lymphatic system until it encounters a helper T-cell, usually in a lymph node or the spleen. The helper T-cell (T_H) binds with the presenting part of the antigen, clones, and then releases chemicals that stimulate the production of antigen-specific B- and T-cells. The activated B-cells are responsible for the humoral

The Inflammatory Response

Pre-capillary Sphincter

Generic Cell

Mast Cell

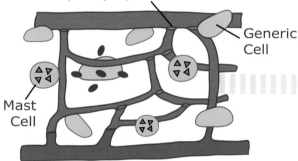

1. Bacteria attack a healthy cell.

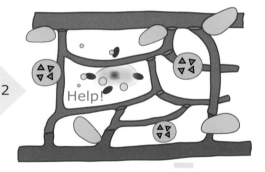

2. The cell calls for help by releasing a chemical alarm.

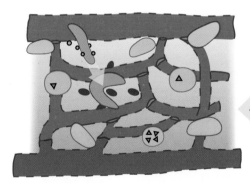

4. Local blood vessels vasodilate and leak causing swelling. Specialized white blood cells (phagocytes) move into the tissue spaces to attack, engulf and destroy the bacteria.

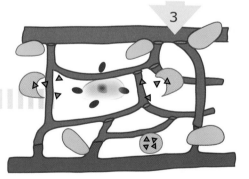

3. Local mast cells respond by degranulating and releasing inflammatory chemicals.

44 Anatomy & Physiology

Activating the Immune System

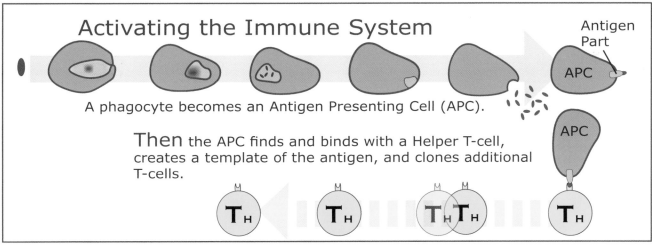

A phagocyte becomes an Antigen Presenting Cell (APC).

Then the APC finds and binds with a Helper T-cell, creates a template of the antigen, and clones additional T-cells.

Immune Responses

The cloned T-cells release chemicals that activate the B- and T-cells responsible for the humoral and cell-mediated immune responses respectively.

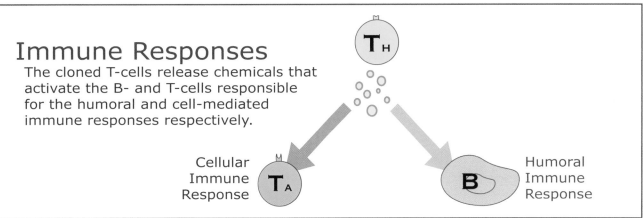

Cellular Immune Response

Humoral Immune Response

Primary Humoral Response

Activated B-cells clone and become either plasma cells or memory B-cells. Plasma cells are responsible for creating antibodies (IgD, IgM, IgG, IgA and/or IgE). IgD binds with a cloned B-cell to produce a memory B-cell while the other antibody classes are produced depending on the location of the antigen and need.

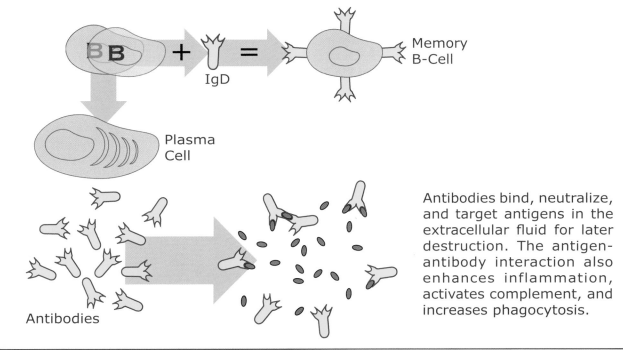

Memory B-Cell

IgD

Plasma Cell

Antibodies bind, neutralize, and target antigens in the extracellular fluid for later destruction. The antigen-antibody interaction also enhances inflammation, activates complement, and increases phagocytosis.

Antibodies

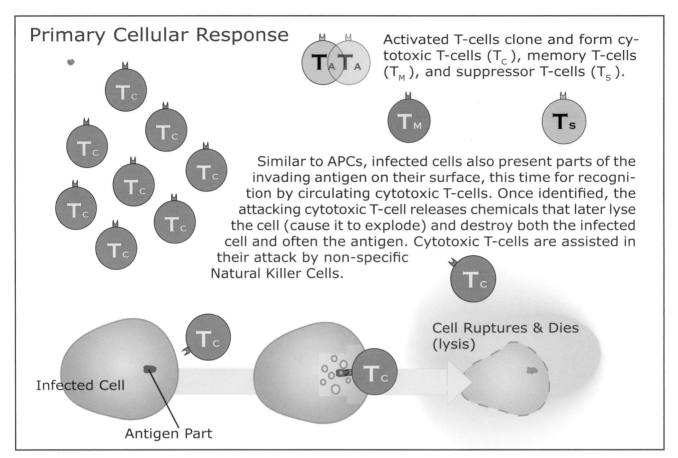

Primary Cellular Response

Activated T-cells clone and form cytotoxic T-cells (T_C), memory T-cells (T_M), and suppressor T-cells (T_S).

Similar to APCs, infected cells also present parts of the invading antigen on their surface, this time for recognition by circulating cytotoxic T-cells. Once identified, the attacking cytotoxic T-cell releases chemicals that later lyse the cell (cause it to explode) and destroy both the infected cell and often the antigen. Cytotoxic T-cells are assisted in their attack by non-specific Natural Killer Cells.

Infected Cell

Antigen Part

Cell Ruptures & Dies (lysis)

immune response while the activated T-cells are responsible for the cellular immune response.

Once activated, B-cells clone to form both memory B-cells and plasma cells. Memory B-cells have long lives (years) and are able to mount a rapid humoral response within hours if they encounter the same antigen at a later date. Plasma cells produce protein molecules called antibodies or immune globulin (Ig) at an astounding rate of about 2000 per second. Most antibodies freely circulate in the extracellular fluid spaces and bind to the antigens they were created to defend against. Once bound, the antigen is neutralized and targeted for later destruction by circulating phagocytes. There are five classes of antibodies (IgD, IgM, IgG, IgA, and IgE). Each class has a slightly different role in the body's humoral defense processes: IgD usually attaches to the surface of B-cells and gives rise to the memory B-cells responsible for immunological humoral memory. IgM circulates in the blood and is the first antibody to be produced by plasma cells during a primary immune response. IgG is the most abundant antibody in plasma and offers protection against viruses, bacteria, and toxins. IgG also crosses the placenta and transfers passive immunity from the mother to the

fetus. IgA is primarily found in body secretions and prevents microorganisms from attaching to the skin and the mucous lining of the lungs and gut. IgE helps to neutralize gastrointestinal parasites. A single plasma cell can concurrently produce multiple classes of antibodies, each specific to the same antigen.

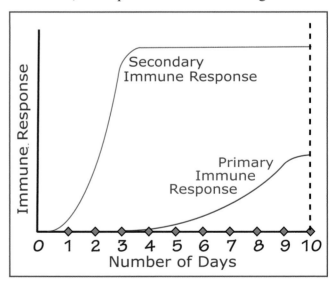

Specialized T-cells are activated at the same time as the B-cells and are responsible for cell-mediated immunity. Cytotoxic T-cells or killer T-cells (T_C) recognize, attack, and destroy infected cells and foreign tissue without damaging healthy cells.

Memory cytotoxic T-cells (T_M) have a long life, potentially years, and are able to mount an attack within hours of a secondary exposure. Suppressor T-cells (T_S) inhibit B- and T-cell activity once the invading antigens have been destroyed.

Problems with the immune system may occur in three separate areas: immunodeficiencies, such as genetic defects or AIDS, autoimmune diseases, such as multiple sclerosis, type I diabetes, and rheumatoid arthritis, and local or systemic allergies. Of these, allergic reactions are the most commonly encountered in a wilderness setting. Acute allergic reactions are caused by "abnormal" IgE antibodies attached to stationary mast cells or circulating basophils and are usually triggered by bites or stings. Acute reactions may be either local or systemic (anaphylaxis) depending on the placement of the IgE. Subacute reactions, usually to food, are caused by "abnormal" IgG or IgM antibodies. Delayed allergic reactions, usually caused by contact with poison ivy, poison sumac, poison oak, or mango skin, are not caused by abnormal antibodies, but by an "abnormal" cell-mediated immune response that produces a skin dermatitis characterized by blisters and weeping. All types of allergic reactions and their pathophysiology are discussed in detail in Section VII, Environmental Injuries & Illnesses.

SECTION IV

Patient Assessment System

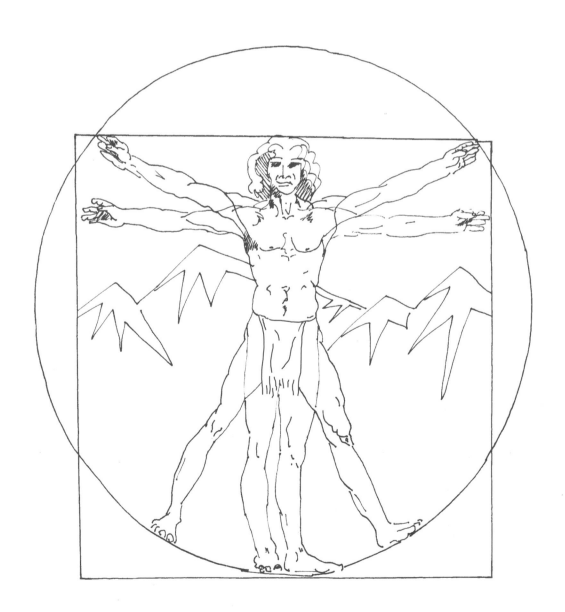

Patient Assessment System

Introduction

There are three interdependent components required for accurate patient assessment: surveys, patient SOAP notes and an MOI-based evaluation process. Precise and realistic assessment is required for effective field treatment, evacuation (when necessary), and ongoing patient monitoring. SOAP stands for Subjective (what you are told), Objective (what you see), Assessment (what you think is wrong), and Plan (what you're going to do about it). The three surveys (Scene Survey, Primary Survey, and Secondary Survey) are done sequentially in order to gather both scene and patient information in an organized and highly efficient manner. Information from the surveys, and the subsequent assessment and treatment plan, are recorded in the patient's SOAP note for easy reference. The evaluation process is based on a clear understanding of the Mechanism of Injury or Illness (MOI). Together the components of the Patient Assessment System offer an integrated and systematic approach to gathering, organizing, and evaluating patient information. Each is necessary to ensure effective treatment.

To complete an accurate assessment and efficiently treat your patient, first size-up and stabilize the scene. Then, complete the Primary Survey and treat your patient's life-threatening problems. Next, document your observations and treatments. After recording the information gathered during the Scene Survey and the Primary Survey, begin a second, more detailed, patient exam. Focus on the patient's history, physical exam findings, and their vital signs. Record, evaluate, and prioritize your findings before continuing to treat your patient. During a prolonged evacuation, monitor your patient by repeating both patient surveys. Revise and update your notes as necessary.

Mechanism of Injury & Illness

There are three basic mechanisms of injury or illness (MOI): trauma, environmental, and medical. For the most part, they are each self-explanatory: Traumatic mechanisms involve getting hit by or hitting something. Environmental mechanisms occur outside. And medical mechanisms focus on disease. That said, there is some overlap and confusion is possible: Allergies may be caused by environmental or medical MOI. A ruptured ear drum could be the result of direct trauma, an abrupt pressure change while SCUBA diving, from rapidly expanding air during a lightning strike, or an ear infection. None-the-less, identifying the MOI is essential to forming an accurate clinical picture that leads to a diagnosis and treatment. The mechanism of injury or illness plus the patient's signs and symptoms yields a possible problem list or differential diagnosis (MOI + S/Sx = DDx).

Most injuries and illnesses on outdoor trips involve minor traumatic injuries (strains, sprains, blisters, and shallow wounds) or over-use; mild environmental illnesses related to dehydration, heat, cold, and sun exposure, and high altitude; and most medical problems tend to be restricted to personal or group hygiene and endemic infectious diseases. When serious injuries or illnesses do occur, it's vital to recognize them quickly. The possible problem list, or differential, for trauma and environmental MOI is rather short, easily remembered, and problems are relatively simple to rule out. In contrast, the differential for medical problems is quite large, often complex, and sometimes impossible to rule out accurately in the field. Diagnostic strategy in a remote setting calls for first ruling out traumatic MOI and then environmental MOI, before considering a medical mechanism. See Patient Evaluation on page 54 and the introduction to each of the problem-based sections.

Patient SOAP Notes

The general story and scene information, relevant patient demographics, subjective information, objective information, the patient's problems, their anticipated problems, and your proposed treatment plan (including evacuation) are recorded in the patient's SOAP note. The SOAP format is the standard practice for documenting patient information within the medical profession. Refer to Section XIII, pages 268-269 for a copy of the Wilderness Medicine Training Center's Patient SOAP Note.

While the SOAP format may initially seem awkward to use, you will find it both efficient and helpful in assessing and treating your patients. Document the story, scene, subjective, and objective information you gathered during the three patient surveys in the first three sections of the SOAP note then begin the evaluation process. Once you have completed the evaluation process, record your assessment (the patient's current problems and their anticipated problems) and your treatment plan (including evacuation) under the Assessment and Plan headings in the SOAP note. During prolonged treatment, repeat the two patient surveys, as needed, to monitor the patient for changes, the development of any new and/or anticipated problems, and how they are responding to your treatment. Revise your SOAP note as it becomes necessary. Transfer a copy of your SOAP note with your patient and keep one for your records.

Patient Surveys

The three patient surveys gather the information you will need to evaluate and treat your patient. Each survey has three components (represented by triangles in the illustration). While you always complete the surveys sequentially, the order of their components varies with each patient and situation. Follow each survey with a treatment phase to address any problems encountered, and if indicated, call for help with the patient's evacuation.

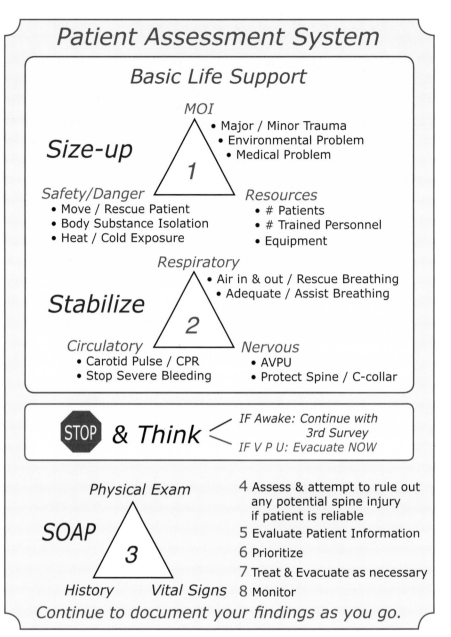

Patient Assessment System

Basic Life Support

Size-up — Triangle 1
MOI
• Major / Minor Trauma
• Environmental Problem
• Medical Problem
Safety/Danger
• Move / Rescue Patient
• Body Substance Isolation
• Heat / Cold Exposure
Resources
• # Patients
• # Trained Personnel
• Equipment

Stabilize — Triangle 2
Respiratory
• Air in & out / Rescue Breathing
• Adequate / Assist Breathing
Circulatory
• Carotid Pulse / CPR
• Stop Severe Bleeding
Nervous
• AVPU
• Protect Spine / C-collar

STOP & Think
IF Awake: Continue with 3rd Survey
IF V P U: Evacuate NOW

SOAP — Triangle 3
Physical Exam
History   Vital Signs
4 Assess & attempt to rule out any potential spine injury if patient is reliable
5 Evaluate Patient Information
6 Prioritize
7 Treat & Evacuate as necessary
8 Monitor
Continue to document your findings as you go.

Record all of your findings in the patient's SOAP note. It may be appropriate to *Call for help!* before entering the scene, after completing your Primary Survey, or after you have fully evaluated the patient.

Scene Survey ~ the first triangle

The Scene Survey is the first of the three surveys. It is divided into three components: mechanism of injury or illness (MOI), safety, and resources. Complete the Scene Survey BEFORE you enter the scene.

Safety/Danger: Your safety and that of other rescuers, bystanders, and your patient is critical. Danger may present itself in numerous ways: rockfall, avalanche, flood, lightning, hazardous materials, violent people or animals, venomous reptiles, etc. Address these physical dangers immediately without endangering yourself or others. If there are potentially dangerous environmental factors present (e.g.: extreme heat, cold, lightning, etc.) remove the patient from them as soon as possible while protecting yourself and others. Medical mechanisms (illness and disease) require additional protection. Consider the following precautions for all patient contact: protective clothing, gloves and glasses. Wear a mask or place one on your patient if you suspect a respiratory disease. Wash yourself and your clothing thoroughly after treating a patient. While impractical in a wilderness environment, in an urban situation, contaminated materials should be deposited in a sealed plastic or metal container and clearly marked for proper disposal. ***It is imperative that you***

do not enter a scene without first assessing and addressing both real and potential dangers.

Mechanisms of Injury or Illness (MOI): The mechanisms are divided into three broad categories: trauma, environmental, and medical. If during the Scene Survey you suspect major trauma, assume that the patient's spine is unstable and *immediately* immobilize it. If movement is necessary, support the patient's spine in the "in-line" position throughout the movement. Immediately address urgent environmental and medical mechanisms that may place you or your patient at risk. Address subtle non-life-threatening environmental and medical problems after the focused history and exam. ***Resources:*** Quickly assess the available resources in light of the scene dangers, MOI, and number of patients. If possible, assess the number and training of the rescuers; the medical, rescue, and evacuation equipment immediately available; the closest medical and rescue assistance, their training and response time; and all communication options.

Primary Survey ~ the second triangle

The Primary Survey is the first of two patient surveys. Begin the Primary Survey after the scene has been stabilized. Quickly check your patient's three critical systems—respiratory, circulatory, and nervous—and treat any immediate life-threatening problems. ***Treatment for problems identified during your Primary Survey is covered in detail in Section V, "Basic Life Support."***

Respiratory System Check: Assess your patient's airway and breathing. Their airway should be open with air moving freely in and out. Breathing should be adequate to perfuse the body tissues with oxygen. Blue-tinged mucous membranes indicate poor perfusion. If either the patient's airway or breathing is compromised, begin rescue breathing.

Circulatory System Check: If your patient is NOT awake, feel for a pulse at the carotid artery in their neck and do a complete body survey looking for external bleeding. If necessary, cut their clothing. They should have a palpable pulse and no severe bleeding. If they do not have a pulse, consider CPR or CCR and defibrillation. If severe external bleeding is present, wipe away excess blood and STOP it with well-aimed direct pressure.

Nervous System Check: Patients with a normal functioning nervous system should be awake and cooperative. If the patient is not awake, consider *calling for help* now. If there is evidence of major trauma during the scene survey, immobilize the patient's spine and maintain in-line stability during any patient movement.

Treat all problems found in the Primary Survey BEFORE continuing onto the Secondary Survey. Record all the information gathered during the Scene Survey and your Primary Survey, including patient demographics and treatments rendered, in the first part of the patient's SOAP note BEFORE beginning the Secondary Survey.

Secondary Survey ~ the third triangle

Begin the Secondary Survey after the Primary Survey has been completed, the patient's critical systems are stabilized, and the findings documented. Record the information gathered during the Secondary Survey as you gather it in the appropriate spaces in the patient's SOAP note. The three components of the Secondary Survey are: the SAMPLE history, the physical exam, and the patient's vital signs. The sequencing of the components will vary depending upon the individual patient and situation.

SAMPLE History: The patient's history is extremely important in identifying and treating illness and disease. The history may be subdivided into components and identified by the acronym SAMPLE. SAMPLE stands for: Symptoms, Allergies, Medications, Past medical history, Last food and fluids, and Events leading up to the illness or injury. The patient's history is considered subjective information because it is told to you by the patient or someone else. Some information for the SAMPLE history may be prerecorded in a medical form.

- ***Symptoms:*** Ask questions relating to the onset, provocation, quality & character, region & radiation, severity, and timing of their symptoms (OPQRST).

> ## OPQRST
>
> *ONSET.* When did the pain/problem start? What were you doing when it started? Was the onset sudden (acute), gradual, or part of an ongoing problem?
>
> *PROVOCATION.* Does anything make the pain/problem better or worse? Is the pain/problem relieved with rest?

- *Allergies:* People can be allergic to proteins in food, plants, pollen, medications, the venom from the bite or sting of insects, reptiles, and marine animals. Ask questions related to the type of allergy the severity of their response, and what type of treatment was required. For example: *Do you have any allergies? If yes, ask: Describe what happens when exposed? How do you prevent and/or treat them?*

- *Medications:* Review all the patient's prescription and over-the-counter medications and dosages for clues to their current problem. When asking questions about medications, consider prescription medications, over-the-counter medications, herbal remedies, homeopathic treatments, and recreational drugs, or alcohol. If the patient is currently taking any drug, follow up with additional questions. Such as: *Why are you taking this drug? What is the route and dose? When did you last take it? Who prescribed it?*

- *Past Medical History:* Review patient's medical form and discuss any prior problems. Examine the patient's history for any potential contact with an infectious disease over the past year. Relate questions about their personal and family medical history to a suspected MOI.

- *Last Food & Fluids:* Carefully evaluate the patient's intake and output as it relates to the MOI and their current hydration, caloric, and electrolytic-statuses. Compare their caloric intake to their energy expenditure. Include questions about their urine color and output and the color and quality of their stool. For example: *What did you have to eat today? Yesterday? Is this your normal diet? How much water did you drink today? What else did you drink today? When? How much? When did you last urinate? What color was your urine? How much was there? When did you last have a bowel movement? What was the consistency and color of your stool? Is the frequency, consistency, and color of your urine and stool normal?*

- *Events:* Ask the patient to describe, in as much detail as possible, all the events leading up to the illness or injury. Try to identify any lapses in the patient's memory if you suspect head trauma is a MOI. For example, ask: *What were you doing immediately prior to the start of the problem? What were you doing in the last 24-48 hours? Have you done this activity before?*

Physical Exam: The physical exam and vital signs are considered objective information because they have been directly observed by you. A detailed physical exam should reveal any skin, soft tissue, or musculoskeletal injuries. A thorough exam should both *look* and *feel* for any abnormalities over the patient's entire body. Essentially you are looking for discoloration, swelling, abnormal fluid loss, and/or deformity. Feel for tenderness, crepitus, and instability.

For traumatic MOI, begin the physical exam at the patient's head and progress to their chest, abdomen, pelvis, back, and extremities. Pressure should be gentle but firm. Ultimately, the depth and speed of the physical exam will depend on a number of factors: the overall severity of the patient's condition, the harshness of the environment, and the skill and resources of the rescuers. *Examine the patient's trunk first—head to pelvis—since the critical systems are housed there; finish with the extremities.*

In most cases, there is no need to physically examine a medical patient head-to-toe; rather, examine only those areas the patient reports as painful. See Section VIII, Medical Illnesses, for details on how to conduct a thorough physical exam on a medical patient.

Vital Signs: If you have the patient's normal vital signs on an expedition medical form, enter them in the space provided on the patient's SOAP note and take a complete set of vital signs as early as possible for comparison and further assessment. Vital signs assist in measuring the function of the three critical systems and are necessary aids in identifying clinical patterns specific to a particular injury or illness. Because you are concerned with identifying patterns, the change in the patient's vital signs over time is more important than any single set. Use the patient's pulse, respirations, mental status and level of consciousness as indicators of clinically significant change. If you notice a ten-point variation in the patient's pulse, respirations that become easier or more labored, the patient's mental status or level of consciousness drops, take and record a complete set of vitals. Mental status and difficulty of respirations are quick and easy to monitor; a pulse takes a bit more time unless you have a pulse oximeter. Once you have identified a clinical pattern, taking further complete sets of vital signs should not hinder treatment and evacuation UNLESS a change in the patient's vital signs would indicate a change in treatment. Because the changes over time reveal a diagnostic pattern, record the time with every set of vital signs taken. If you do not take a vital sign, note that as well. The seven vital signs are: pulse, respiration appearance, oxygen saturation, blood pressure, skin, core temperature, and mental status. Record the patient's vital signs in the vital sign chart in the patient's SOAP note.

- **Pulse:** Take your patient's pulse rate and regularity at their radial (wrist) or carotid (neck) arteries. Rate is measured over one minute. Limit the adjectives describing your patient's pulse to *regular* or *irregular*. Use a pulse oximeter if it is available.

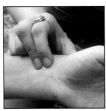 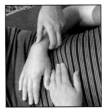 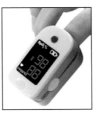

- **Respirations:** Take your patient's respiratory rate over one minute. You may find it easier to time the interval between respirations and divide the result into sixty than to actually count each respiration. Describe the quality of their respirations. Limit your adjectives to *easy* or *labored*.

- **Oxygen Saturation (SpO_2):** Use a pulse oximeter to measure the percent of oxygen available in the patient's blood. In the field it can help to identify poorly oxygenated patients and avoid unnecessary oxygen therapy. Readings are unreliable if the patient has low blood flow or decreased perfusion. A pulse oximeter cannot detect hypoventilation when the patient is on supplemental oxygen. Most pulse oximeters also quickly and reliably measure the patient's pulse. Choose a small durable unit for field use; use lithium batteries in cold environments.

- **Skin:** Assessing the color, temperature, and moisture content of a patient's skin conveys information about their peripheral circulation. Normal skin—regardless of the patient's race or pigmentation—is pink, warm, and dry.

- **Blood Pressure (BP):** Taking a patient's blood pressure, although valuable for assessing the status of their circulatory system, is often a rare event in a remote field situation; most land-based expeditions cannot afford the weight or space for a cuff and stethoscope. In emergency medicine, the systolic (top number) pressure is more important than the diastolic (bottom number) to measure the patient's perfusion status. Take their systolic blood pressure by auscultation (listening with a stethoscope) or palpation (feeling at the radial artery). If you don't have a blood pressure cuff, closely monitor the patient's mental status and level of consciousness.

Taking Blood Pressure

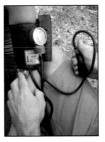

By Auscultation

1. Place stethoscope over brachial artery.

2. Pump cuff until no heart sounds.

3. Deflate slowly.

4. First heart sound is systolic pressure.

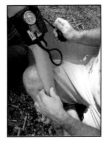

By Palpation

1. Locate radial pulse.

2. Pump cuff above until pulse disappears.

3. Deflate slowly.

- **Core Temperature:** The most accurate core temperature is measured with an esophageal probe (may be carried by Advanced Life Support); the next best option is a rectal temperature; both are used in hypothermic patients. Axillary (under the arm) and oral temperatures are one degree less than rectal temperatures. Use an oral or axillary temperature if your patient is alert, cooperative, and their injuries or illness is minor. Because of battery limitations, a digital thermometer is better suited to warm and hot environments. Winter expeditions are best served by carrying a mercury hypothermia thermometer; package it well, glass breaks.

- *Level of Consciousness/Mental Status:* Level of consciousness is measured using the AVPU scale. AVPU stands for Awake, Voice responsive, Pain responsive, and Unresponsive.

A patient is *awake* if they are asking questions, volunteering information, and/or responding to their environment appropriately. Mental status is a more detailed measurement of an awake patient. If your patient is awake, describe their behavior: cooperative, irritable, combative, drunk, anxious, tired, sick, etc. Changes in mental status may indicate a minor problem with the brain and often precede level of consciousness changes.

A *voice-responsive* patient responds to the stimulus of the rescuer's voice. Within the voice-responsive range, patient responses may vary from abbreviated sentences or words to moans to directed movement. A high voice-responsive patient will respond verbally but will not ask questions or volunteer information. A voice-responsive patient may respond with single words or groans. A low voice-responsive patient will not respond verbally but may move an arm, leg, fingers, etc. upon request (e.g.: "Squeeze my hand if you can hear me.").

A *pain-responsive* patient will respond to a painful stimulus by groaning and/or moving (contracting) away from the pain while an *unresponsive* person will not respond to any stimulus.

Patient Evaluation

Once you have completed the surveys and recorded the information in the patient's SOAP note under the subjective and objective headings, you need to evaluate it. The evaluation process is algorithmic in nature. Begin the evaluation process by identifying the specific MOI within each of the three categories: trauma, environmental, and/

or medical, then follow the algorithm for that category. Since there may be more than one category of MOI, it may be necessary to work through more than one algorithm. *Trauma and environmental mechanisms are easier to rule out than medical mechanisms; therefore, begin with trauma, move to environmental, and finish with medical.* Each mechanism will have a problem list associated with it; together, they form a complete list of your patient's problems and anticipated problems. Use this list to prioritize and develop a treatment plan, including evacuation. Continue treating your patient after you have recorded your assessment, evaluation, and treatment plan in their SOAP note.

Trauma Algorithm

When you are evaluating traumatic injuries, first identify what part of the patient's body, such as the head, chest, abdomen, spine, or extremities, was impacted by the traumatic mechanism. Next, for each part, identify the major system(s) housed within that part and its components. Each system component will have a limited number of problems associated with both the component and the specific mechanism. This is your possible problem list. Use the patient's signs and symptoms to rule out problems from your possible problem list to create the current problem list.

Environmental Algorithm

When you are evaluating the potential for environmental problems, first examine the environmental conditions and mechanisms over the past few days to the present. Environmental conditions or mechanisms can only yield a few related problems. These problems form your possible problem list. Use the patient's history, signs, and symptoms to rule out problems from your possible problems list to create the current problem list.

Medical Algorithm

Medical problems are diagnosed based on the patient's signs, symptoms, and history. Accurate diagnosis requires an in-depth knowledge of specific illnesses and disease. Many medical problems cannot be diagnosed without the clinical procedures and knowledge available to physicians in a hospital setting. When evaluating the potential for medical problems, a thorough history and physical exam, including all vital signs, are necessary. If flu-like signs and symptoms, eye pain, skin rash, or respiratory distress are present, review the patient's potential contact history for the past 3-6 months for endemic infectious diseases. Create a possible problem list based on your findings. Rule out problems through specific diagnostic testing. If a problem cannot be identified, consider treating the patient's signs and symptoms. Closely monitor the patient for any anticipated problems, drug reactions, and improvement. Rule out problems based on successful treatment. Modify the problem list, anticipated problem list, and treatment plan as necessary.

Patient Monitoring

Monitor your patient for changes, the development of new problems, anticipated problems, and response to treatment. Monitor by repeating all or part of the two patient surveys. Evaluate and record any new information in the patient's SOAP note. Revise your treatment and evacuation plan as it becomes necessary.

Evacuation Guidelines

The need for evacuation depends on the severity of the problem and your resources. The type of evacuation depends on the mobility of the patient, the size of your party and its resources, the difficulty of the terrain, the distance involved, and the cost. Evacuations are dangerous and often expensive; consider rescue and evacuation insurance. Any evacuation, regardless of the type (helicopter, plane, car, snowmobile, 4-wheeler, boat, horse, carry, etc.) should not endanger either you or your patient beyond your capacity to safely manage the risk. In most cases, your field treatment for minor non-life-threatening injuries will be effective and rapid evacuation will not be necessary. By contrast, your field treatment for most life-threatening illnesses or injuries will simply buy you and your patient some time. In these situations, focus on a quick, accurate assessment and fast evacuation. The "effective treatment window" for life-threatening problems is often specific to the particular illness or injury. If a rapid evacuation is not possible and your patient has a life-threatening injury or illness, your field treatment options are often ineffective and your patient may die. In general, any problem that causes a drop in the patient's AVPU is very serious. If a patient reaches definitive medical care (major hospital) while they are still awake, they have a reasonable chance for complete recovery. If they reach definitive care with a significantly decreased level of consciousness—voice responsive, pain responsive, or unresponsive—their chances for a complete recovery, or a recovery at all, are respectively reduced. A general guideline for making evacuation decisions follows: any apparently minor problem that is persistent, uncomfortable, and not relieved

Evacuation Levels & Criteria

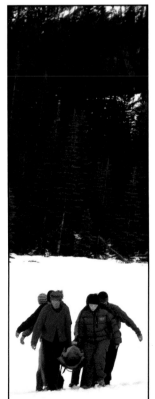

Level 1: Extremely Urgent Evacuation.

This level is reserved for immediately life-threatening injuries and illnesses; the patient may die.

Level 2: Urgent Evacuation.

This level is reserved for injuries and illness that are NOT immediately life-threatening but have the potential to become so. It also includes those injuries and illnesses that may result in permanent disability without rapid hospital intervention.

Level 3: Non-urgent Evacuation.

This level is reserved for injuries and illnesses that are not life-threatening or likely to result in permanent disability, where your field treatment is effective, however, the patient is unable to continue with the expedition without putting themselves or other group members at risk, and/or, where further evaluation is warranted.

No Evacuation.

No evacuation is needed for injuries and illnesses that are not life-threatening or likely to result in permanent disability, where field treatment is effective, further evaluation is unwarranted, and the patient is able to continue with the expedition without putting themselves or other group members at risk.

by your field treatment requires an evacuation. The urgency of the evacuation depends on the degree of involvement, or potential involvement, of any critical system(s). The greater the degree or potential, the more urgent the evacuation. Any problem that is immediately life-threatening, has the potential to become life-threatening, or could result in permanent disability without hospital intervention IS urgent and requires an immediate evacuation. *It is vitally important that all expedition members know the availability, resources, limitations, and how to contact the organizations, if any, responsible for rescue and evacuation in their expedition area as well as the resources available at both local and regional clinics and hospitals. A detailed Emergency Action Plan should be designed prior to leaving for the expedition. Organizations responsible for clients should know the limitations of their communication equipment within their operation areas and plan accordingly.*

In practice, there is little logistical difference between Level 1 and Level 2 evacuations. Some injuries and illnesses are difficult to place within any evacuation framework. When in doubt, it's often better to choose the higher level. When deciding on an evacuation level in today's world of instant communication, it's appropriate, whenever possible, to seek consultation with an outside expert. Keep in mind that an increase in urgency is often accompanied by a corresponding increase in stress and stress hormones in both rescuers and patients. Increased stress may lead to lapses in judgement and decision-making ability that may in turn lead to further injuries. The phrase, "Slow down, we're in a hurry." is usually sound advice when applied to evacuation decisions in a wilderness environment.

Helicopter Use

Helicopters serve two primary purposes in wilderness medicine: 1) early treatment and rapid evacuation of the critically injured; and 2) the controlled evacuation of minor injuries where other methods of evacuation would be more difficult, more costly, and potentially more dangerous to rescuers.

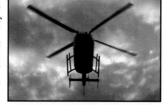

"Go" and "standby" requests are usually made via radio, cell phone, or satellite phone. Most aeromedical helicopters are dispatched directly from their base, by Search and Rescue (SAR) teams on the scene, or through local law enforcement (sheriff's office). *Rescuers should immediately request a helicopter to standby if they suspect a critical need;* in most cases there is no charge for a standby request. Map or GPS coordinates insure that the pilot will find you.

Helicopters have limitations. Most fly under "Visual Flight Rules" (VFR) and require a minimum of one-half mile of visibility and a 500-foot ceiling during the day; the minimum required visibility increases to three miles at night. Larger helicopters often have greater VFR minimum requirements. Some helicopters, usually military, are equipped with specialized instruments that permit them to fly in more difficult conditions. Even with a helicopter en route to your scene, weather and air turbulence at the landing site could pose a significant problem and prevent landing. *Never assume that a helicopter dispatched for you will arrive; always have a backup plan.*

While helicopters require less space than fixed-wing aircraft to land, they too have their limitations. A safe landing zone is FLAT and approximately 100 feet x 100 feet depending on the size of the helicopter. It should permit the chopper to land and take off into the wind; a light breeze is preferable to no wind, heavy wind, or gusts. At night, use head lamps to illuminate the landing spot and any hazards. Rotors generate extremely high wind; hold down or anchor any loose gear. In below-freezing conditions, be aware of wind chill; exposed skin can freeze in moments. Direct everyone near the landing site to cover their eyes or look away. Most pilots circle the landing zone before landing. *Avoid waving your hands above your head to attract attention; this is the universal "wave-off" signal that tells a pilot NOT to land.* While it is helpful to know the hand signals used to guide a helicopter to a safe landing, you do not NEED to know them; if possible, contact and follow the pilot's instructions via radio or phone. Once the helicopter has landed, wait for the rotors to come to a FULL STOP. Continue to wait until you receive a clear signal from the pilot (or crew member) before approaching any helicopter. Stay within the pilot's (or crew member's) line of sight and follow their directions. Do not smoke within 200 feet of any helicopter.

SECTION V

Basic Life Support

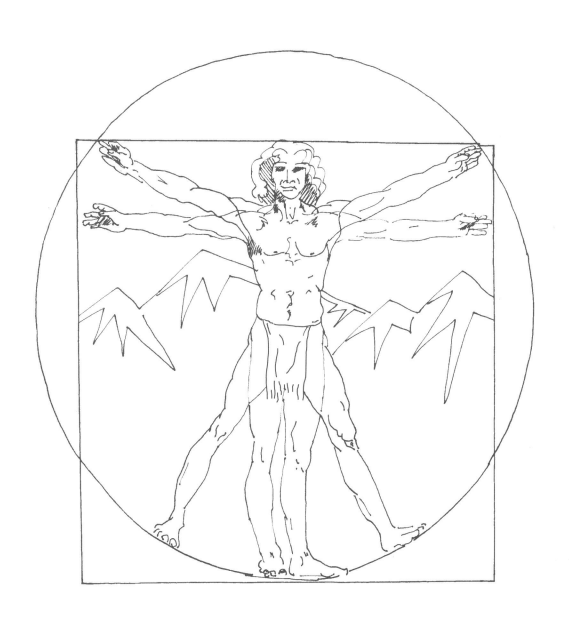

Basic Life Support

Introduction

Basic Life Support (BLS) generally refers to *noninvasive* emergency assessment and treatment of the problems encountered during the Scene and Primary Surveys, while Advanced Life Support (ALS) refers to *invasive* treatments usually reserved for EMT intermediates, paramedics, nurses, and physicians.

Respiratory Arrest & Severe Respiratory Distress
Pathophysiology

Upon your arrival at a scene, a patient may not be breathing. Even if they are breathing, they may not be breathing well enough to oxygenate their brain and vital organs. Respiratory mechanisms for inadequate perfusion include: respiratory infection, asthma, respiratory burns, exposure to inhaled toxins, traumatic damage to the respiratory center, and chest trauma. Under normal conditions, brain cells will die within four to six minutes without oxygen. ***You do not need to know the specific mechanism to begin emergency treatment; however, the mechanism will affect the outcome of the treatment.***

Assessment

- If a patient is talking, they are breathing and their air exchange is adequate for perfusion.
- If a patient appears unresponsive, place your hand or cheek over their mouth to determine if they are breathing. If they are breathing, you will feel warm, moist air against your cheek or hand.
- A voice-responsive, pain-responsive, or unresponsive patient who is breathing needs assistance if the mucous membranes of their mouth and lips are blue (cyanotic). Peel their lip back and look.

BLS Treatment

- Begin positive pressure ventilations (rescue breathing) and ventilate until the patient's chest begins to rise. Do not overinflate the patient's lungs; overinflation forces air into the patient's stomach and increases their likelihood of vomiting. Use mouth-to-mouth or mouth-to-simple-face-mask breathing; both methods are safe and effective.
- Supplemental oxygen at high-liter flow. Plug the oxygen line into the oxygen port on the face mask or use with a bag valve mask.
- Anticipate vomiting. If you are alone, work from the patient's side or if you are working with a partner, work from the top of the patient's head. Remove the mask between breaths to effectively monitor the patient's airway; maintain spine stability if the MOI includes trauma.

Breathing Check
Feel for warm, moist air on exhalation. Watch for chest rise and fall.

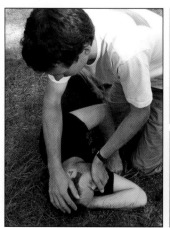

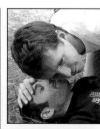

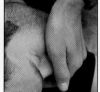

Rescue Breaths
Breathe until the patient's chest starts to rise. Stop. Breathe again after chest falls.

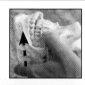

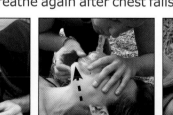

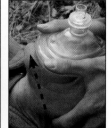

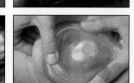

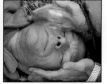

Obstructed Airway

Pathophysiology

Any blockage that significantly reduces the patient's ability to exchange air requires immediate intervention. There are four ways that a patient's airway can be blocked: foreign objects, kinks, swelling, and/or fluid. Foreign objects physically obstruct the upper airway; common objects are food, gum, chewing tobacco, and the patient's teeth. If the patient's neck is twisted or flexed at an odd angle, the airway may be kinked, like a garden hose, and therefore blocked. In an unresponsive person, the muscles that make up the tongue may relax, causing it to block the air passage. Trauma, anaphylaxis, or burns may cause local swelling of the soft tissue and subsequent blockage. Fluids, such as blood, vomitus, and water, may also block the airway and be aspirated.

Assessment

- If the patient is NOT exchanging air, give a rescue breath (as described previously). If the air does not go in, reposition the airway and try again. If the air still does not go in, the patient's airway is blocked. Closely examine the upper airway for foreign objects, kinks, fluids, and swelling; treat as described below.

BLS Treatment

Foreign Objects

- Do not intervene with an alert patient who is coughing and actively trying to clear their own airway.
- With **adults and children**, use abdominal or chest thrusts. Chest thrusts are identical to those used in CPR or CCR. Chest thrusts are also indicated for adults who are pregnant, extremely obese, or V, P, or U (defined on page 54). Be prepared for vomiting. Use one hand with small children as illustrated in the photo below, use alternating back blows and chest thrusts with infants.

Kinks

- Align the patient's head to open their airway. Maintain spine stabilization if the MOI is major trauma.
- Use a jaw thrust (see photo on previous page) or similar maneuver in patients having a depressed level of consciousness (V, P, or U).
- Consider inserting an oral or nasal airway.
- If the patient is on their back, consider rolling them onto their side. Maintain spine stabilization if the MOI is major trauma.

Fluids

- Reposition the patient so that gravity assists fluid drainage. Maintain spine stabilization if the MOI is major trauma.

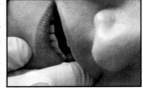

- Look inside the patient's mouth. Finger sweep for objects, if necessary. Use extreme caution; keep your fingers outside the patient's teeth.

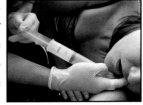

Abdominal Thrusts

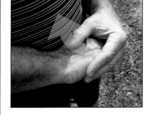

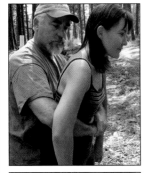

For adults, use two hands. For small children, use only one.

Push the abdominal organs up into the diaphragm to forcefully expel air thereby clearing the obstruction.

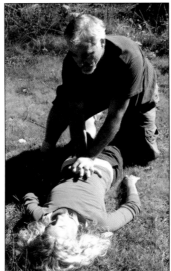

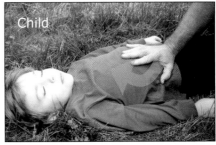
Child

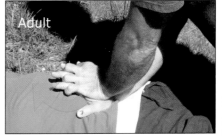
Adult

- Suction fluids from the patient's cheek.
- Call ALS for insertion of an endotracheal tube if it appears that the patient may remain V, P, or U and begin or continue to vomit.

Swelling

- If anaphylaxis is the MOI, administer SQ or IM 1:1000 epinephrine immediately. Pediatric dose: 0.15 cc. Adult dose: 0.3-0.5 cc. Follow with an antihistamine to prevent rebound (see *Allergic Reactions* in Section VII).
- For trauma and burn patients, align the patient's airway and call ALS. Advanced life support treatment includes the insertion of an endotracheal tube or preforming an emergency tracheotomy.

Cardiac Arrest

Pathophysiology

Normothermic Patients

A normothermic patient with no pulse is not perfusing and their brain cells will die within four to six minutes without oxygen. Unlike the sensitive cells of the central nervous system, both striated and smooth muscle tissue can live hours without oxygen. Because of this disparity in cellular survival times, it is possible to restart a patient's heart after their brain has died. Numerous mechanisms may cause a cessation in pulse. All are extremely serious.

Cardiopulmonary resuscitation (CPR) uses a combination of chest compressions and rescue breathing to delay brain death and extend the resuscitation window while cardiocerebral resuscitation (CCR) utilizes chest compressions only; both are potentially life-saving techniques. It takes approximately 10-12 chest compressions to build enough intrathoracic pressure to start circulating blood. The same intrathoracic pressure that circulates the patient's blood also brings in a small amount of fresh air and oxygen. If there is residual air and oxygen in the lungs, as occurs in cardiac arrest caused by a heart attack, then chest compressions are more effective in the short term for delaying the onset of brain death than when combined with rescue breathing because they maintain a consistent intrathoracic pressure. That said, a combination of chest compressions and rescue breathing (CPR) is more effective than CCR for patients whose arrest stems from a primary respiratory problem and lack of available oxygen, as

occurs in near drowning, lightning, and a complete snow burial. The effect of both techniques decreases rapidly over time and cannot save or prolong the life of a pulseless patient for greater than 20 minutes.

For CPR or CCR to be effective the patient's circulatory system must be intact and their core temperature above 90° F (32° C); your chest compressions must be hard and fast (ideally 100 per minute) and delivered in the lower third of the patient's sternum; your weight must be centered directly over the patient and the patient's chest must be allowed to fully recoil between compressions. If rescue breathing is indicated, ventilate until the patient's chest begins to rise; do NOT over inflate, over inflation forces air into the patient's stomach and increases the likelihood of vomiting. ***While CPR alone may be effective in resuscitating a patient in arrest from a primary respiratory problem, neither CPR nor CCR will restore a pulse in major-trauma patients whose arrest stems from increased ICP, significant lung damage, or volume shock.***

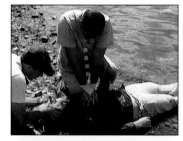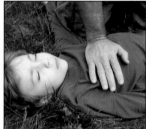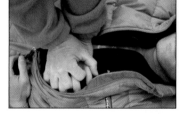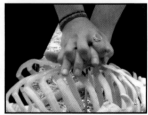

In settings where rapid defibrillation, advanced cardiac life support, and rapid transport to a major hospital are not possible, the overwhelming majority of patients in cardiac arrest will die. It is important that all rescuers understand the limits of CPR and CCR and when it is appropriate to start and stop them in both the wilderness and urban environment.

Abnormal Cardiac Rhythms & Defibrillation

There are four abnormal cardiac rhythms associated with cardiac arrest: asystole (flatline), ventricular fibrillation (VF), pulseless ventricular tachycardia (VT), and pulseless electrical activity (PEA). If a patient's heart is in asystole, there is no electrical

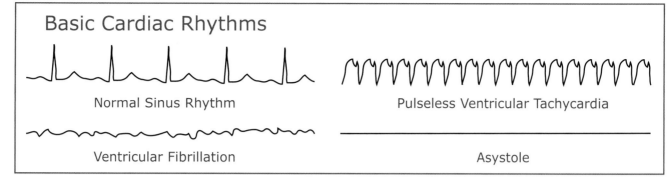

Basic Cardiac Rhythms

Normal Sinus Rhythm

Pulseless Ventricular Tachycardia

Ventricular Fibrillation

Asystole

activity and no pulse. In ventricular fibrillation there is uncoordinated electrical activity, the heart quivers and does not contract, and there is no pulse. In pulseless ventricular tachycardia there is coordinated electrical activity; however, the contractions are ineffective because the ventricles do not have enough time to fill, and there is no pulse. In PEA there is also coordinated electrical activity—an electrocardiogram indicates the rhythm *should* be producing a pulse but the heart muscle does not respond—and again, no pulse. PEA is always caused by a severe cardiac insult: severe prolonged hypoxia or acidosis, extreme hypovolemia, or a flow-restricting pulmonary embolus. Treatments vary according to the rhythm and the root cause: asystole may be converted to ventricular fibrillation via aggressive basic life support and/ or drugs; ventricular fibrillation and pulseless ventricular tachycardia may be converted to a normal sinus rhythm via defibrillation and drugs; PEA may respond to CPR or CCR combined with drugs and/ or IV fluids that address the root cause. Asystole and PEA will not respond to defibrillation.

Defibrillation is the definitive treatment for ventricular fibrillation and pulseless ventricular tachycardia. A defibrillator works by sending an electrical current through the patient's heart. The current depolarizes the heart, disrupts the arrhythmia, and provides an opportunity for the heart's pacemaker to reestablish a normal sinus rhythm. The external defibrillators used by rescuers in pre-hospital settings may be manual or automated. A rescuer using a fully automated external defibrillator (AED) has little interaction with the device beyond following the auditory and visual prompts and placing the shock pads. A semi-automatic or manual defibrillator requires advanced training and typically has an electrocardiogram (EKG or ECG) display and readout, user override capabilities, and rhythm analysis software. Advanced Life Support personnel tend to

carry semi-automatic or manual units, while AEDs are readily available in many public places. AEDs occasionally appear in a wilderness environment with clients who are at risk for heart attacks, for example at ski areas, in remote lodges, on rafting trips, on professional development courses, and where reliable communication and transport to a hospital are possible.

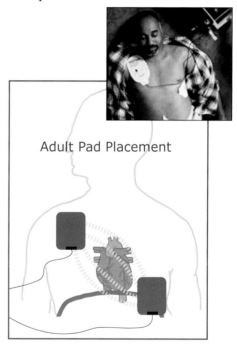

Adult Pad Placement

Most AEDs may be used in light rain or snow. Current models will instruct you to give 5 cycles or 1-2 minutes of CPR or CCR between each shock. At most, there are three buttons to push on an AED: power, analyze, and shock. Some have only two: power and shock. Many have a single power or shock button, while a few are fully automated, turn on when opened, analyze when the pads are correctly attached, and deliver a shock without prompting. Protocols require that users avoid touching the patient while the AED is analyzing a rhythm, in order to assure that inadvertent movement on the part of the rescuer does not disrupt the analysis. You should

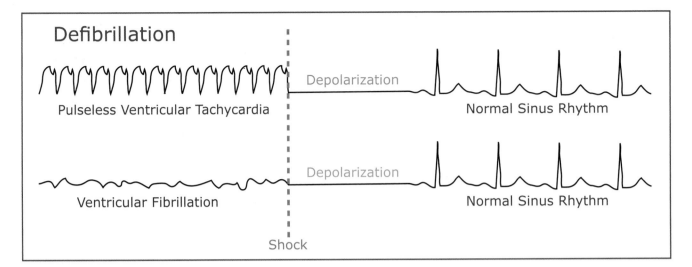

Defibrillation

Pulseless Ventricular Tachycardia — Depolarization — Normal Sinus Rhythm

Ventricular Fibrillation — Depolarization — Normal Sinus Rhythm

Shock

also avoid touching a patient while the machine is delivering a shock to ensure that no electricity is accidently diverted into your body. There must be good electrical connections between the AED pads and the patient's chest for the AED to function properly; many AEDs are packaged with a safety razor, so that you can remove excessive hair from a patient's chest to ensure good conduction. Because children have strong and healthy circulatory systems, it's rare for them to need defibrillation. That said, an AED may be safely used on children older than one year. While pediatric pads are preferred, adult pads may be used if pediatric pads are unavailable; place adult pads on the front and back of the child's chest with the heart in the middle.

If a defibrillator that displays a tracing of the patient's cardiac activity is available and you are trained in its use, you will be able to determine if there is organized electrical cardiac activity or not. In all cases, a signal to shock means that the cardiac rhythm is either ventricular fibrillation or pulseless ventricular tachycardia. A signal not to shock means that the patient has a cardiac rhythm which would not benefit from defibrillation: asystole or PEA. It is always important to assess the patient's pulse and treat accordingly. When purchasing an AED for use in a cold environment with potential hypothermia patients, consider buying one that displays a tracing of the patient's cardiac rhythm.

Hypothermic Patients

You may not be able to palpate a pulse in a severely hypothermic patient; definitive assessment often requires a cardiac monitor. If a functioning heart rhythm exists, chest compressions may cause

ventricular fibrillation and death. Severely hypothermic patients can survive for up to three hours without a pulse. Before starting CPR, check for a pulse for a full 60 seconds. If the patient doesn't have a pulse, begin rescue breathing at roughly 12 breaths per minute; the additional oxygen may stabilize the myocardium and make their pulse palpable. Take care not to hyperventilate the patient; low blood CO_2 levels increase the possibility of spontaneous ventricular fibrillation. If supplemental oxygen is used with a bag valve mask, it must be pre-warmed to between 100º F (38º C) to 108º F (42º C) and humidified; ventilate at roughly six breaths per minute. After three minutes of rescue breathing, recheck for a pulse for a full 60 seconds. IF the patient does not have a pulse and definitive care is available *within* three hours, DO NOT start CPR. Handle the patient gently, place them carefully in a full hypo-package, and transport. IF the patient does not have a pulse and definitive care is *greater than* three hours away, hypo-package (refer to the photos on the next page) and begin CPR. Discontinue resuscitation efforts after 30 minutes with a physician consult and after 60 minutes without. If possible, do chest compressions through the full hypo-package.

Whether or not you use an AED on a hypothermic patient depends on their core temperature. Core temperature is more accurate if taken with an esophageal probe (an ALS skill); in the absence of an esophageal probe, use a mercury or extended-range digital hypothermia thermometer to take a rectal temperature. If the patient's core temperature cannot be determined or is above 86º F (30º C), follow the AED protocols for a normothermic patient. If the patient's core temperature is below 86° F (30° C) and the device states that shocks are indicated, shock the patient once. If unsuccessful, discontinue use of the AED after the initial shock. Begin CPR and rewarming until the patient's core temperature has reached 86° F (30° C). For every degree above 86° F (30° C), the likelihood of successful defibrillation increases. (see Section VII, Hypothermia for specific instructions regarding when and how to safely rewarm hypothermic patients in the field.).

In a cold environment, begin warming and resuscitation efforts concurrently. Roll the patient onto a ground cloth or into a bivy sack, onto an insulation pad, and then into a sleeping bag or bags.

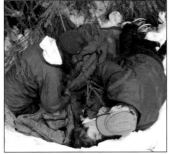

BLS Hypothermia Packaging

Fold tarp under pad accordion style. Fold edge of sleeping bag under pad. Roll patient on side and lay out tarp, pad, and sleeping bag.

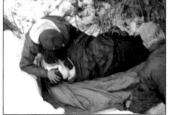

Brush any snow off patient if they are wearing standard winter gear and remove any wet clothes.

Roll patient to opposite side and pull out the tarp and sleeping bag edges.

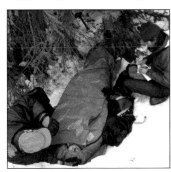

Roll patient into bag and zip, then fold the tarp over the bag to protect it. Do your physical exam through the sleeping bag.

Avalanche Victims

Roughly 65% of victims who perish in an avalanche die from a lack of oxygen (hypoxia); 15% from a combination of hypoxia, high levels of carbon dioxide (hypercapnia), and hypothermia; and, 20% die from traumatic injuries. Several factors determine the victim's ultimate chances of survival, including burial time, presence and size of an air pockets, the density of the snow, and the severity of any traumatic injuries. According to current research, there is a 91% probability of survival if the victim is recovered within 18 minutes; this is called the survival phase. The chance of survival drops to 34% over the next 22 minutes during the asphyxia phase, drops again to 28% between 35-90 minutes, and even further to 7% between 90-120 minutes. ***In the asphyxia phase, all persons without an air pocket die.*** Hypothermia and hypercapnia are only concerns with complete burials exceeding 90 minutes. NOTE: While rare, patients having a large air pocket or access to outside air have survived up to two hours.

Once the victim has been located, take care to preserve any air pocket by digging diagonally from downhill rather than vertically along the probe. Clear the patient's mouth and nose ASAP to establish an open airway. The presence of an air pocket and no snow in the patient's airway indicate that the victim was still breathing after the avalanche. Most air pockets are small and sickle-shaped, with ice on the inner surface of the pocket next to the patient's mouth and nose. In complete burials exceeding 35 minutes, the patient may be moderately to severely hypothermic. Excavate a large hole, move the victim as little and as slowly as possible, and place them in a hypothermia package. Warming and resuscitation efforts, if necessary, should occur concurrently.

If a patient is not breathing, has no signs of circulation after a 60-second pulse check, and burial time is known or estimated to be less than 20 minutes, begin CPR. If an AED is available, follow the guidelines for a normothermic patient. If a pulse does not return within 30 minutes of resuscitation efforts, STOP CPR.

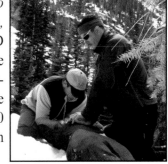

If an air pocket is present or uncertain, the patient is not breathing, has no signs of circulation after a 60-second pulse check, and burial time is estimated to be between 18-35 minutes, BEGIN CPR. If an AED is available, follow the guidelines for a hypothermic patient. If a pulse does not return with 30 minutes of resuscitation efforts, STOP CPR.

If there is NO air pocket, the patient is not breathing, has no signs of circulation after a 60-second pulse check, has snow in their mouth and/or nose, and burial time is estimated to be greater than 35 minutes, DO NOT START CPR; the victim is dead.

Drowning Victims

Because CPR alone may be effective in resuscitating a drowning victim and a victim's core temperature rarely falls below 90° F (32° C) even in cold water, aggressive BLS is indicated and hypothermia is a lower priority. As with hypothermia, it is important to check the patient's pulse for a full 60 seconds before starting CPR. It's important to note that drowning victims have occasionally been successfully resuscitated after prolonged submersion (greater than 30 minutes but less than one hour) in cold water (less than 50° F/10° C), but ONLY with ALS intervention. This means that resuscitation should begin immediately if the victim has been submerged for less than an hour and rescue attempts should continue for a full hour before downgrading to a body recovery. If the patient's core temperature is above 86° F (30° C) and a defibrillator is available, follow the protocols for a normothermic patient. If the patient's core temperature is below 86° F (30° C) and the device states that shocks are indicated, shock the patient once. If unsuccessful, discontinue use of the AED after the initial shock; begin CPR and rewarming until the patient's core temperature has reached 86° F (30° C). For every degree that the patient's core temperature is above 86° F (30° C), the likelihood of successful defibrillation increases. **STOP CPR if a pulse does not return within 30 minutes of beginning CPR. If resuscitation is successful, evacuate all near-drowning victims to a hospital; life-threatening pulmonary edema can occur any time within the next 24 hours.**

Lightning Victims

Lightning victims may suffer from traumatic or electrical injuries. Lightning may take a superficial pathway over the victim's body causing few injuries, or it may travel deeper via the victim's nerves and blood vessels causing respiratory arrest that may lead to cardiac arrest. CPR alone is often effective and should be started immediately on all pulseless lightning victims. Respiratory paralysis may persist for hours after the victim's pulse returns; serious, immediate and delayed neurological, renal, cardiac and muscular sequelae are possible (see Section VII, Lightning Injuries for details).

Assessment

Normothermic Patients

- **No pulse.** For the purpose of initiating CPR or CCR, the patient's pulse is checked at the carotid artery for a **maximum** of 10 seconds. The patient's neck should be in alignment during the pulse check.

Hypothermic Patients

- **No pulse.** For the purpose of initiating CPR or CCR, the patient's pulse is checked at the carotid artery for a **minimum** of 60 seconds. The patient's neck should be in alignment during the pulse check.

Treatment

Always follow state law and your protocols. If communication is available, call for ALS support and/or physician consult. If resuscitation is successful, transport the victim to definitive care.

Begin Resuscitation Efforts

- **Begin CPR** if the patient's arrest is due to a primary respiratory problem, OR if defibrillation and ALS intervention may be delayed for more than five minutes. Compress the patient's chest hard and fast. Ventilate until the patient's chest begins to rise; do NOT overinflate. The ratio of compressions to ventilations is thirty compressions to two breaths. Use high-flow supplemental oxygen, if available. Be prepared for vomiting.

- **Begin CPR** if the patient is hypothermic and definitive care is greater than three hours away.

- **Begin CCR** if the patient's arrest is due to heart attack, defibrillation is less than five minutes away, and ALS intervention is possible. Compress the patient's chest hard and fast.

- **Defibrillate** if ventricular fibrillation or pulseless ventricular tachycardia has been confirmed regardless of core temperature; the AED will advise shock.

Do Not Begin CPR or CCR

- IF the patient's core temperature is below 90° F (32° C) and definitive care is available within three hours. The patient may survive with definitive hospital care and CPR may precipitate ventricular fibrillation or pulseless ventricular tachycardia; avoid chest compressions, handle gently, hypo-package, and transport.

- IF obvious signs of death are present (e.g.: dismemberment, rigor mortis, frozen chest, ice formation in the airway, etc.), the patient is dead.

- IF the patient's core temperature is less than 50° F (10° C), the patient is dead.
- IF the patient has been submerged in cold water for more than one hour, the patient is dead.
- IF the MOI is major trauma and the patient's arrest stems from increased ICP, significant lung damage, or volume shock, the patient is dead.
- IF initiating and/or continuing CPR or CCR puts you or others at risk.
- IF the patient has a standing DNR (Do Not Resuscitate) order.

Stop Resuscitation Efforts

- IF the patient's core temperature is above 90° F (32° C) and there has been a documented 30 minutes of pulselessness and resuscitation efforts, the patient is dead.
- IF the patient's core temperature is below 90° F (32° C), a defibrillator is available and a shock or shocks have been delivered, CPR has been initiated, the patient's pulse does not return after 30 minutes of rewarming and resuscitation and communication is available, consult a physician. If communication is not available, continue rewarming, CPR, etc. for 60 minutes; if patient remains pulseless after 60 minutes, STOP all resuscitation efforts, the patient is dead.

Severe Bleeding

Pathophysiology

While common in military and para-military tactical situations, terrorist attacks, and explosions, and somewhat common in motor vehicle and farm machinery accidents, life-threatening bleeding is rare in a recreational wilderness environment. Chainsaws, ice-climbing tools, tree stubs, motorboat props, etc. can elicit significant injuries. Rescuers should assess all trauma patients for external bleeding that, if not immediately controlled, may rapidly lead to volume shock and death. Most life-threatening bleeding is arterial; however, severe venous bleeding is possible. Hemophiliacs and patients taking anticoagulant medications may be at extreme risk from even small lacerations.

Assessment

- Closely examine *all* trauma patients for significant bleeding. Remove or cut clothing and visually inspect the wound. If necessary, wipe away excess blood. Maintain spine stabilization and feel for blood in areas that are difficult to see.

BLS Treatment

- Wipe away blood to identify the source.
- Immediately apply well-aimed, direct pressure. Use a trauma dressing to distribute the pressure, if possible. Maintain the pressure until the bleeding has stopped. Normal clotting requires 10-20 minutes.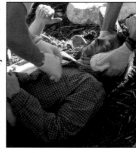
- With severe bleeding, consider using hemostatic agents to promote clotting.

Pressure Bandages

Consider applying a pressure bandage. A wide elastic bandage makes an excellent pressure bandage. Apply the bandage with enough force to stop the bleeding. Write the time that the bandage was first applied on the bandage and remove the bandage within thirty minutes of application. **Monitor** the patient's circulation, sensation, and motor function below the injury site (distal CSM) and consider loosening the bandage early if CSM becomes severely compromised.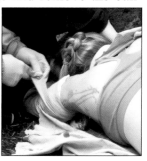

Wound Packing

If the wound is arterial, use gauze to blot excess blood from the cavity and locate the bleeding artery, then, pulling from the center of a gauze roll, completely fill the cavity with gauze and secure with a pressure bandage.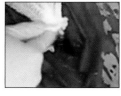

Tourniquets

Tourniquets are difficult to improvise quickly. If you anticipate a need for a tourniquet, purchase and carry a commercial one. Continuous application of a tourniquet for greater than two hours can result in permanent nerve injury, muscle injury, vascular injury, and skin death. The application of cold packs to the bleeding site during a long transport may reduce the damage associated with a tourniquet.

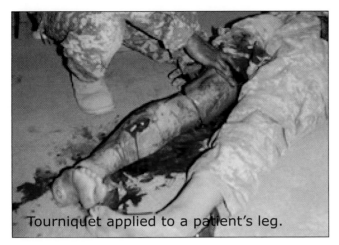
Tourniquet applied to a patient's leg.

Commercial Tourniquets

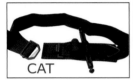
CAT

MAT

SOF

- If necessary, apply a tourniquet approximately two inches above the wound site, when neither direct pressure nor a pressure bandage are able to stop severe life-threatening bleeding. Do not place a tourniquet over a joint. Tighten the tourniquet until bleeding stops and *begin a Level 1 or 2 Evacuation depending on the patient's overall condition.*

- *Do not remove the tourniquet in the field if an amputation or near-amputation is present, if the patient exhibits S/Sx of volume shock, or if the patient's condition is unstable due to a different MOI.*

- Reassess the patient after 30 minutes. If no red flags for removal are present, place a pressure bandage over the wound site, and, while leaving it in place, loosen the tourniquet. If there is significant bleeding from the site, retighten the tourniquet. If there is no significant bleeding from the site, remove the tourniquet. If appropriate, downgrade the evacuation level. *DO NOT clean the wound.*

Unstable Spine
Pathophysiology

If you find or suspect major trauma as a MOI during the scene size up (see Section IV, Patient Assessment System), immediately immobilize the patient's spine. Movement of unstable vertebrae may cut the spinal cord causing irreversible loss of motor function and sensation below the injury site. A high cord injury may cause death. Unstable movement may be caused by the traumatic event, voluntary patient movement, or by the rescuers. Damage to the tissue surrounding the spinal cord may cause pain, tenderness, and swelling. Cord damage resulting from swelling may be temporary or permanent. When working with a patient with a suspected spine injury, your treatment goal is to avoid all unstable spinal movement.

Assessment

- Assume all patients with an uncertain or positive mechanism for major trauma to have an unstable spine and immobilize them.

BLS Treatment

- Use your hands to stabilize the patient in the position found.

- If necessary during your initial treatment, you may safely align the patient's spine to anatomical position using traction. Once the movement has been completed, traction is no longer required. Continue to stabilize and support the patient's spine.

- If rapid movement is necessary, you should maintain the patient's spinal alignment by firmly controlling their weight centers (head, shoulders and hips). Their head is best controlled using your hands or the patient's arms to form a "head sandwich." Their shoulders and hips are best controlled by using leverage and lots of hands.

- Improvise a cervical collar to help prevent cervical flexion as soon as possible; a SAM splint works well. Secure with an elastic wrap, vet wrap, or scraps of cloth; use tape only as a last resort.

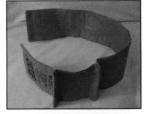

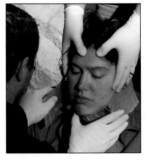
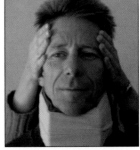

- Roll your patient onto their side with their knees bent and head supported in a spine-stable position; use a pack, clothing, or another person to support them if you have to leave for any reason.

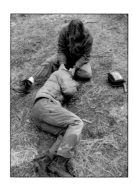 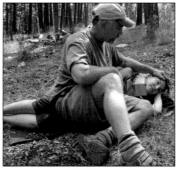

Spine-stable Hypothermia Packaging

It's not unusual to need to shelter a patient from the environment due to a combination of excessive heat or cold and the severity of their injuries or illness. When trauma is a MOI, it's vital to maintain the stability of the patient's spine as you work to protect them from the environment.

SECTION VI

Traumatic Injuries

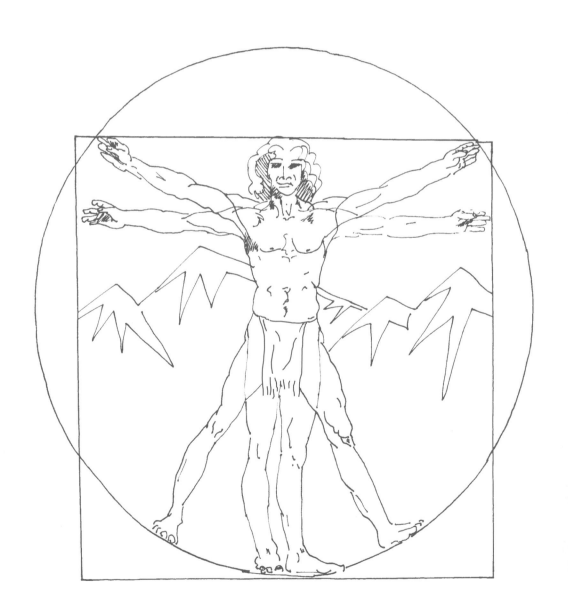

Traumatic Injuries
Assessing Traumatic Mechanisms

Each MOI has a different thought process associated with its assessment. When the MOI is trauma, there are two critical questions:

1. How MUCH kinetic energy was generated during the event?

Kinetic energy can be calculated by multiplying half the mass of the moving object times its velocity squared: $KE = 1/2\ M \times V^2$. Conceptually, this means that a slight increase in speed means a large increase in kinetic energy. Consider the following incidents involving sea kayaks:

Sea Kayak Incident 1: A group of beginning solo sea kayakers were playing sea kayak polo in empty boats. During the game, a student accidentally hit another student with the nose of his kayak on his lower left rib cage from a few feet away, causing his victim to capsize.

Sea Kayak Incident 2: A group of solo sea kayakers were floating outside a surf zone, contemplating if they could make a safe landing on the beach; their boats were fully loaded with camping gear for a four-day trip; the waves were two to three feet in height. During the ensuing discussion, two members of the group unknowingly drifted into the swells and started to surf towards shore. Unable to control their kayaks, one paddler was hit hard by the nose of his friend's boat on his lower left rib cage as she surfed down the wave behind him. Although hurt, the victim managed to safely land his boat on the beach.

Even though the victims in both incidents were hit in the same place on their bodies—their left lower rib cages—they had very different injuries. When victim one surfaced, he had a slightly tender side that showed traces of a bruise the next day; his injury completely healed within a week. Victim two also had a tender side, but the additional mass of a fully-loaded boat, combined with the speed and force of the wave, ruptured his spleen. Victim two required emergency surgery to remove his spleen and eventually recovered months later to live the rest of his life without a spleen.

2. Where did the kinetic energy go?

Was any kinetic energy dissipated during the event? If so, how much? How much went into the victim's body? If it went into the victim, what part of the victim's body was impacted and what organs were potentially damaged? Consider the following incidents involving a mountain bike crash:

Cyclist Incident 1: A female cyclist was speeding down a steep gravel road when she accidentally laid her bike down sideways in the loose gravel. She slid about twenty feet on her left side with her bike, before gradually coming to rest against a large rock.

Cyclist Incident 2: A female cyclist was speeding down a hill when she hit soft sand, her front wheel dug in and turned, and she was thrown head-first over her handle bars into a large rock.

The kinetic energy generated in both incidents was identical; however, in the first incident the energy was dissipated during the slide and transferred over time to the victim's skin. As a result, the cyclist in the first incident suffered abrasions along her left side and, while painful, they healed with minimal scarring over the next three to four weeks. In the second incident, the kinetic energy was abruptly transferred into the cyclist's head and neck. In this case, she suffered a concussion and a fracture of her fifth cervical vertebra. She was extremely lucky and fully recovered over the next seven months.

Once you have established how much kinetic energy was generated and how the energy was distributed during a given traumatic incident, identify what part of the patient's body was hit or damaged and attempt to locate the exact spots where the impact occurred. Pain and tenderness are clues, but often take time to appear (see ASR below). If in doubt, include all of the possible problems and rule them out later as you gather more information. Once you know where the impact occurred, identify the major system(s) and the anatomical components of each that are housed in that part of the patient's body. Each system component will have a limited number of possible problems associated with it. Once you have defined a possible problem list, use the patient's signs and symptoms to rule out possible problems and arrive at an accurate current problem list.

Autonomic Stress Response (ASR)

Most traumatic incidents are stressful for both patients and rescuers. You'll recall that the autonomic nervous system responds to stress by stimulating either its sympathetic or its parasympathetic division; both patients and rescuers are candidates for an autonomic stress response (ASR).

If the sympathetic nervous system is engaged, the body prepares for "fight or flight": Pupils dilate to increase vision; pulse, respiratory, and blood pressure rates rise to meet an intense physical demand; awareness, often viewed as anxiety, increases; sweating increases, while vasoconstriction leaves the skin pale, cool, and moist; and, endorphins are released to block pain. *A patient experiencing sympathetic ASR cannot give accurate information about their injuries. In most cases the patient is unaware of any physical problems and may not exhibit abnormal signs or symptoms upon physical examination. Their vital sign pattern may mimic or mask volume shock. A rescuer experiencing sympathetic ASR may not think clearly and may make poor decisions.*

If the parasympathetic nervous system is stimulated, the patient becomes nauseated, dizzy, and may faint; blood pools centrally around their digestive tract; their pulse, respiratory and blood pressure rates fall; their skin is pale and cool; and, if they had an altered consciousness, upon awakening, the patient is often confused. *Parasympathetic ASR may mimic the signs and symptoms of a concussion and make accurate assessment of a traumatic head injury difficult. A rescuer who is experiencing parasympathetic ASR, similar to a patient, may become nauseated, lightheaded, and faint.*

Internal Bleeding and Plasma Exudate

Everything in the body is contained in a membrane and connected to the whole with connective tissue. If a rupture or leak occurs at any level, the leak is contained within the next larger stuff sack. This concept is perhaps the single most important concept in understanding the pathophysiology of most traumatic injuries. Practically speaking, this means that when damage occurs at the cellular level, blood and plasma leaks may be contained within the tissue membrane. If the tissue membranes rupture, blood and plasma leaks may be contained by the organ membrane. If an organ membrane ruptures, blood and plasma leak into the body cavity. Blood leaking into the closed compartment of the skull will cause an increase in in-

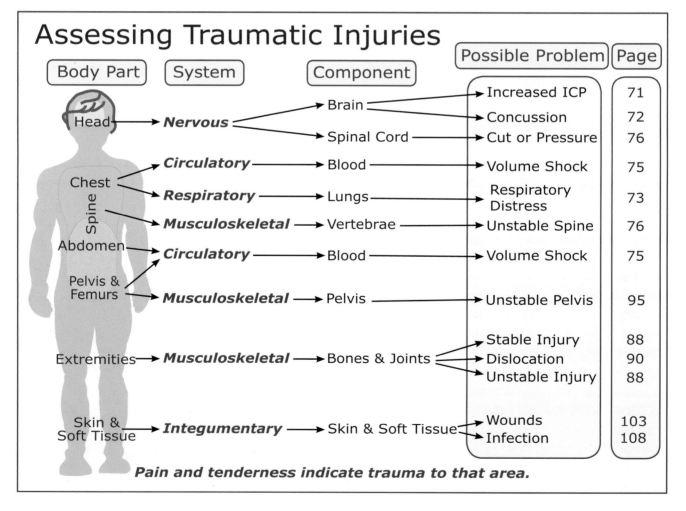

70 *Traumatic Injuries*

tracranial pressure that if not controlled, will lead to brain stem herniation and death. Blood leaking into the chest cavity may compress the heart and lungs causing respiratory distress and systemic perfusion problems; if not controlled, it will lead to respiratory and cardiac arrest. Blood leaking into the abdominal cavity will cause pain, tenderness, and guarding; if not controlled, it will lead to volume shock and death. Signs and symptoms of internal bleeding generally present within a few minutes or hours of the traumatic incident. Signs and symptoms of plasma leaking into a tissue, organ or body compartment typically present within 24 hours of the precipitating event.

Once your patient's possible problems have been identified, they are ruled out based on their signs and symptoms, leaving the patient's current problem list. Build your anticipated problem list from the patient's current problems and treat both the current and anticipated problems. For traumatic injury assessment, refer to the chart on the previous page.

Increased ICP
Pathophysiology

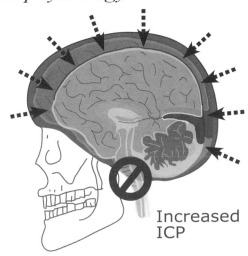

Increased
ICP

Head trauma may injure brain cells and activate the inflammatory response, leading to edema and swelling during the first 24 hours. A blow to the head may also damage blood vessels and cause localized bleeding. Any fluid—blood or plasma—leaking into the closed compartment of the skull causes an increase in pressure. Increasing pressure leads to decreased perfusion and subsequent injury to otherwise healthy brain tissue. This, in turn, causes more leakage and progressively increasing pressure. If the pressure is not relieved, it will lead to death from brainstem herniation, which causes mechanical

compression and subsequent loss of vital functions. The body has no compensatory mechanism for increased ICP; field care is limited to early recognition and immediate evacuation to a major trauma center.

Prevention
- Wear a correctly fitted, well-padded helmet that is specifically designed for the activity, such as climbing, bicycling, paddling, etc.

Assessment
General
- The MOI is head trauma. While positive signs and symptoms for musculoskeletal injuries to the head indicate head trauma, they do not necessarily indicate increased ICP.
- Patients with increasing ICP are assumed to have an unstable spine injury unless previously cleared (see Spine Injuries on page 76).
- Patients may present with a late clinical pattern.

Early Clinical Pattern
- The patient is awake, but becomes increasingly tired and lethargic, or increasingly irritable; irritability may progress to active combativeness. Patients with the early clinical pattern for increased ICP often appear drunk.
- The patient has a headache that worsens, rather than improves over time; similar to a migraine or bad hangover.
- The patient exhibits multiple episodes of vomiting.

Late Clinical Pattern
- The patient becomes voice-responsive, pain-responsive or unresponsive over time (minutes or hours depending on the severity of damage.)
- Vomiting eventually stops and the patient's respirations become irregular. Seizures are common, as the patient approaches cardiac arrest and death.

Field Treatment
- Maintain and protect the patient's airway. Consider side packaging, if a spine injury is suspected ,and the patient is actively vomiting.
- Maintain spine stability unless it has been previously cleared.
- Begin rescue breathing and oxygen therapy, if the patient's respirations are slow or absent.
- Position the patient on their back or side with their head slightly higher than their feet.

• Begin a Level 1 Evacuation.

• Cardiac arrest denotes death. CPR is not indicated.

Concussion

Pathophysiology

A concussion is a minor brain injury that occurs when a blow to the head disrupts normal brain function, causing mild neurologic signs and symptoms. Most concussed patients exhibit no structural damage when their brain is viewed using advanced imaging techniques (MRI, CT). Most patients completely recover within 24 hours; however, a few take longer, sometimes much longer, to heal. Severe blows to the head may damage blood vessels, injure brain tissue, and lead to increased ICP during the first 24 hours. Although rare in a wilderness context, a slow venous bleed into the space beneath the dura, may lead to a subdural hematoma, and the signs and symptoms of increased ICP over the next seven to ten days. For field evacuation purposes, a concussion may be defined as a temporary loss of consciousness or amnesia due to a blow to the head.

That said, most minor concussions DO NOT involve a loss of consciousness, amnesia, seizures or vomiting; however, those that do are considered significantly more severe. Symptoms vary with each individual, can be difficult to recognize, and typically fall into four categories: physical, cognitive, emotional, and sleep-related. (Refer to table at the bottom of the page.)

Both cognitive and physical rest is required for healing of minor concussions; surgery is required to treat those that progress to increased ICP.

Symptoms may take minutes, hours, days, weeks, months, or even longer in rare cases, to fully resolve. Recovery is typically longer in children and adolescents. Symptoms should resolve with time; if they linger or worsen, it is cause for immediate alarm/concern. It is imperative that all concussed patients be symptom free at rest and with exertion BEFORE gradually returning to normal activity.

A rare condition, called second impact syndrome (SIS), may rapidly lead to increased intracranial pressure and death if a recently concussed patient receives a second, even minor, blow to the head before their symptoms fully resolve. SIS should not be confused with repetitive head injury syndrome where a person suffers from repetitive head injuries over a long period of time and experiences a progressive loss of cognitive abilities.

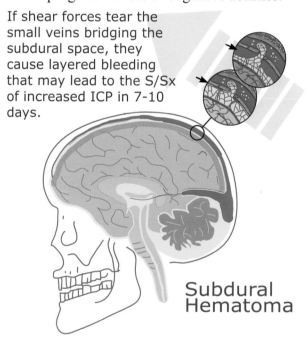

If shear forces tear the small veins bridging the subdural space, they cause layered bleeding that may lead to the S/Sx of increased ICP in 7-10 days.

Subdural Hematoma

Signs & Symptoms of a Concussion

Physical	Cognitive	Emotional	Sleep
• Headache	• Feeling mentally "foggy"	• Irritable	• Drowsy
• Nausea	• Feeling slow	• Sad	• Trouble falling asleep
• Balance problems	• Difficulty concentrating	• Emotional	• Sleeping more than usual
• Dizziness	• Difficulty remembering	• Nervous	• Sleeping less than usual
• Visual problems	• Forgetful		
• Fatigue	• Confused		
• Light sensitivity	• Answers questions slowly		
• Noise sensitivity	• Repeats questions		
• Numbness/tingling			
• Dazed/stunned			

Prevention

- Wear a correctly fitted, well-padded helmet that is specifically designed for the activity, such as climbing, bicycling, paddling, etc.

Assessment

- The MOI is head trauma. While positive S/Sx for musculoskeletal injuries to the head indicate head trauma, they do not necessarily indicate a concussion.
- Patient is alert and cooperative following a blow to the head, with or without showing the S/Sx described in the table on the previous page, and may have experienced a temporary loss of consciousness.
- Concussed patients often cannot remember what happened prior to the precipitating event (retrograde amnesia) and/or show short-term memory loss following the event (anterograde amnesia). If you cannot determine if the patient has had an episode of altered mental status and if either type of amnesia is present, assume the patient has a concussion.
- A mild headache is common and typically gets better with time and both physical and mental rest.
- Nausea may be present due to parasympathetic ASR. A single episode of vomiting is not uncommon immediately following the event.
- Many concussed patients are tired and wish to sleep.
- Increased ICP may develop within 24 hours of the traumatic event.

Field Treatment

- If the injury occurred with no loss of consciousness, monitor the patient for two hours. If S/Sx DO NOT develop, no further treatment is necessary.
- Begin a Level 3 Evacuation for all patients who experience a temporary loss of consciousness, amnesia, or seizures.
- Monitor for the early S/Sx of increased ICP.
- If the patient's signs and symptoms worsen, upgrade to a Level 2 Evacuation. If the complete clinical pattern for early increased ICP develops, upgrade to a Level 1 Evacuation.
- Encourage the patient to sleep. Sleep is healing; however, because of the potential for developing increased ICP, do not leave your patient alone during the first 24 hours and awaken them every two hours to an alert status if they fall asleep. Closely monitor them for vomiting while they are sleeping.

Respiratory Distress
Pathophysiology

A blow to the chest can easily knock the wind out of a patient. If severe enough, it may fracture a rib—or ribs—and/or damage the patient's lungs. All may cause respiratory distress. The initial respiratory distress seen from "getting the wind knocked out" of a patient will disappear within a few minutes; it may continue or return if there is lung damage.

Although painful, simple rib fractures usually heal without further complications; however, multiple rib fractures often destroy the integrity of the chest wall (flail chest) and damage the lungs. Damage to the lungs will result in respiratory distress if the blow tears either pleura and permits air and/or blood to leak into the pleural space. If each subsequent inhalation forces more blood or air between the pleura, it will prevent the lung from fully inflating. A "collapsed lung" is known medically as a pneumothorax, hemothorax, hemopneumothorax, or a tension pneumothorax, depending on the type and severity of the leaking blood and/or air. Prognosis is generally good with minor damage to one lung. If both lungs are involved and ALS is not readily available, the patient may die. The bruising of lung tissue may occur independently from or in addition to a pleural delamination, if blood vessels and alveoli are ruptured during the traumatic episode. Although rare, blood leaking into damaged alveoli may cause productive coughing and pink foam as the blood is expelled.

Assessment
General

- The MOI is chest trauma. When chest pain and tenderness are present after a blow to the chest, anticipate and monitor for respiratory distress.
- A sharp, knife-like pain upon inhalation indicates a fractured rib. A rib fracture is usually accompanied by point tenderness and occasionally crepitus at the fracture site. If the patient's lungs remain intact, the respiratory distress triggered by a broken rib will resolve with abdominal breathing.
- Patients may present with a late clinical pattern.
- A pink, foamy, productive cough indicates damage to the alveoli and/or respiratory mucosa.

Early Clinical Pattern

- The patient is awake and anxious or irritable.

- The patient complains of difficulty breathing, may assume a standing or sitting tripod position, and will have difficulty speaking in full sentences.
- The patient exhibits both increased respiratory and pulse rates.
- Blood pressure may vary and is NOT clinically helpful in assessing the presence of respiratory distress; however, a stable or falling blood pressure, coupled with a rising pulse, indicates internal bleeding that may lead to volume shock. A rising blood pressure, respiratory rate, and pulse usually indicates an intact circulatory system.
- Prognosis is generally good with minor damage to one lung and rapid evacuation.

Late Clinical Pattern

- The patient continues to experience and exhibit greater and greater difficulty breathing, and over time, as blood oxygen levels drop, becomes voice-responsive, pain-responsive, and unresponsive.
- Both pulse and respiratory rates continues to rise and patient may arrest.
- Blood pressure may vary and is NOT clinically helpful in assessing the presence of respiratory distress; however, a stable or falling blood pressure, coupled with a rising pulse, indicates internal bleeding that may lead to volume shock. A rising blood pressure, respiratory rate, and pulse usually indicate an intact circulatory system.
- No lung sounds are present in the injured part of the patient's lung.
- Cyanosis (blue color) may be present in mucous membranes and skin, as the patient's condition deteriorates.
- A complete delamination of both lungs or pressure on an intact lung from a tension pneumothorax will result in death, if ALS is not readily available.

Field Treatment

Basic Life Support Treatment

- Assist awake patients to a sitting position while maintaining spine stability.
- Position voice-responsive, pain-responsive, and unresponsive patients on their injured side to permit the lung on the uninjured side to expand normally.
- Reassure and coach awake patients to breathe with their diaphragm (belly breathe).
- Consider applying a cervical collar if the patient will remain in a sitting position.

Treatment of Isolated Rib Fractures

- Administer pain medication.

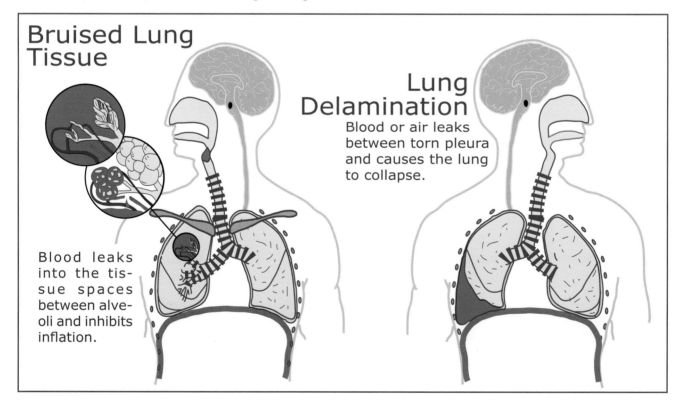

Bruised Lung Tissue

Blood leaks into the tissue spaces between alveoli and inhibits inflation.

Lung Delamination
Blood or air leaks between torn pleura and causes the lung to collapse.

- To avoid pneumonia, **do not** tape or bandage the patient's chest; instead, encourage them to take a deep breath, even though it will be painful, once every 20 minutes or, at a minimum, once per hour.
- Begin a Level 3 Evacuation and monitor for lung damage.
- If respiratory distress is present or returns, begin a Level 1 Evacuation.

Treatment of Flail Chest

- The patient has multiple ribs broken in two or more places, creating an unstable chest wall. Because of the force required, lung damage is likely.
- Begin a Level 2 Evacuation and monitor the patient for respiratory distress due to lung damage.
- Begin a Level 1 Evacuation if respiratory distress is present or returns.

Treatment of Lung Damage

- Continue to reassure awake patients.
- Awake patients prefer to remain in a sitting or semi-reclined position where gravity helps to hold the abdominal organs away from the diaphragm and aid in breathing.
- Position voice-responsive, pain-responsive, and unresponsive patients on their injured side in order to permit the lung on the uninjured side to expand normally.
- Begin positive-pressure ventilations (PPV), if the patient becomes cyanotic and unresponsive. Note that rescue breathing may not be effective as pressure increases within the pleural space.
- Administer oxygen.
- With penetrating trauma, cover the wound site with an occlusive dressing (Vaseline® impregnated gauze or plastic) as soon as possible. Remove the dressing and reapply if the patient's respiratory distress dramatically increases after application. Hold the dressing in place with tape or an ace wrap.
- Begin a Level 1 Evacuation.
- Cardiac arrest denotes death. CPR is not indicated.

Internal Bleeding & Volume Shock
Pathophysiology

Trauma to the chest, abdomen, pelvis, and upper leg may result in damage to large blood vessels, highly vascular organs (lungs, liver, spleen, pancreas, kidneys), and large bones. Serious damage to any of these components may result in internal bleeding and a progressive loss of systemic perfusion (volume shock) ultimately affecting the brain and often leading to death. Although protected by the ribs, the spleen and liver are prone to injury from blunt trauma. If the bleeding is contained by the organ's membrane, the organ swells and the surrounding area is tender. With continued bleeding or rough handling, the stuff sack may rupture and the patient may die. External bleeding from any major artery may also lead to volume shock; however, external bleeding is relatively easy to assess and successfully treat in the field.

Assessment
General

- The MOI is trauma to the major vessels, vascular organs, and/or large bones. While local pain and tenderness are positive signs and symptoms for musculoskeletal injuries to the chest, abdomen, pelvis or femur(s) and a body compartment large enough to bleed into, they do not necessarily indicate volume shock.
- Blood inside the abdominal cavity irritates the lining of the peritoneum causing pain and guarding. The patient typically presents on their back with their knees bent and with tense abdominal muscles.
- The patient may present with a late clinical pattern.

Early Clinical Pattern

- The patient is either awake, anxious, and irritable, or lethargic with increased pulse and respiratory rates.
- The patient's skin is usually pale, cool, and moist.
- Blood pressure is within the normal range.
- *A patient can show the early clinical pattern for volume shock and "stabilize" if the bleeding is contained within an organ membrane. These patients MUST be handled gently to avoid a rupture of the stuff sack and development of severe volume shock.*
- Young, fit patients remain awake then deteriorate rapidly as their compensatory mechanisms are overwhelmed. *Monitor their pulse closely.*

Late Clinical Pattern

- The patient becomes voice-responsive, pain-responsive, and unresponsive.
- Pulse and respiratory rates continue to increase.

- The patient's skin is pale or cyanotic, cool and moist.
- Blood pressure drops.
- Progressive internal bleeding will lead to the late stages of volume shock and culminate in cardiac arrest and death.

Field Treatment

- ***Stop external bleeding with well-aimed direct pressure and pressure bandage.***
- A tourniquet may be required in tactical situations. Military and police personnel should train and carry a commercial tourniquet; when a tourniquet is required, there is generally not enough time to improvise one.
- Position the patient on their back, with or without the legs and feet slightly elevated.
- ***If internal bleeding is suspected, handle the patient gently and restrict movement (no exercise)***

to prevent rupturing a swollen organ stuff sack.
- Administer supplemental oxygen.
- Begin a Level 1 Evacuation.
- Cardiac arrest indicates death. CPR is not indicated.

Spine Injuries
Pathophysiology

While the human spine is well-engineered and quite strong, spinal trauma may fracture vertebrae and/or damage the soft tissue surrounding the spinal cord. Movement of unstable vertebrae may cut the spinal cord, causing irreversible loss of motor function and sensation below the injury site. A high cord injury may cause death. ***Unstable movement may be caused by the traumatic event, voluntary patient movement, or by rescuers.*** Damage to the tissue surrounding the spinal cord may activate the inflammatory response, causing spinal pain, tender-

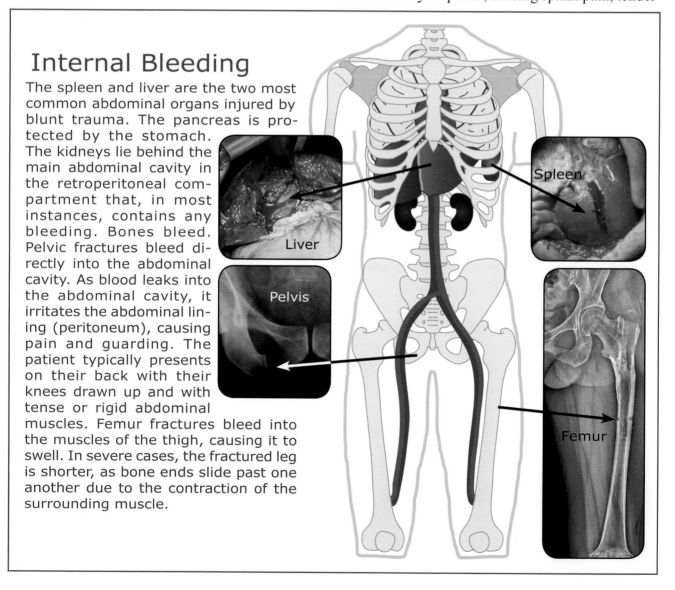

Internal Bleeding

The spleen and liver are the two most common abdominal organs injured by blunt trauma. The pancreas is protected by the stomach. The kidneys lie behind the main abdominal cavity in the retroperitoneal compartment that, in most instances, contains any bleeding. Bones bleed. Pelvic fractures bleed directly into the abdominal cavity. As blood leaks into the abdominal cavity, it irritates the abdominal lining (peritoneum), causing pain and guarding. The patient typically presents on their back with their knees drawn up and with tense or rigid abdominal muscles. Femur fractures bleed into the muscles of the thigh, causing it to swell. In severe cases, the fractured leg is shorter, as bone ends slide past one another due to the contraction of the surrounding muscle.

Liver

Spleen

Pelvis

Femur

ness and swelling. Swelling may cause cord damage if undue pressure accumulates within the closed space of a vertebra. Cord damage, resulting from swelling, may be temporary or permanent.

Initial Spine Assessment & Patient Handling Guidelines

The MOI is direct trauma to the spine or trauma to any part of the body that may indirectly damage the spine. ***Initially, because the anticipated problem is a cord injury, assume all patients with an uncertain or positive mechanism for a spine injury have an unstable spine. Immobilize their spine as soon as possible.*** Later, IF they meet the criteria for ruling out an unstable spinal injury, you may remove the immobilization. Your initial spine stabilization is best accomplished with "hand stability" in the position the patient is found, UNLESS there is immediate danger to the scene and/or the patient presents with a primary respiratory or circulatory problem. In either case, you will need to move the patient quickly. ***Rapid movement of patients suspected of having an unstable spine, increases the risk of spinal cord damage. Avoid rapid movement, unless there is a life-threatening situation that requires it.*** Slow, controlled movement of a spine-injured patient into anatomical position is safe and required for both patient packaging and comfort. The goal for moving a patient with an injured spine is to prevent any unstable spine movement. ***Movement towards normal anatomical position is generally considered safe; however, immediately STOP any movement that causes spine pain or any electric or shooting pain that appears to originate from the spinal cord and travels down any limb.*** Adhere to the following guidelines:

- ***Move the patient as little as possible*** to get the job done.
- ***Break down all movement into small increments.***
- ***Avoid large, unsupported movements.***
- ***Gentle axial traction is safe; axial compression or lateral movement is unsafe.*** Gentle axial traction in line with the patient's spine is considered safe; however, spinal compression may damage the spinal cord. Lateral movement creates shear forces that are easily transmitted to other parts of the spine and may cause cord damage.
- ***If the movement is rapid, the rescuers limited in number, or the terrain extremely difficult, you will need to focus your attention and strength on protecting the cervical spine first, the thoracic spine second, and then, if possible, the lumbar spine.***
- ***As soon as possible, apply a cervical collar around the patient's neck to help prevent cervical flexion and excessive side bend combined with rotation.*** Hand stabilization using a "head sandwich" must remain in place even when a cervical collar is securely applied until a spine injury has been ruled out or the patient is completely secured in a backboard or litter. Cervical collars are not considered a splint.
- ***Firmly control the patient's weight centers*** (head, shoulders, hips). Control the head using your hands and/or the patient's arms to form a "head sandwich." Control the shoulders and hips through leverage and lots of hands.
- ***Move one weight center at a time*** into alignment while supporting the others. Once one weight center is in normal anatomical position with respect to another, maintain that alignment throughout the movement process. The person controlling the pa-

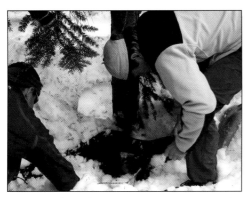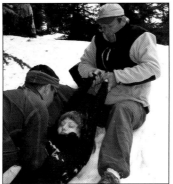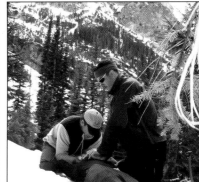

Avalanche Rescue: Locate & Recover ~ Axial Drag with Cervical Support ~ CPR

tient's head *follows* the movements of the patient's shoulders in order to maintain cervical alignment.

- **When multiple rescuers are involved, there must be one leader and many supporters.**
- **Avoid carrying a spine-injured patient to a backboard or litter; a slip or fall could be fatal.**
- When using a litter or backboard, focus your attention on how to move the backboard closer to the patient rather than how to move the patient closer to the backboard.
- **Axial loading is preferable to horizontal loading.** In most cases a patient may be lifted, the litter or backboard slid axially under them, and the patient lowered onto the litter or board. The entire procedure is quick with little rescuer or patient movement.
- **Rolling is safe. Roll patients onto a board or litter, if they present on their stomach.**
- If a spine injury can be localized to the cervical spine, the patient's legs may be extended or flexed safely; avoid lateral movement. If the injury can be localized to L-4 or below, the patient's head and neck do not need to be immobilized.

Criteria for Ruling Out Unstable Spine Injuries

Not all trauma patients have an unstable spine injury; in fact, most do not. However, because the consequences are so severe—paralysis or death—and patients are often unreliable in the short term, all patients in urban settings with a positive MOI are fully immobilized and transported to a hospital for evaluation. Because full spine immobilization and evacuation from a remote environment is difficult and often dangerous for all concerned, careful field assessment of a potential spine injury is warranted before making a decision to board a patient. Prior to and during the spine assessment, the patient should remain supported in a spine-stable position. If your patient is lying down, roll them onto their side so that they face you; support their chest and hips with your upper legs. The assessment may also be done with the patient in a sitting or standing position; in most cases, regardless of the patient's position, a second rescuer should support the patient's head. **Begin a formal spine assessment using the crite-**

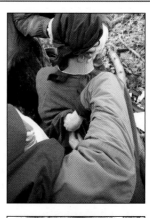

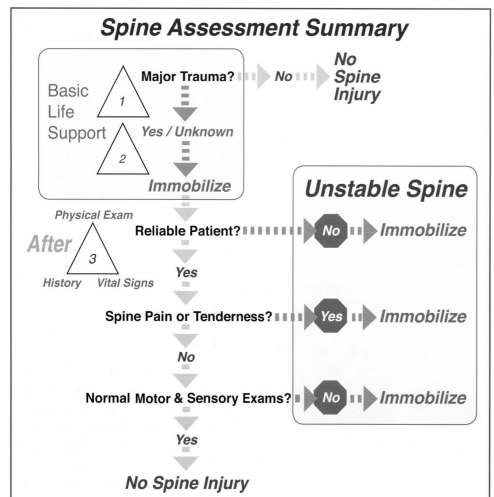

Spine Assessment Summary

Basic Life Support

1

2

Major Trauma? ▶ No ▶ **No Spine Injury**

Yes / Unknown

Immobilize

After

3

Physical Exam

History   Vital Signs

Reliable Patient? ▶ No ▶ *Immobilize*

Yes

Spine Pain or Tenderness? ▶ Yes ▶ *Immobilize*

No

Normal Motor & Sensory Exams? ▶ No ▶ *Immobilize*

Yes

No Spine Injury

Unstable Spine

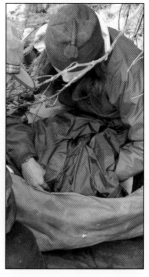

ria outlined below AFTER you have completed the third triangle of the patient assessment system (see page 50); use the patient's SAMPLE history and physical exam to determine if the patient is reliable and has no distracting injuries.

Spinal Fractures

- If the spinal cord is completely cut by a traumatic MOI, the patient will not be able to feel or move below the damaged level. Partial damage is rare, but possible, and may be detected during thorough motor and sensory exams of the patient's hands and feet.

- Vertebrae are essentially bony circles that surround and protect the spinal cord. Vertebrae, like all bones, are surrounded with a highly enervated stuff sack. Spinal nerves originating in the lower cervical spine and upper thoracic spine enervate the forearms and hands. Spinal nerves originating in the lower lumbar spine and sacrum enervate the lower legs and feet.

- Patients with a significant fracture anywhere in the bony circle surrounding the spinal cord will usually present with spine pain.

- Spinal fractures are tender, when pressure is exerted on the spinous process.

Focused Spine Assessment

The focused spine assessment has five components:

- **Reliable patient.** The patient must be reliable and have a normal pain response. They must be alert, calm and cooperative. A spine injury cannot be ruled out in patients who present with ASR, painful and distracting injuries, intoxication, or an altered mental status.

- *No spine pain.* A patient's spine cannot be cleared if, when questioned, they complain of spinal pain.

- *No spine tenderness.* A patient's spine cannot be cleared if, upon a thorough spinal exam, they indicate any spinal tenderness. During the spinal exam, each spinous process must be individually palpated. This is a safe procedure as long as gross spinal movement is prevented.

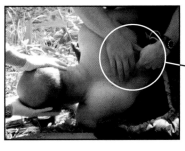 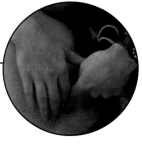

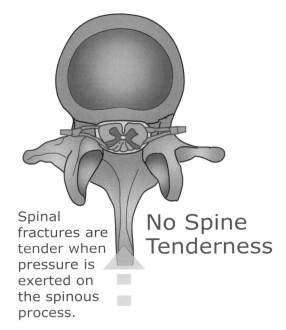

Spinal fractures are tender when pressure is exerted on the spinous process.

No Spine Tenderness

- ***Normal motor and sensory exams.*** The patient must have normal motor and sensory exams, as described below. An abnormal finding in either exam indicates a possible injury to the patient's spinal cord and the patient must be immobilized. Incomplete cord damage is possible (anterior cord syndrome, central cord syndrome, Brown-Sequard syndrome) and can be discovered through the following motor/sensory examinations.

Normal Motor Exams

The motor examinations described below test motor nerve roots in the cervical and lumbar spine; a normal exam indicates intact motor function at the level of the cervical and lumbar spine. If all motor tracts are intact, a patient will demonstrate equal strength on both the right and left sides during the motor exams. There are two motor exams for each hand and foot. ***If a local injury limits movement in a hand or foot, the motor exam may be considered normal with a minimum of one normal test result for each hand and foot.*** If neither exam can be conducted because of local injuries on a hand or foot, the motor exam is considered abnormal and the patient's spine must be immobilized.

- First, have the patient spread the fingers of one hand and offer resistance by trying to keep them spread as you squeeze the index and ring fingers together (1st and 3rd). With a normal exam their resistance should be equal and feel "springy." With an injured wrist, support the hand during the test. ***Supporting and testing must be done in the same manner on each*** *side.* This exam tests nerves servicing the adductor muscles in the patient's hand and the C-8 nerve root.

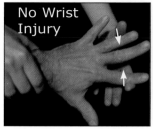
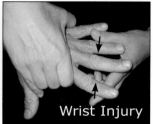

No Wrist Injury

Wrist Injury

• Next, while holding the patient's wrist with one of your hands, have them extend the supported hand and offer resistance as you push downward on the extended fingers. Again, with a normal exam their resistance should be equal and feel "springy." This test can be performed on a patient with a local wrist, hand, or digit injury in the following manner: For a wrist or hand injury, support the hand and push down on the fingers; for a digit injury, support the wrist and push down on the hand.

Supporting and testing must be done in the same manner on each side. This exam tests the extensor muscles in the patient's forearm and the C-7 nerve root.

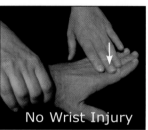

No Wrist Injury

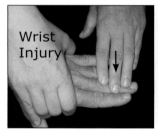

Wrist Injury

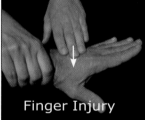

Finger Injury

• Moving to the patient's feet, place your hand against the bottom of the patient's foot and ask them to push against it. Repeat the test with the other foot. With a normal exam, the pressure will be strong and equal. This exam can be performed in the presence of a local injury to the ankle or foot, by using the patient's big toe in place of their foot.

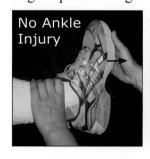

No Ankle Injury

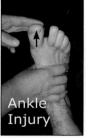

Ankle Injury

Supporting and testing must be done in the same manner on each lower extremity. This exam tests the flexor muscles in the patient's calf or foot and the S-1 and S-2 nerve roots.

• Finally, while holding the top of the patient's foot, ask them to pull up against your fingers. With a normal exam, the pressure will be strong and equal. This exam can also be performed in the presence of a local injury to the ankle or foot, by using the patient's big toe in place of their foot. *Supporting and testing must be done in the same manner on each lower extremity.* This exam tests extensor muscles in the patient's lower leg or foot and the L-5 nerve root.

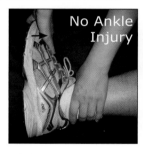

No Ankle Injury

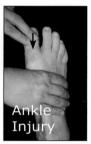

Ankle Injury

Normal Sensory Exams

Sensory tracts on the sides (lateral) of the cord carry incoming signals for pin-prick pain and temperature, while sensory tracts on the back (posterior) carry incoming signals for light touch and joint proprioception. A patient with an intact cord will be able to distinguish between pin-prick pain and light touch in each extremity. A partially damaged or compressed cord or spinal nerve due to a fractured vertebra may present with electric, tingling, or shooting pain down one, or both, arms or legs. It would be extremely unusual to have an abnormal sensory exam without an abnormal motor exam. Carry a safety pin in your first aid kit.

• *Immobilize the patient's spine if they report weakness, numbness, tingling, electric or shooting pain, or no sensation in any extremity.*

• The sensation for pain is carried in lateral (spinothalamic) tracts of the anterior cord, while the sensation for light touch is carried in the tracts of the posterior cord. Testing sites on the back of the hand correspond to the C-7 or C-8 dermatome; testing sites on the shin or top of the foot correspond to the L-5 or S-1 dermatome. (See page 35 for more information on dermatomes.)

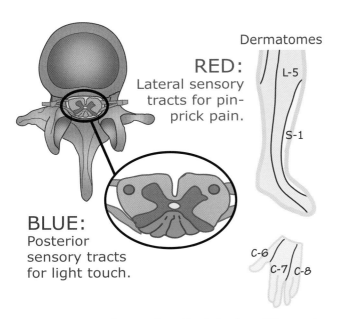

Dermatomes

RED: Lateral sensory tracts for pin-prick pain.

BLUE: Posterior sensory tracts for light touch.

L-5

S-1

C-6

C-7 / C-8

Pin-prick Pain & Light Touch

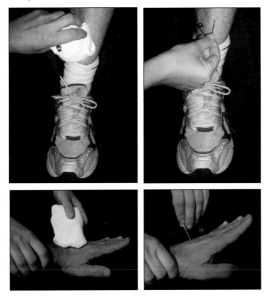

- Choose a testing site on the back of the patient's hand and demonstrate the pin-prick and light touch exam to them with their eyes open; avoid drawing blood. Once they understand the exam, ask them to close their eyes. Using the same testing site, prick the skin on the back of the patient's hand and ask them to tell you if they felt the pin or the cloth. After they answer, touch their hand in the same spot using a soft object; and again ask, if they felt the pin or the cloth. Repeat the pin-prick and light touch tests on the opposite hand; use the same testing site. Then, move to the patient's feet. Choose a testing site on the patient's shin or top of their foot and perform pin-prick and light-touch exams at the same location on each side; after each test,

ask the patient if they felt the pin or the cloth. ***The patient MUST be able to distinguish between pain (pin-prick) and light-touch (cloth).*** The exam is considered abnormal and the patient must remain immobilized if they are unable to tell the difference.

Field Treatment for an Unstable Spine & Cord Injury

- The treatment goal is to immobilize all potentially unstable vertebrae to prevent spinal cord injury. Field treatment for a spinal cord injury is the same as the field treatment for an unstable spine injury.

- Patients with unstable spines MUST be handled very carefully during the splinting process to avoid causing a spinal cord injury or causing additional damage if they are already cord injured.

- In alert and reliable patients, pain or tenderness at a specific site indicates potential instability at that site. If the suspected injury can be localized to the lower lumbar spine (L-4, L-5), hip or pelvis, the patient's head may remain free during the evacuation, significantly increasing their comfort. If the injury can be localized to the cervical spine, the patient's legs may be safely extended or flexed, although lateral movement should be avoided because it is easily transmitted up to other parts of the spine; this small freedom also increases patient comfort during a long evacuation. Injuries to the thoracic spine require complete spinal immobilization. ***When in doubt, immobilize the entire spine.***

- All litters or backboards should provide a light-weight, rigid platform for the patient to be attached to. Improvising effective spine splits is extremely difficult with severe consequences in the event of equipment failure; use commercial litters, commercial backboards, or pre-tested, homemade backboards specifically designed for that purpose. There are numerous commercial litters available; the most popular are the Stokes litter (a steel or aluminum wire-basket litter), the Thompson litter (a fiberglass or plastic shell with aluminum rails), and the SKED litter (a lightweight, flexible, plastic litter that can be rolled up to fit into its own backpack). In addition, there are numerous fiberglass litters designed for ski evacuation. The most common is the Cascade toboggan. With the exception of the SKED litter, it is unnecessary to use both a litter and backboard in combination.

For the additional weight, little extra support is gained. The most versatile and easiest litter to transport is the SKED; it is used in conjunction with a thin lightweight backboard, a KED or OSS, or a total-body vacuum splint. It excels in all technical evacuations and carry-outs, especially those that require maneuvering in confined spaces, as required for caving rescues. Both the Stokes and Thompson litters are encountered more frequently in the field than a SKED. The Stokes works well in technical situations and in water, which flows through the wire mesh, while the Thompson litter easily slides over snow. Both work equally well in a carry-out. Backboards are commonly used with commercial ski toboggans to facilitate the transfer of the patient into a waiting ambulance or clinic. The practical and visual differences between a litter and a backboard are huge. A litter has sides, offering the patient increased stability and comfort over difficult terrain, while a backboard does not. If the evacuation is technical and/or the carry out long and arduous, it is infinitely preferable to use a litter, rather than a backboard. Unfortunately, backboards, especially poorly designed ones, are much more common. If an improvised backboard is truly needed, one may be built by lashing poles together to form a strong, lightweight, axially rigid "board." It should be 12-18 inches wide and cut to the length of the patient. Its serviceability will depend upon the choice of materials, preferably strong and lightweight, and the lashing ability of the builder. Always test improvised spine splints on an uninjured person before using.

Backboard & Litter Packaging Guidelines

The long-term care of a spine-injured patient is extremely difficult. Rescuers must provide food, water, and waste elimination. Psychological problems related to claustrophobia or immobilization may arise with alert patients at any time. All packaging systems must be constructed with these issues in mind. The following guidelines apply to all litter packaging techniques, regardless of the style of litter or backboard:

- The packaging system should immobilize the spine injury in all directions (side-to-side, up-and-down). Keep the area above the patient's head clear to avoid spinal compression.

- In the absence of severe environmental conditions that demand immediate protection for the patient, packaging material should be assembled and prepared before the patient is moved onto it.

- The packaging system should be well padded and should protect the patient from the rigors of the evacuation. A minimum of two sleeping pads should be used to line the bottom of the litter. Pad the spaces between the patient's side and the litter straps, by rolling and tying sleeping pads or bags together with strips of cloth or by rolling extra clothing, grasses, or other suitable materials into a ground cloth or tarp. To secure the cervical spine, extend the rolls beyond the patient's head and anchor them to the top of the litter using the "Go Beyond" principle (see photos on page 84). Use

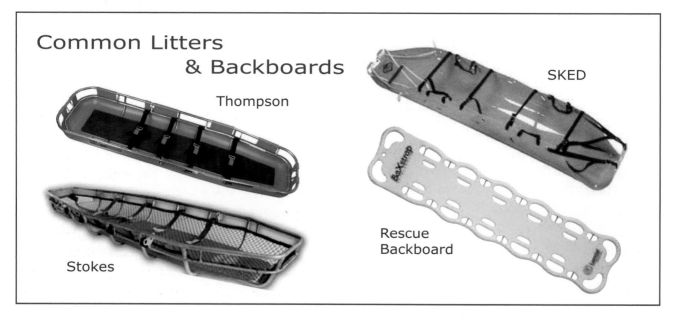

Common Litters & Backboards

Thompson

Stokes

SKED

Rescue Backboard

foot stirrups, a climbing harness groin anchor, or rigid padding, to prevent the patient from sliding towards the foot of the litter. Use narrow, in-line shoulder straps to prevent movement towards the patient's head. Slightly flex the patient's knees and support them with soft firm padding, such as a rolled jacket or stuff sack filled with soft materials.

- The packaging system should provide adequate thermoregulation. ***Consider a hypothermia package for all patients immobilized in a litter, regardless of the environmental conditions; the package may be left open and unsealed, if currently unneeded.*** Remember that it is easier to keep your patient warm than to warm them up. Restricted movement, traumatic injury, illness, available calories, and their hydration level. All affect the ability of patients to self-regulate their temperature; monitor their core temperature.

- Consider diapering patients in preparation for waste elimination; if ALS is present, consider a urinary catheter and drainage bag.

- To help prevent vascular damage from long-term immobilization, massage the patient's limbs, especially their legs, for a few minutes each hour.

- The attachment system should be simple, strong, and easily adjustable. It should provide easy access to the patient's airway. Aside from commercially manufactured "Spiders," there are only two rigging systems that are effective enough to be used during an extended evacuation: the ✕ System and "Shoe Lace" attachment systems.

In the ✕ ***System,*** individual straps with sturdy quick-release buckles, including seatbelt buckles or cam straps, are used to create a ✕ over the patient's shoulders. Two-inch wide straps are preferred. The center of the shoulder ✕ should be over the center of the patient's sternum, with the upper edges ending above the patient's shoulders. Secure the patient's hips using single or multiple straps in one of the following configurations: ✕, X, or — ; the strap or straps should firmly anchor the patient's pelvis to the litter or backboard. The patient's thighs and lower legs may be secured using a horizontal strap instead of an X. The strap over the patient's upper legs should be midway between the patient's knees and hips. The strap over the patient's lower legs should be midway between the patient's knees and ankles.

All of the straps should be attached to the litter as low as possible, to help eliminate lateral space and decrease the amount of padding. The ✕ system is typically used with backboards and fiberglass litters.

In the ***"Shoe Lace" System,*** a rope or one-inch webbing about 30 feet in length is laced through the vertical posts of the litter; take care to keep the rope or webbing below the main rails of the litter to avoid damaging the rope during a technical rescue. To avoid cutting full-length ropes, feed enough rope through the posts to secure the patient and tie a "stopper" knot at the foot of the litter. Then, beginning at the patient's feet, carefully "milk" the slack out until the patient is secure; the ends are tied off at the patient's shoulders. Completely tie the patient's body to the litter or board before securing their head.

- Immobilizing the patient's head is best done by using the "Go Beyond" principle (see photos on page 84). Duct tape may work well if securely applied across the patient's forehead and eyebrows in dry conditions. Take care to ensure easy access to the patient's airway, in the event that the patient vomits.

- All patients suspected of a cervical or thoracic spine injury should have a cervical collar in place prior to loading. ***Continue to stabilize the patient's head, even with a cervical collar in place, until the patient is completely immobilized in the litter or board.*** Cervical collars are not considered a splint.

- ***Completely secure the patient's body prior to strapping their head, in case vomiting occurs during packaging.*** It is easier to support the patient's head during a roll, than their body, thus offering less chance for unstable movement of the cervical spine during the roll.

- If a ***hypothermia package*** is used, it may be prepared for loading by pre-assembling the individual layers, followed by rolling all the layers lengthwise into two connected rolls. Temporarily secure each end of the package using a piece of cloth, cord or a quick-release strap. The entire package can then be slid, either with the litter or backboard, or separately, under the patient. Quickly release each end, before the patient is lowered. The hypothermia package can then be sealed and the patient secured to the litter or backboard. Head blocks or lateral sleeping bag rolls can be placed and secured either

Loading a Hypothermia-packaged Patient into a Litter

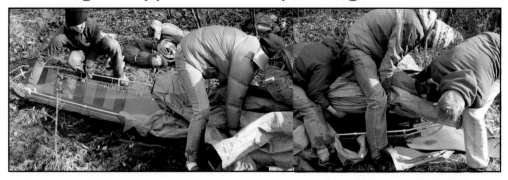

Lift the patient and the hypo-thermia package together and slide the litter under; leave any unwanted material on the ground.

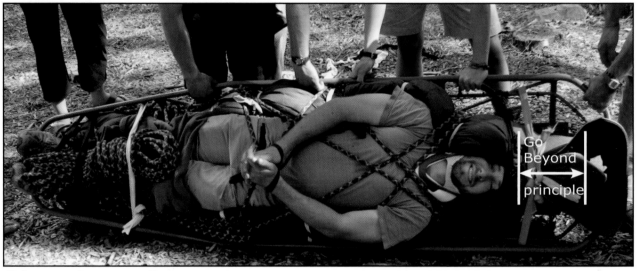

Shoe Lace System
With a Stokes litter, use climbing rope and the "Go Beyond" principle to secure the patient's head. Extra rope is coiled, tied, and stored on top of the patient's legs.

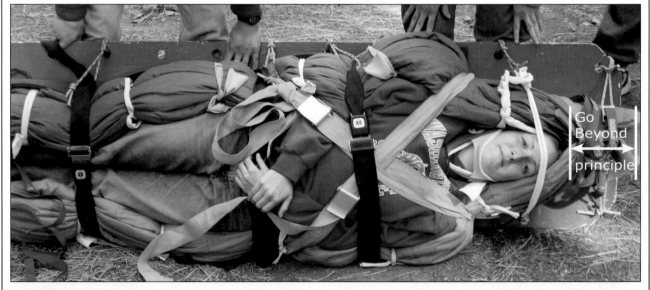

✘ System
With a wooden backboard, use individual straps and the "Go Beyond" principle to secure the patient's head. The sleeping pad helps to hold the rolled sleeping bags in place.

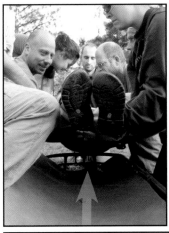
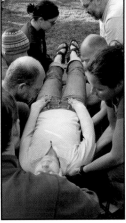
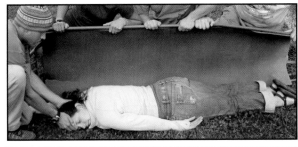
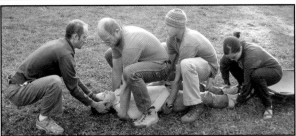
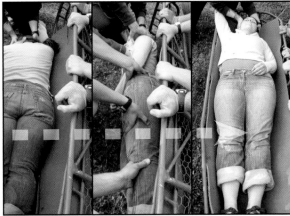
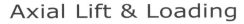

Axial Lift & Loading

Rolling

inside or outside of the external vapor barrier.

- *Axial loading is preferable to horizontal loading.* In most cases a patient may be lifted, the litter or backboard slid axially under them, and the patient lowered onto the litter or board. The entire procedure is quick, with little rescuer and patient movement.

- *Roll* patients into a litter, or onto a backboard, if they present on their stomach or if you do NOT have enough people for an axial load.

Improvised Litters

Effective litters may be improvised in a number of ways. While spine-stable litters can be constructed, they are complex and the consequences of a failure are severe; if possible, stabilize the patient and wait for a commercial litter to be brought in. That said, a "Daisy Chain" rope litter can be quite useful to evacuate a spine-injured patient after a mountaineering accident when inclement weather is moving in.

Guidelines for Litter Use in Non-Technical Terrain

Non-technical litter use is defined according to the steepness and stability of the terrain. If a rescuer falls and is both quickly and safely able to arrest their fall without prior training or equipment, then

the terrain is considered non-technical. Even on non-technical terrain, a litter may require a belay if it cannot rest securely without support.

- Once the rigging process is complete, carrying straps may be added along the sides of either a litter or backboard to facilitate long-distance carrying; three straps per side is common. To decrease the possibility of dropping the litter, rescuers should not tie into the litter or attach themselves to the carrying straps in any way.

- *Passing the litter* is the fastest way to move a litter though short stretches of difficult or unstable terrain or over an object directly in your path.

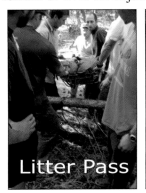
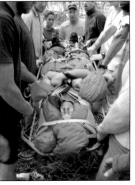

Litter Pass

Rescuers form two opposing lines facing one another and pass the litter slowly along the aisle

Daisy Chain Rope Litter

Replace the internal back-pack frame stays with poles to provide spinal support. Put the patient in a hypo-pack and carry them to the preset rope. Position them on the rope so that their head will be immobilized by the hip belt.

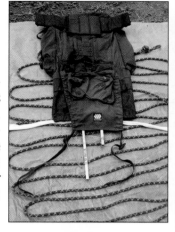

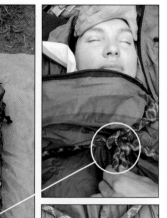

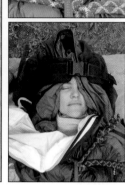

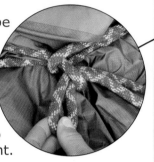

The top end of the rope is tied with an overhand knot on a bight. The loops are tightened and pulled through one at a time, similar to a daisy chain, and tied off at the ankles with two half-hitch knots on a bight.

Position a folded sleeping pad so that it goes beyond the hip belt to secure the patient's head. Attach a C-collar to the patient prior to lifting them into the hypo-pack and maintain manual head stabilization until the litter is chained through the patient's hips. The white cloth strap attached to the poles, helps to stabilize the poles during packaging. Extra rope is coiled and slid under the lower-leg straps. The litter may be carried by holding directly onto the rope on the side of the patient or by attaching carrying straps.

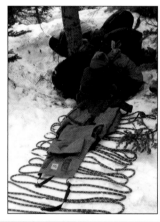

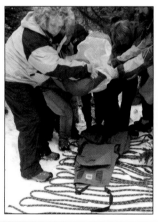

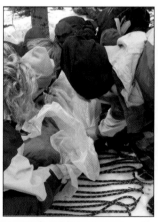

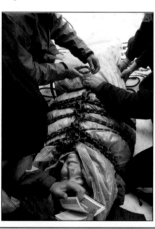

between them. As the litter passes by them, pairs of rescuers peel off and move to the front of the line to await the litter once again. Each rescuer must assume a stable position upon reaching the front of the line. The process continues until the litter is past the difficult or unstable terrain. At any time, a rescuer should be able to call "STOP!" to reassess a situation or give time for the line to reform. Rescuers may choose to alternate sides

as they move to the front of the passing line. ***Rescuers MUST remain secure and immobile in their position when in contact with the litter.*** Litter passes are also a quick, safe, and easy way to change litter bearers. This is the most efficient method of litter travel, especially during long evacuations. It is desirable to have a minimum of 36 people for extended litter evacuations.

• *"Toe-nailing"* is a carrying method used in steep or

rugged terrain, where either litter passes are impossible or the number of rescuers is limited. It involves resting the uphill end of the litter securely against the hill, on a rock, etc. while the downhill end is supported on the knees of one or two rescuers. The four remaining litter bearers step slightly uphill to a secure new, comfortable, and stable position. On command, they lift the litter up and forward to a new "Toe-nail" position. The process is repeated until the obstacle is passed and litter carrying or passing can begin again. Although less stable, the same toe-nail process may be used in reverse for descents.

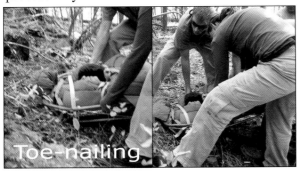
Toe-nailing

• *Consider a belay if the litter cannot rest securely while unsupported, on the terrain being crossed.* A belay is most effective when the rope and the litter remain in the fall line; avoid traversing with a belay. A tree wrap is the simplest and most efficient form of litter belay; choose a strong, healthy tree. Simply tie one end of the rope to the head (or tail) of the litter using any traditional climbing knot; the rope should be "rolled" a few times around the chosen rail to help maintain an even pressure on the litter and to prevent rotation when in use. Then wrap the other end once or twice around the tree and you're ready to belay or lower the litter. Use a static rope designed for rescue. More wraps increase the friction. The bigger the tree, the fewer the number of wraps needed to generate the same amount of friction. It is often easier to manage the belay, if you stand on the downhill side of the tree. If you leave a long tail when tying the belay rope into the litter, the tail may be used to secure the litter when you need to raise or lower the belay. This is usually referred to as "tailing off" the litter. Consider all of the patient's problems when deciding which end of the litter to tie the belay rope into. An alert and cooperative patient is most comfortable with their head pointing uphill.

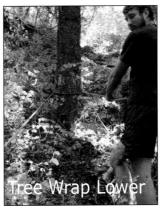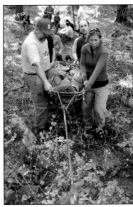
Tree Wrap Lower

If a tree wrap is used to lower a litter, be prepared to add or subtract wraps, depending upon the friction required to support both the litter and its attendants. When lowering a litter, the attendants may face either up or downhill, whichever is more comfortable, and lean downhill using the belayed litter for support. The litter bearer's legs should be perpendicular to the slope, as if rapelling.

• *The simplest way to assist litter bearers in climbing a steep hill, while belaying the litter at the same time, is to use a counterweight raising system.*

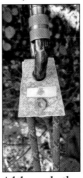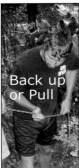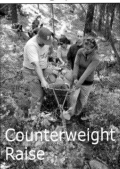
Back up or Pull
Counterweight Raise

• Although the counterweight raising system does require a rescue pulley, it is not considered a true haul system because there is no mechanical advantage; however, it does make climbing a slippery hill *much* easier and safer. It is also easy to remember how to set up and use. The principle is identical to the system used to raise old-fashioned windows or heavy garage doors. Simply run the haul rope uphill and through a well-anchored rescue pulley, then have three or four rescuers back up holding the rope, as the litter attendants carry the litter uphill. An additional rescuer can act as a belayer, using a tree wrap located directly below, and as near to the anchor and pulley as possible. It's amazing how helpful this simple system can be.

• *Rescuers who are unfamiliar with the use of the litter and rope systems described in this text should not try to use them during a real evacuation without prior training.*

Extremity Injuries
Pathophysiology

Trauma to the extremities may damage bones, cartilage, ligaments, tendons and/or muscles. It may also damage nearby nerves and blood vessels resulting in a loss of distal perfusion and innervation. Musculoskeletal injury to the extremities rarely involves enough internal damage to blood vessels to cause volume shock, although it is possible in the case of a severely angled femur fracture. Musculoskeletal damage to the head, chest, and pelvis indicates the possibility of critical injuries. Damage, done to the musculoskeletal system itself, heals according to the development of its vascular bed. Bones and muscles are highly vascular and heal quickly, tendons more slowly, and ligaments and cartilage very slowly, if at all. As with all tissue injuries, the local inflammatory response is stimulated. After a few days, the process of rebuilding the damaged structures begins and, in most cases, proceeds without serious complications. Complications occur when a large amount of tissue is damaged, the swelling is severe, and distal perfusion is compromised. If circulation is not restored within a few hours, the cells will die, gangrene may follow within days, and the limb will require amputation to save the patient's life. Deep wounds associated with underlying structural damage are at high risk for infection.

Field assessment of extremity injuries is based on distinguishing between *stable* and *unstable* injuries, rather than between types of fractures and degrees of sprains or strains. All stable injuries and many unstable injuries may be successfully treated in the field and may not require an evacuation. Since minor extremity injuries are common in wilderness settings, great detail is given to their assessment and treatment in the following pages.

Assessment Criteria for Long Bones & Joints

Stable Injury Assessment

- Range of motion (ROM) and distal circulation, sensation, and motor function (CSM) are intact.
- The patient experiences mild-to-moderate pain and tenderness at the injury site.

- Although painful, the patient is able to bear weight on or use the affected limb shortly after the injury; the injured limb has near-normal strength.
- The injured limb initially presents with mild swelling that may become severe over the next 24 hours due to inflammation caused by tissue damage; the greater the damage, the greater the swelling.

Unstable Injury Assessment

- The injured limb's range of motion (ROM) is significantly decreased and distal circulation, sensation, and motor function may be impaired.
- The patient is unable to bear weight on or use the affected limb; the limb is noticeably weaker compared with the unaffected limb.
- The patient reports moderate-to-severe pain, tenderness and swelling immediately after the injury.
- Crepitus—a crunching feel and/or sound—may be present.
- The patient may report hearing a "snap" or "pop" on impact.
- The limb may be deformed.

Stable   Unstable   Unstable

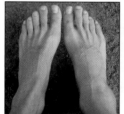 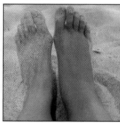 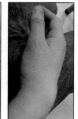

Field Treatment for Stable Injuries

- The goal of field treatment for a stable injury is to prevent additional damage and allow time for healing. Treatment is usually definitive and an evacuation may not be necessary. ***Begin a Level 3 Evacuation*** if the patient cannot safely continue with the trip.
- The patient should rest and avoid using the injured limb. The limb should be splinted if the patient must use it. The splint may be removed when there is no further chance of additional injury. Refer to the discussion of improvised splints later in this Section.
- Administer OTC ibuprofen or naproxen sodium for pain and inflammation. Either medication helps to reduce local swelling and to improve circulation. They encourage faster healing by increasing the delivery of nutrients and the removal of waste.

- Cool the affected area to help reduce swelling and pain. Use ice for 20 to 30 minutes at 90-minute intervals, to allow local reperfusion. If ice is not available, cold water immersion will help. In a hot, arid environment, take advantage of evaporative cooling, by lightly wrapping the injury in cotton and keeping it wet. However, DO NOT immerse or apply wet wraps to an open wound.

- Herbal remedies include arnica and comfrey. Comfrey contains allantoin and helps promote the growth of connective tissue; it is easily absorbed through the skin. Arnica appears to stimulate the circulatory system and help reabsorb internal bleeding. Other herbs useful in the treatment of stable musculoskeletal injuries include rue and witch hazel. Use the herbs externally in salves or as compresses over intact skin. Do not take internally.

- Stop administering pain medications and reassess after 48-72 hours. Start, and gradually increase, range of motion and strengthening exercises. Patients *must* not overexert and *must* stop if they feel pain. Begin pain-free activity, after range of motion and strength return to normal. Pain medications may mask pain during use and should be avoided. If swelling and pain return during or after exercise, the pain and anti-inflammatory medications may be resumed; exercise should be discontinued and the limb rested until the swelling subsides once again.

Field Treatment for Unstable Injuries
General Treatment Guidelines

- The goal of field treatment for unstable injuries is to position and immobilize the injury for protection during the evacuation and to promote healing; surgery may be necessary in difficult cases.

- Open wounds associated with unstable injuries are at high risk for infection and, if possible, should be thoroughly cleaned prior to realigning the limb.

- Administer OTC ibuprofen or naproxen sodium for pain and inflammation. Prescription (Rx) pain medications may be required for severe pain.

- Cool the affected area to help reduce swelling and pain. Use ice for 20 to 30 minutes at 90-minute intervals to allow local reperfusion.

- Monitor the injury site for swelling and decreased distal circulation, sensation, and motor function (CSM) during the next 24 hours.

Evacuation Guidelines

- In-line closed fractures are not considered an emergency; begin a Level 3 Evacuation.

- Ligament repair may be done at any time and is not an emergency; begin a Level 3 Evacuation.

- Tendon repair is best done within 5-10 days and is not an emergency; begin a Level 3 Evacuation.

- Muscle repair is best done within 6 hours or 4-5 days later, after inflammation has subsided. Muscle repair is not an emergency; begin a Level 3 Evacuation.

- Closed dislocations are best reduced within six hours, but are not typically considered an emergency; if reduction is successful and CSM is intact, consider a Level 3 Evacuation. Begin a Level 2 Evacuation if reduction is unsuccessful or CSM is impaired.

- Begin a Level 2 Evacuation, for all open fractures; ideally, the injured patient should be at a major hospital within 24 hours, because of the high probability of developing a bone infection.

- Begin a Level 2 Evacuation if there is no CSM distal to a suspected fracture site for a period greater than two hours.

Treatment Guidelines
for Unstable Long-bone Injuries

- ***Traction angulated long bones into anatomical position. STOP traction if the patient complains of severely increased pain or if physical resistance is felt during realignment.***

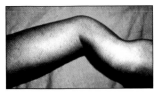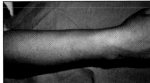

- Stabilize and support the injured limb with hands, as many as required, until the splint is in place.

- Immobilize in a splint. Refer to the discussion of improvised splints later in this Section.

- Monitor the CSM distal to the injury and adjust the splint as necessary to maintain good local perfusion.

Treatment Guidelines
for Unstable Joint Injuries

- ***Unstable joints should be splinted in the position they are found, UNLESS the deformity is severe enough to impede safe packaging and transport or if the patient's distal CSM is impaired.***

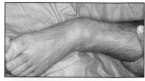

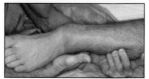

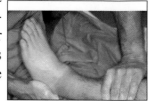

- Joints with severe deformity or impaired distal CSM should be tractioned towards mid-range position and splinted as soon as the deformity is corrected or the distal CSM has returned. Discontinue traction and splint the joint in position if you encounter physical resistance or if the patient complains of extreme pain during the repositioning process.

- Monitor the CSM distal to the injury and adjust the splint as necessary to maintain good local perfusion.

Treatment Guidelines for Musculoskeletal Injuries to the Head, Chest, Hip, Pelvis & Femur(s)

- ***With chest trauma, rule out respiratory distress secondary to lung damage.***

- ***With trauma to the chest, abdomen, pelvis, and femur(s), rule out volume shock secondary to internal bleeding.***

- ***Rule out volume shock secondary to internal bleeding with trauma to the chest, abdomen, pelvis and femur(s).***

- ***Consider spinal immobilization on a backboard or in a litter.***

- Avoid wrapping rib fractures. Patients with musculoskeletal injuries to the chest wall should be encouraged to inhale deeply at regular intervals. Deep inhalation maintains air exchange in the entire lung, which helps to prevent respiratory infections during healing.

- ***With an extremely painful, isolated, and angulated mid-shaft femur fracture AND a total evacuation time less than six hours, consider a femur-traction splint, in combination with a backboard or litter.*** With a total evacuation time greater than six hours, a sandwich-style splint in combination with a backboard or litter is usually a better choice. Eventually, all models of femur-traction splints cause a loss of distal perfusion to the injured leg. Refer to the discussion of improvised splints later in this Section.

Dislocations
Pathophysiology

A dislocation is the partial or complete displacement of one or more of the bones that make up a synovial joint. The immediate reduction of all dislocations helps to prevent additional damage and to promote healing by returning the joint to its anatomical position. ***The MOI for simple dislocations is INDIRECT TRAUMA.*** Direct trauma causes complicating fractures that usually require surgery and classify the dislocation as complex. Complex dislocations are treated in the field as an unstable joint injury. The field reduction of simple dislocations to digits, patellas and shoulders is relatively easy, and is therefore encouraged. If reduction is successful, the joint should be splinted for a minimum of 10 days and then treated as a stable injury. If reduction is unsuccessful or CSM is not restored following a successful reduction, treat the dislocation as an unstable joint injury. In either case, follow-up care with a physician is recommended.

Assessment of Simple Digit Dislocations

- The MOI is indirect trauma, often from falling while climbing with a finger trapped in a crack.

- Compare the injury with the same digit on the opposite (uninjured) hand or foot.

- The patient presents with an angulated finger or toe.

Field Treatment
of Simple Digit Dislocations

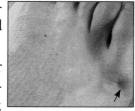

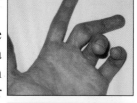

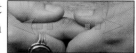

- Isolate the injured joint between the index fingers and thumbs of your hands.

- Support the injured finger against your chest or the injured toe against your thigh; traction the joint quickly into anatomical position.

- Splint the digit in mid-range position-of-function for a minimum of 10 days and then treat as a stable injury. Refer to the discussion of treatment for stable injuries, earlier in this Section.

- Administer OTC ibuprofen or naproxen sodium for pain and inflammation.

- Cool the affected area to help reduce swelling and pain. Use ice for 20 to 30 minutes at 90-minute intervals to allow local reperfusion.

Assessment of Patellar Dislocations

- The MOI is indirect trauma, usually as a result of a sudden twist or pivot. Dislocations of the patella commonly occur while descending in deep, heavy snow or on slippery talus and occasionally occur while telemark or alpine skiing in breakable crust or heavy snow.

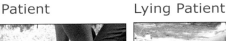

- The patient commonly presents on their side or back, holding the injured knee; the knee is slightly bent and the patella is displaced laterally.

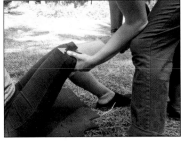

Field Treatment of Patellar Dislocations

- During the relocation process, maintain a right angle between the patient's thigh and their hip/pelvis.

- Support the injured leg at the knee and ankle. Encourage the patient to breathe deeply and RELAX.

- Guide the patella into anatomical position with your thumb, as you straighten the injured knee. Some range of motion should now be present in the knee joint; however, motion may be slightly decreased and painful.

Sitting Patient   Lying Patient

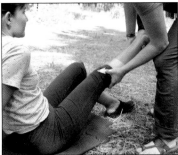

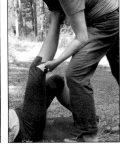

- Splint the knee in mid-range position-of-function for a minimum of 10 days and then treat as a stable injury. Refer to the discussion of improvised splints earlier in this Section.

- Administer OTC ibuprofen or naproxen sodium

for pain and inflammation.

- Cool the affected area to help reduce swelling and pain. Use ice for 20 to 30 minutes at 90-minute intervals, to allow local reperfusion.

- ***Prevention:*** Wrap the knee below the patella, above the upper calf, using a self-adhering wrap (Coban® or Vet Wrap®) to put pressure on and tighten and shorten the quadriceps tendon.

Assessment of Simple Anterior Shoulder Dislocations

- The MOI is indirect trauma. Shoulder dislocations often occur while paddling a canoe or kayak in whitewater, from rolls, hole riding, or eddy turns and peel outs in strong current, during a fall from a fist jam, during a fall onto a single tool while ice climbing, while bump skiing, or in any fall that is broken with an outstretched arm.

- The patient typically presents sitting with the elbow on their injured side supported, often with self-traction, and held away from their body.

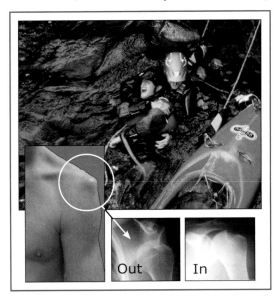

Field Treatment of Simple Anterior Shoulder Dislocations

There are numerous methods for reducing simple dislocations of the shoulder. All use traction to relieve pain and fatigue muscles; all use external rotation to reduce the dislocation. The two methods shown below are easy to understand and implement. The baseball method is active, while the hanging traction method is primarily passive. Both require relaxation to succeed.

Anterior Shoulder Reduction Techniques

Hand Position 1

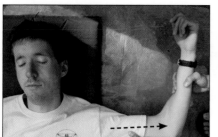

Hand Position 2

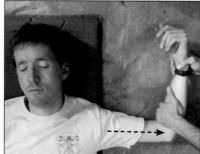

Hand Position 3

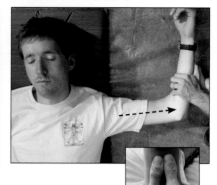

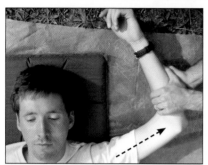

Baseball Method

Baseball position (above) is: shoulder, shoulder, elbow.

High baseball position (left) is: ear, ear, elbow.

Continue traction until you hear/feel the joint reposition and the patient completely relaxes. If relocated, pain will be almost gone and the patient will be able to touch their opposite shoulder with the hand on their injured side.

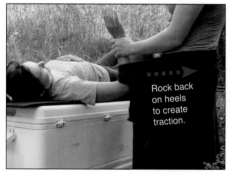

Rock back on heels to create traction.

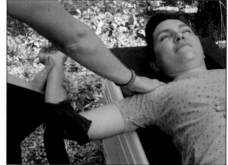

Alternately, place the patient on a waist-high platform then tie a soft piece of material around your hips and hook it through the patient's arm. Traction is applied by rocking back on your heels.

Hanging Traction

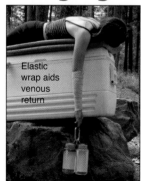

Elastic wrap aids venous return

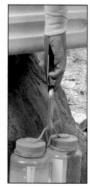

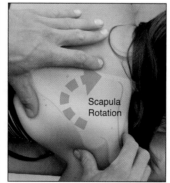

Scapula Rotation

As traction is maintained by the hanging weight, gently rotate the patient's shoulder blade (scapula) medially. If an assistant is available, they can apply external rotation to the humerus until the shoulder reduces. The elastic wrap aids venous return.

Water Bottles   Hook   Scapula Rotation

"Baseball" Method

- Assist the patient in moving to a flat, padded area.
- Check distal CSM in the hand on the injured side.
- Check for sensation in the axillary nerve by pinching the deltoid muscle on the patients "injured"

arm. If they can't feel your pinch, there is pressure on the axillary nerve.

- Help position the patient on their back.
- Apply traction at the elbow to relax the shoulder muscles and relieve pain using one of the hand

positions shown on the previous page. Maintain traction throughout the treatment process until the reduction is successful or abandoned.

- If the patient is lying on a slippery surface, such as snow or wet leaves, an assistant should hold the patient's jacket—or a tarp or ground cloth wrapped around their chest—to prevent the patient from sliding when traction is applied.

- While maintaining traction, rotate the "injured" arm to "baseball" position and WAIT. If during this process the patient complains of severe pain while tensing their shoulder muscles, stop the rotation—while maintaining traction—and wait for them to relax once again. While continuing to maintain traction, resume rotation until the patient's shoulder is in the "baseball" position. After maintaining traction in the "baseball" position for a minimum of five minutes, move the arm to "high baseball" position.

- While still maintaining traction, WAIT for the patient's shoulder muscles to relax and the shoulder to relocate (reduce). If you are able to get the patient to relax, most shoulders will reduce within 5-20 minutes. When the shoulder relocates, you will feel a bump (or series of bumps) and the patient will smile.

- If the patient's shoulder has in fact relocated, they will feel no pain as you SLOWLY release the traction. If pain is present, resume traction and wait for the shoulder to relocate. If the patient does not complain of pain as you release the traction, assist them in moving the arm to their side; the elbow should rest comfortably against the patient's body.

- Recheck distal and axillary CSM as described above.

- Administer OTC ibuprofen or naproxen sodium for pain and inflammation.

- Splint the injured shoulder against the patient's body for a minimum of 10 days and then treat as a stable injury.

- Cool the affected area to help reduce swelling and pain. Use ice for 20 to 30 minutes at 90-minute intervals, to allow local reperfusion.

- If the patient's shoulder does not reduce within 30 minutes, try the "Hanging Traction" method described below and shown on the previous page. If unsuccessful, pad and splint the shoulder in position and begin a Level 3 Evacuation; consider a Level 2 Evacuation if there is no distal CSM.

"Hanging Traction" Method

- Check the patient's distal and axillary CSM as described previously.

- Assist patient to a padded "platform" both tall and flat enough to permit their arm and a suspended weight to hang freely. Place patient face down on the "platform" with their "injured" arm hanging down as shown on the previous page.

- Attach duct tape to the skin of the "injured" arm to create an "eye hook" large enough for a carabiner or rope to pass through easily; you may also tape the weighted sack directly to the patient's arm. Lightly wrap the taped arm using an ace bandage to increase the patient's venous return.

- Using a carabiner or rope, attach a weighted container such as a stuff sack filled with rocks, or filled water bottles, through the taped "eye hook." Add weight until the patient's pain is relieved; use the smallest amount possible to maintain pain-free traction; 5-10 pounds is typically sufficient.

- Rotate the scapula inward and slightly up to facilitate the reduction. If an assistant is available, they may apply external rotation to the humerus, until the shoulder reduces.

- If shoulder reduces (usually within one hour), splint it and treat it as a stable injury for a minimum of 10 days, as described previously.

- If the patient's shoulder does not reduce within the hour, pad and splint the shoulder in position and begin a Level 3 Evacuation; consider a Level 2 Evacuation if there is no distal CSM.

Assessment of Jaw Dislocations

- The MOI is typically due to extreme mouth-opening while yawning, vomiting, or during a seizure.

- The patient complains of pain and difficulty opening their mouth.

- With a unilateral dislocation, the patient's jaw moves away from mid-line. With a bilateral dislocation, the patient presents with an underbite.

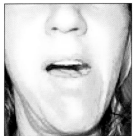

Unilateral   Bilateral

Field Treatment of Jaw Dislocations

- Pad your thumbs; cloth or gauze works well.
- Stand in front of the seated patient to increase leverage.

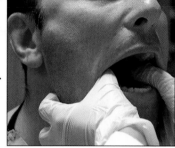

- Place gloved, padded thumbs over both of the patient's lower molars, as far back as possible. Curve fingers around the patient's jaw as shown above.
- Use your thumbs to press firmly down and back on the patient's molars, until their jaw relocates.

Assessment of Posterior Hip Dislocations

- The patient presents on their back or side with the leg on the affected side shorter than on the unaffected side and rotated inward.

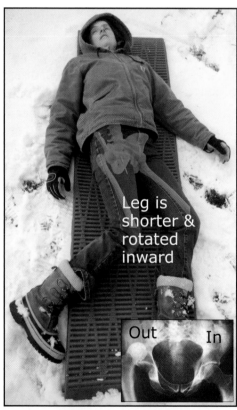

Leg is shorter & rotated inward

Out   In

- The patient may have fractures to the knee, patella, and/or the femoral head, neck, shaft, or socket (acetabulum).
- The patient reports moderate-to-severe pain.
- Associated nerve injury and loss of nerve function are possible.

94 Traumatic Injuries

Field Treatment of Posterior Hip Dislocations

- If the leg on the side of the dislocation has no significant fracture, one rescuer stabilizes the patient's hips, while a second squats with arms crossed under patient's knee and lifts, using their legs, until the femoral head relocates.

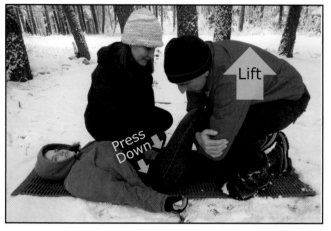

Lift

Press Down

- If reduction is successful and there is no nerve damage, begin a Level 3 Evacuation.
- Begin a Level 2 Evacuation for patients with an unreduced posterior hip dislocation; death of the femoral head and permanent nerve damage may occur any time within the following 24 hours without reduction.

Improvising Effective Splints

The goal of splinting is to immobilize the injury in all directions. All splints should be:

- Well Padded
- Easily Adjustable
- Strong
- Simple
- Lightweight
- Comfortable

There are four concepts central to improvising effective splints: casts, jelly rolls, sandwiches, and buddy splints. All are discussed below.

Cast Splint

Cast splints are used to immobilize digits, forearms, wrists, ankles and knees. Carefully mold, pad and attach a SAM® splint to the injured limb with a cloth roll; a conforming bandage (Coban® or Vet Wrap®) will also work. When forming the splint, take care to remove all pressure points. Avoid elastic bandages because it is very difficult to control the pressure during application. Too much pressure causes

CSM problems, while not enough permits unwanted movement. Padding should be thick and smooth; it may consist of the patient's heavy pile sleeve, thick sock(s), etc. An improvised SAM® splint can be made from heavy foil, such as a windscreen from a backpacking stove.

Sandwich Splint

Sandwich splints may be used to immobilize in-line femur fractures or Tib/Fib fractures. The splint has rigid "boards" on the outside, thick padding on the inside, and is held in place with straps. When completed, the two "boards" are parallel and distribute the compression forces evenly. A "board" may be a real board, snowshoe, etc. or one constructed with finger-thick poles (tent poles, ski poles, green sticks, internal pack stays, etc.) taped together. Suitable strap material can be webbing, cam straps, strips of strong cloth, or rope. Thick padding can be made from carefully folded clothing, sleeping pads, tarps, or sleeping bags. Effective padding may also be made by filling a small stuff sack with soft objects. Sandwich splints may utilize the "Go Beyond" principle when securing an ankle within the splint. Use a sock roll or knit hat to pad under the knee.

Jelly Roll Splint

Jelly roll splints effectively immobilize unstable knees and ankles and offer better protection during the evacuation than a cast splint. You will need a long, FIRM sleeping pad and thick padding. Roll the padding into the sleeping pad from both ends. Hold each side to prevent the jelly roll from unrolling as it is attached; it is held in place using straps. Use the "Go Beyond" principle when splinting an ankle.

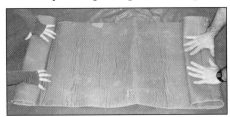

Loosely roll towards the center from both ends.

Buddy Splint

A buddy splint is simple and quick to assemble. The injured limb is simply splinted against another part of the body. For example, the shoulder, upper arm, elbow, and forearm can be splinted against the chest by rolling and knotting, or taping the patient's shirt or jacket around the injured upper limb. A sim-

ilar result can be obtained by pinning the sleeves of the patient's jacket to the body of the jacket or by using cravats or cloth strips to tie the limb in place. Other common uses of buddy splints are taping two fingers together or tying two legs together. Both of the latter splints may be reinforced by adding a well padded "board."

Femur Traction Splint

All femur traction splints are complicated splints that MUST be used with a backboard or litter. Femur traction splints should ONLY be used on an extremely painful, isolated, and angulated mid-shaft femur fracture and ONLY if the total evacuation time is less than six hours. All require an anchoring strap in the groin area that eventually compresses the femoral artery and reduces distal circulation. Use as little traction as possible to reduce the patient's pain; if possible, use a sandwich splint instead.

Unstable Pelvis & Pelvic Splint

An unstable pelvis typically requires a significant MOI, is extremely painful, and 40% of the time, causes internal bleeding that leads to volume shock. S/Sx of a pelvic fracture include pain in the pelvic area, lower back, groin, and/or hips, with or without instability, S/Sx of volume shock, blood in the urine, which is colored red/brown, and bladder and bowel incontinence. If an unstable pelvic injury is suspected, apply a pelvic splint (see page 101) and immobilize the patient on a backboard or litter. Carefully lift the patient and center a folded tarp over the femoral trochanters and pubis. Pull, maintain tension, and securely pin or tie in place. Place a thin inflatable sleeping pad between the tarp and the patient; inflate the sleeping pad after pinning to increase stability. Move the pelvis as little as possible; avoid rolling the patient.

The Splints

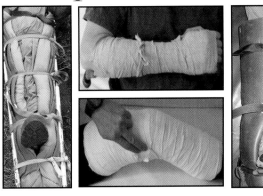

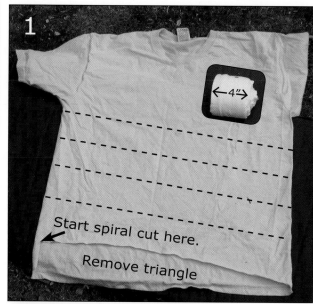

3 Cut the underarm seams on each side and unfold. Then round the corners.

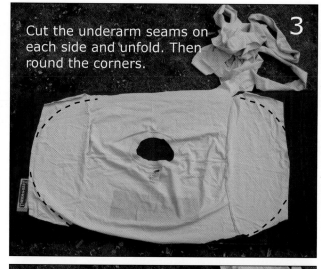

4 Continue to spiral cut until you run out of room.

END

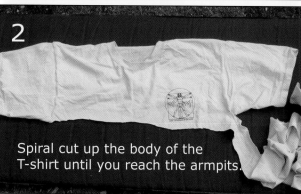

1 ←4"→

Start spiral cut here.

Remove triangle

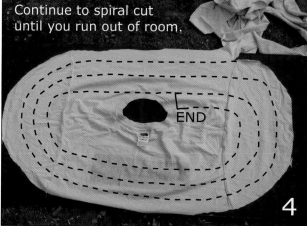

2 Spiral cut up the body of the T-shirt until you reach the armpits.

T-Shirt Cutting 101: How to turn a T-shirt into a cloth roll for splinting.

Improvising Cloth Rolls

Cloth rolls are used with SAM® splints to improvise casts. An effective roll can be made from most pieces of clothing using the spiral cutting principle illustrated above. Although simple, practice a few times on an old shirt to work out the kinks before you need the skill. T-shirts, long-sleeved T-shirts, shorts, long pants, and jackets all work. Ideally, the clothing used should be in reasonably good condition and the material should be strong, non-elastic, and free of holes, zippers, and buttons. Tarps, blankets, and rain flies can also be used.

Short strips of cloth used to tie sleeping bags in a tight roll for immobilizing a spine-injured patient in a litter or backboard can be cut from a long roll. Alternatively, they can simply be cut from the legs of a pair of pants or the body of a shirt, by first cutting up the side seam and then across. In this case, a spiral cut is not needed.

Knee Cast

The knee cast may be used for a stable or unstable knee. Cut a 36-inch SAM® splint in half and pad. Mold the lower half of each side of the splint into a curve to fit the patient's lower leg; refer to the photographs on the next page and use your leg as a template, not the patients. Align the center of the splint with the top of the patient's knee cap on each side; keep the edges of the splint away from the knee cap. Begin wrapping the splint with the cloth roll just below the patient's knee and continue downward. Once the lower half of the splint is covered, go back up. Make sure that the patient's knee is bent slightly in the position of comfort. Gently mold, curve, and fold the upper halves of the splint to the patient's upper leg and wrap. Continue wrapping until the entire splint is covered. Use two cloth rolls to secure the splint with an unstable knee, particularly if the patient is tall or if their leg is heavily muscled.

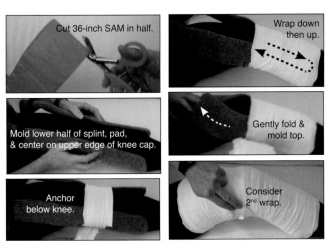

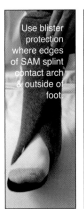 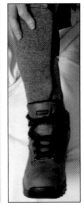 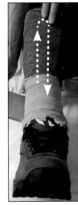 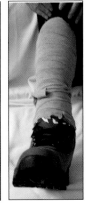

Ankle Cast

Use this splint for an unstable ankle; it is NOT a walking cast. Using your leg as a template, mold the SAM® splint into a stirrup shape and pad as shown below. Place the splint over the boot and anchor at the ankle. Figure 8 wrap around the ankle and foot; have the patient pull up on the top of the splint as you wrap. Once the entire bottom of the splint is wrapped, continue up the lower leg. Split the ends and tie.

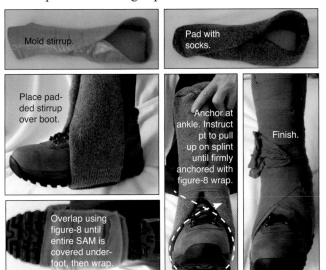

Ankle Walking Cast

Use this splint for a stable ankle when the patient needs to walk out. Remove the insole and place the padded splint over the insole and foot. Beware of blisters; use ENGO® on the edges of the splint, where it comes in contact with the bottom of the patient's foot, especially the arch, and place the splint in the boot. Gently work the foot into the boot and splint. Anchor the splint at the ankle and wrap up and down the lower leg. Split ends and tie. The splint will loosen as it is used. *Use caution during the evacuation, as forces normally absorbed or countered by the ankle will transfer directly to the patient's knee.*

Forearm & Wrist Cast

A forearm and wrist cast can be used for splinting both stable and unstable injuries. Remove all jewelry, watches, or wrist bands. Form the splint, as shown below, using your forearm as a template. Anchor the splint at the patient's wrist and lightly wrap towards their elbow. Make sure to reverse direction before reaching their elbow; allow enough space for the elbow to bend freely. Firmly wrap the patient's knuckles to immobilize the wrist. The patient's thumb can be in or out; most patients will put their thumb in their best position of comfort without asking. Split the cloth roll at the end and tie securely. Consider buddy splinting the arm to the patient's chest.

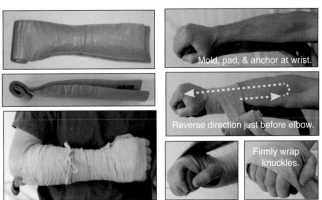

Finger Cast

A finger cast is used to immobilize an unstable finger. Stable fingers are usually taped to an adjacent uninjured finger using a buddy splint. Using a pair of trauma scissors, measure and cut a section from the end of a SAM® splint. Fold and mold the splint to the patient's injured finger and an adjacent uninjured finger using your own hand as the mold; do not form the splint on the patient's hand. Padding is not usually necessary. Anchor the splint at the base of the patient's injured finger and lightly wrap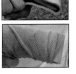

towards the tip. Reverse direction when you come to the end of the splint. Split the cloth roll at the end and tie securely.

Ankle Jelly Roll Splint

The ankle jelly roll splint is used for splinting an unstable ankle injury; it is too awkward to use as a walking splint. Roll a sleeping pad loosely to the center as depicted in the photographs below. Keep the center edges together, support the leg, and slide into place; 8-10 inches of the pad should "Go Beyond" the end of the patient's foot. Ask the patient or a second rescuer to hold the splint in place as you strap. Fasten the ankle strap first, followed by the one above it; cinch the "Go Beyond" section last. If the patient has long legs or the pad is soft, add another strap to the lower leg.

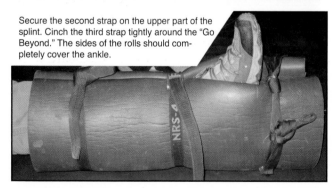

Keep the center of the rolls close together and place the lower leg into the fold. The splint should "Go Beyond" the boot by 8-10 inches. Pinch the upper edge, and tie the first strap around the ankle.

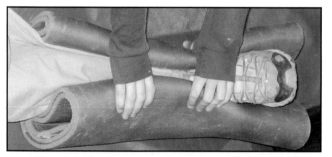

Secure the second strap on the upper part of the splint. Cinch the third strap tightly around the "Go Beyond." The sides of the rolls should completely cover the ankle.

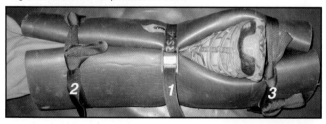

Knee Jelly Roll Splint

Use the knee jelly roll splint to support an unstable knee; it is too awkward to use as a walking splint. Roll the pad loosely to the center. Keep the center edges together, support the leg, and slide into place. Place some soft material (sock roll, knit hat, etc.) under the knee to keep it slightly flexed. Ask the patient or a second rescuer to hold the splint in place as you strap. Fasten the ankle strap first. Then spread the top of the roll wide enough to fit the patient's upper leg and strap. The order of fastening the center straps doesn't matter; however, avoid placing a strap over the knee cap. The finished splint should conform to the patients leg with its sides parallel to one another. Refer to the photograph below.

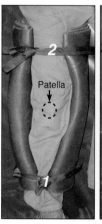 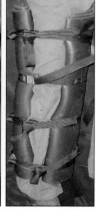 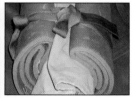

Keep the center of the rolls close together and strap the ankle first. Then spread the top of the roll wide to fit the upper leg and secure the second strap. The order of the center straps doesn't matter; avoid placing a strap over the knee cap. The rolls should conform to the leg.

Knee Sandwich Splint

Use a knee sandwich splint to support an unstable knee when other materials are unavailable. If possible, remove any snow crampons. Tie the bottom of the splint together being careful to leave enough space for adequate compression once the top has been tied. Pad the inside with a sleeping pad and place a sock roll under the patient's knee. Secure the top edges of the splint to finish in the manner illustrated below.

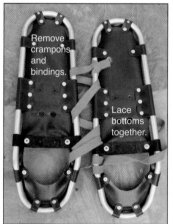 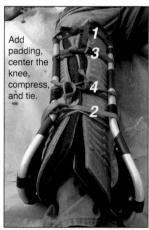

Lower-Leg Sandwich Splint

Use a lower-leg sandwich splint to support an unstable femur or tibia/fibula (lower leg). The splint may also be used for an unstable knee injury by using shorter poles and a jacket for padding in place of the sleeping pad. Fold a sleeping bag and pad in half lengthwise with the bag on top of the pad, support the leg, and slide into place; 8-10 inches of the bag and pad should "Go Beyond" the end of the patient's foot. Ask the patient or a second rescuer to hold the splint in place as you strap. Tape two sets of finger-thick poles together (ski poles, sticks, tent poles, etc.). Secure the poles on the outside of the pad and align them with the long bones of the patient's leg. Fasten the groin strap first, followed by the ankle strap. Take a full turn around poles at each end of the splint to make sure they stay aligned with the bone. Secure the center straps next; avoid placing a strap directly over the knee cap. Cinch the "Go Beyond" section last. Secure and evacuate the patient in a litter; immobilize their hips in the litter if they have an unstable femur.

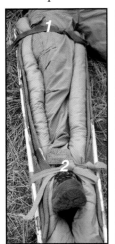

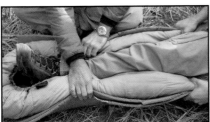

Fold a sleeping bag and pad in half lengthwise and place under the injured leg; "Go Beyond" the boot. Support the knee with a sock roll or knit hat .

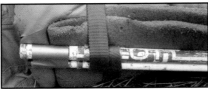

Place two taped poles on the outside of the pad on both sides of the injured leg. "Go Beyond" the boot 8-10 inches. Secure the top of the splint first, then the ankle.

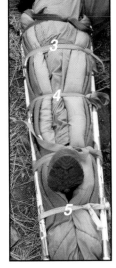

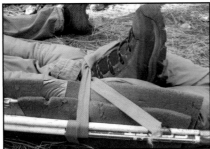

Take a full turn around both sets of poles at both ends of the splint before tying. Secure the center straps next; avoid placing a strap directly over the knee cap. Cinch the "Go Beyond" section last.

Upper Limb Buddy Splint

Use the upper limb buddy splint for supporting a stable or unstable injury to the elbow, upper arm, or shoulder. Pull the hem of the patient's shirt up and over their forearm and elbow. Cut the back corner of the shirt behind the elbow and tie the two tails firmly together.

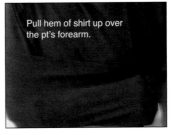

Pull hem of shirt up over the pt's forearm.

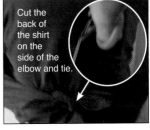

Cut the back of the shirt on the side of the elbow and tie.

A second shirt may be added over the first for more support. Tie a knot on the side; there is no need to cut the second shirt. Use any shirt, jacket or vest. Zip all zippers. If you are using a button-down shirt, there is no need to cut the back; unbutton the bottom buttons and tie the tails together in the front.

Lower-Limb Buddy Splint

Use the lower-limb buddy splint to support an unstable lower leg when there is no deformity, when splinting materials are unavailable, or when an urgent evacuation is required and transportation is readily available. Loosely roll a sleeping pad and place it between the patient's lower legs. Fold a second sleeping pad in half lengthwise and place under both legs. Secure with cloth ties as illustrated below.

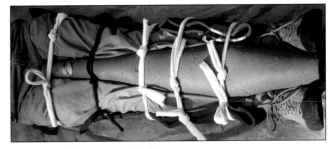

Femur Traction Splint

All femur traction splints are complicated splints that MUST be used with a backboard or litter. Femur traction splints should *only* be used on an extremely painful, isolated, and angulated mid-shaft femur fracture and *only* if the total evacuation time is less than six hours. All require an anchoring strap in the groin area that eventually compresses the femoral artery and reduces distal circulation. Use as little traction as possible to reduce the patient's pain; if possible, use a sandwich splint. If possible, hold manual traction from the patient's knee until the splint is in place. Applying a traction splint takes multiple people. Refer to the photographs on the following page.

1. Locate a rigid support for the leg that is strong enough to withstand the traction pressure without bending or breaking. Use duct tape to create a "board" or pole 1-3 inches wide and 6-10 inches longer than the patient's leg as measured from the top of the pelvis to the sole of the foot; use the patient's uninjured leg as a template to measure the correct pole length. Multiple tent poles, a single Megamid pole, two ski poles, two paddle shafts, or multiple green sticks can make good supports.

2. Two sections of 1-inch webbing, or other material of similar strength, each at least 30 inches long, will separately form the "groin anchor" and the traction device. Tie an overhand loop in one end of both sections or use cam straps. Using one section at a time, place the knot (or cam) as close as pos-sible to one end of the rigid support, fold the other end over the top of the support, and tape in place, creating a pocket for the support to rest in. Repeat the process on the other end of the support using the other section of webbing.

3. Use webbing and a cloth roll to make an ankle hitch. Pad the leg with a sleeping bag and pad as per a sandwich splint. Place a 2-3 foot piece of webbing across the sole of the patient's footwear and align it with the malleolus (bone) on each side of the ankle; the ends of the webbing will be along the side of the patient's leg near the knee. Begin-ning at the ankle, wrap the sleeping bag, pad, and webbing firmly around the patient's ankle with the cloth roll. Go about halfway up the lower leg, split the end of the cloth roll and tie it off. Pull firmly

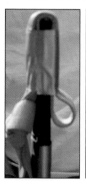
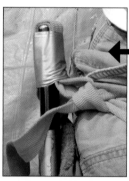
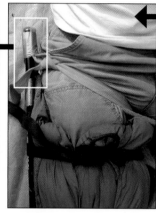
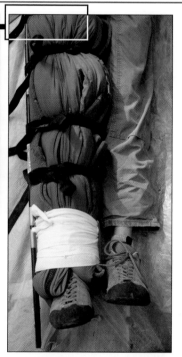

Tape poles together to form a "board." Then fold an overhand knot with a long loop over the ends and tape to create anchor points for the groin strap and traction system. Thread the strap through the webbing at the bottom of the patient's foot and back through the loop. Pull and tie.

Pad and anchor at the patient's groin. Pad the patient's leg as per a sandwich splint.

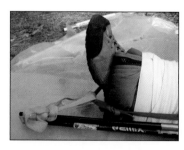
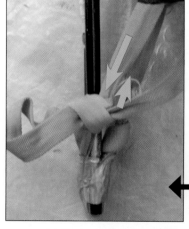
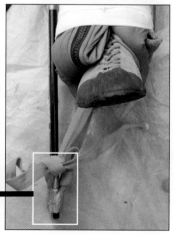

Mid-shaft Femur Traction Splint

down on the webbing and tie the ends under the patient's foot to form a loop.

4. To apply the splint, pad and tie one section around the patient's upper thigh (proximal anchor). Make sure that it is resting snugly in their crotch with the rigid support on the outside of the patient's leg aligned with the axis of that leg. Using webbing or cloth strips, loosely secure the splint to the patient's thigh and lower leg. Pass the webbing on the other end of the rigid support through the bottom of the ankle hitch and back through the loop or cam to create a mini pulley system. Slowly apply traction until the limb is aligned and the patient's pain is reduced. Use as little traction as possible to accomplish this task. The higher the traction pressure, the faster the patient's distal CSM will decrease. Tighten the "straps" tying the patient's legs and support together until snug.

- The splint is finished when the patient's hip and legs are immobilized in a litter or backboard.

- Monitor the patient's distal CSM. If it becomes compromised, convert the traction splint into a sandwich splint and then remove the traction OR immobilize the patients pelvis in a Stokes litter and apply traction, using the same system as described above with the foot rail as the anchor.

Pelvic Splint

To improvise a pelvic splint, carefully lift the patient and place them on a backboard or litter with the center of a folded tarp over the femoral trochanters and pubis. Move the pelvis as little as possible; avoid rolling the patient. Pull, maintain tension, and secure the splint by pinning or tying as shown below. Place a thin inflatable sleeping pad between the tarp and the patient; inflate after pinning to increase stability. Immobilize the patient on backboard or litter.

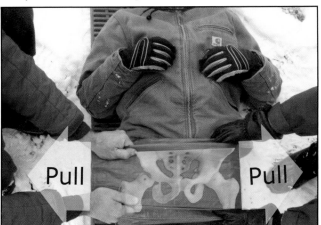

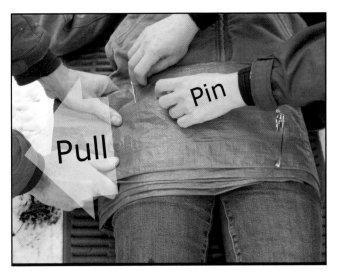

Alternate Splints

You can also apply the cast and sandwich concepts to improvise splints from natural materials. A few ideas are illustrated below: green sticks can be lashed together to create a "board," padded, and secured as with a sandwich or cast splint. Sections of old or green bark may be used to cast a forearm. Light-weight, hanging moss of the Usnea family, for instance, Old Man's Beard, can be used as a padding.

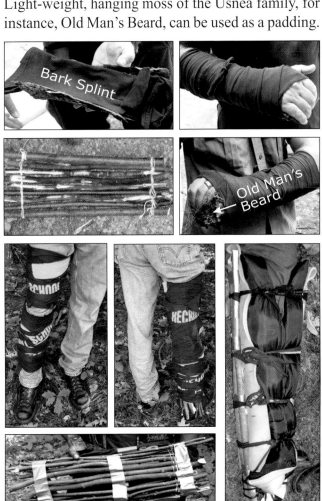

Improvised Patient Carries

For patients whose injuries, such as an unstable ankle or knee, require them to be carried during the evacuation, you will need to improvise a backpack or split-coil carry. If you or a party member are strong and fit enough, a single patient backpack carry is typically your best choice; it may be your only option for carrying a patient on a narrow trail. If you have a wide or open area such as beach, dry wash, forest service road, and only need to transport someone a short distance, you might prefer a two-person carry.

Backpack Carries

There are two simple methods for a single rescuer backpack carry. In either case it's easier to load the patient, if they sit on something that is slightly higher than the rescuer's waist.

• Cut the bottom side seams of your expedition pack and have the patient pull it on like a pair of pants; pad the groin area. Cut the seams carefully and they can easily be repaired later. If your carry-out is long, it is worth the extra time to get out your sewing kit and bar-tack the seam so that it doesn't tear further during use. While the patient may sit facing forward or backward, most patients and rescuers prefer to have the patient facing forward. A forward-facing position provides better balance for the rescuer and allows the rescuer to support the patient's legs behind the knees when terrain permits; it is similar to giving a piggyback ride. The advantage to using a backpack is that you can take advantage of the padded hip and shoulder belt system.

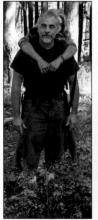
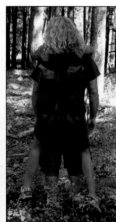
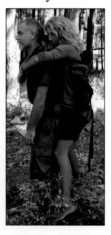

• If a backpack is unavailable, consider using a standard or improvised split-coil carry. Coil a climbing rope into a single coil (not a butterfly coil) and finish by wrapping one end around and through a bight of rope from the other end. Then, carefully split the coil and place the two loops on the ground. Help the patient put a leg through each coil and slide the knot into the small of their back. With the patient facing forward, put your arms through the rope coils in the same manner that you would shoulder a backpack; make sure that the weight is evenly distributed across the coils before lifting. A properly sized coil will hold the patient above your hips, similar to a properly adjusted backpack. Use a bandana or a piece of webbing to improvise a sternum strap to help keep the patient's weight on your shoulders; you may need to pad the rope coils for comfort. Almost anything can be used to make this carry if a rope is not available, including a tarp, tent fly, strong sleeping pads, which are quite comfortable, and two pairs of long pants. Pattern the improvised carry after the two loops of the split coil carry; remember to tie/fix the loops together if using a long tarp in a figure-8 pattern. Test all improvised carries on an uninjured member of your party before using with a patient.

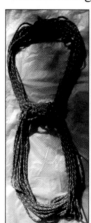
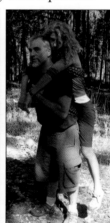
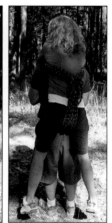

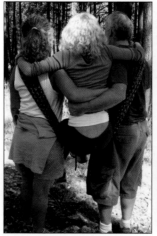
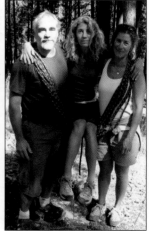

A standard or improvised split coil system may also be used for a two-person carry. Each rescuer puts their head and arm through a loop of the coil and kneels. The patient sits on the knot between the two rescuers and puts their arms around the rescuer's necks. The patient's back is supported by the rescuer's arms.

Wounds
Pathophysiology

All wounds damage tissue, bleed, or ooze plasma. If bleeding occurs, arteries and arterioles constrict and the clotting cascade is activated. If it is successful, bleeding will stop within 5-15 minutes. Within hours, cellular debris from the damaged tissue stimulates the inflammatory response to help prevent infection and begin healing.

Wounds are classified according to their depth and potential for bacterial infection. Superficial and partial-thickness wounds such as abrasions, superficial and partial-thickness burns, shallow cuts, scrapes, and friction blisters, are at low risk for bacterial infection and heal rapidly. Clean, full-thickness wounds with neat edges (lacerations) are at low-to-moderate risk for infection; and while they take a bit longer to heal, healing is complete with little to no scarring. Deep, full-thickness wounds with dirty, ragged edges and damaged bones, ligaments, tendons, or muscles, including puncture wounds and bites, are at high risk for infection; healing is slow and may be incomplete.

Superficial & Partial-Thickness Wounds

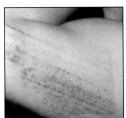
Abrasions

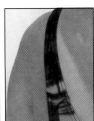
Sun Burn

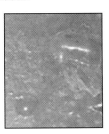
1º & 2º Burns

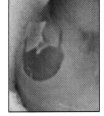
Blisters

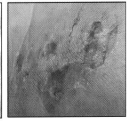
Shallow Cuts

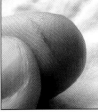
Scrapes

Pathophysiology

In both superficial and partial-thickness wounds, damage is confined to the epidermis or epidermis and upper dermal layers. Bleeding indicates damage to the dermis; the greater the bleeding, the greater the damage. The more damage, the greater the inflammatory response. Capillaries in the dermis, together with fibroblasts, secrete collagen. New skin cells are constructed from the collagen and migrate over the dermis, building from the inside out. Collagen forms faster in a moist, as opposed to dry, environment.

Treatment of Superficial & Partial-Thickness Wounds

- Use aloe vera gel and vitamin E on damaged, but intact, skin (sunburn and superficial burns).

- Wash partial-thickness wounds and the surrounding skin with soap and clean water. Remove all foreign debris by gentle scrubbing and/or by careful picking with tweezers. Vigorous scrubbing may cause minor bleeding and should be avoided if possible. Open closed blisters and remove dead skin prior to cleansing. Pat or air dry.

- Keep the wound moist with a micro-thin film dressing (Tegaderm®) or hydrogel (Second Skin®). Micro-thin film dressings are clear, occlusive and protect the wound from further contamination while promoting healing. Do not use ointment under the dressing. Leave the dressing in place until healing has occurred. Monitor for infection through the dressing. Do not use micro-thin film dressings over joints.

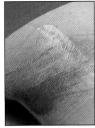
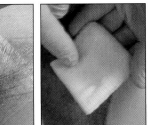
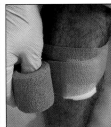

Micro-thin Film Dressing

Ointment Impregnated Gauze Dressing & Coban® bandage.

- If a micro-thin film dressing is not available, use white/light petroleum jelly and a thick gauze dressing; bandage with self-adhering bandage or a cloth roll. Re-clean twice a day. Although commonplace, topical antibiotic ointments—silver sulfadiazine (Rx) or petroleum-based antibiotic ointments—while commonly used, are typically not necessary.

• Glue shallow cuts—often caused by excessive exposure to wind, dry air and cold water—together with super glue BEFORE they begin to bleed.

Friction Blisters

Pathophysiology

Friction and pressure combine to create shear forces that first stretch and irritate the connective tissue between the epidermis and dermis, creating a "hot spot." Later, when the connective tissue finally tears, the skin delaminates and plasma leaks between the torn layers and a blister forms. As long as friction and pressure are present, the skin continues to delaminate and the blister grows until it breaks. More pressure—due to a heavy pack or persistent hiking downhill—will cause deeper damage and a more painful blister. Both the prevention and treatment of friction blisters focus on reducing shear forces within the skin; in many cases, this requires adding an external sliding layer.

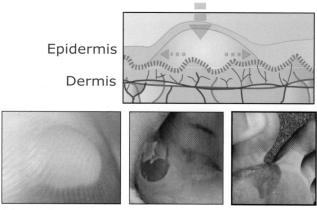

Shear forces and pressure within the skin create "friction" blisters.

Contributing Factors & Prevention

• **Dirty skin increases surface friction.** Wash skin, and socks on a regular basis. Wear gaiters over boot tops and laces to keep dust and dirt out.

• **Wet, saturated skin weakens the epidermis, making it more susceptible to shear forces.** Keep skin, socks, and gloves dry. Change socks regularly. Sleep in clean dry socks. For some people a antiperspirant helps keep feet dry.

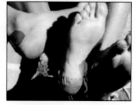

• **A rapid increase in shear forces beyond those normally encountered, doesn't permit enough time for connective tissue to adapt.** Increase load/pack weight and distance slowly to allow the skin to adapt to new forces. Avoid continuous downhill hiking until skin has had time to strengthen.

• **Poor-fitting footwear creates pressure spots.** Make sure footwear, gloves and clothing fit well.

• The absence of an external sliding layer predisposes skin to blisters. Anticipate blisters by treating hot spots BEFORE they become a blister, add an external sliding layer (ENGO® and/or tape) to reduce shear forces within the skin.

Treatment for Friction Blisters

• **At home:** Leave the blister closed and wear footwear that does not irritate the blister. Alternatively, pad the blister with a mole-foam doughnut, until it is reabsorbed (3-10 days).

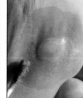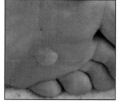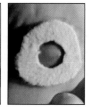

• **To complete a day hike:** Drain the blister, by nicking it using a clean scissors or a scalpel; leave skin cover intact. Pad with doughnuts of mole skin or mole foam to relieve pressure. Add an ENGO® blister patch to footwear or socks.

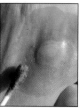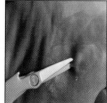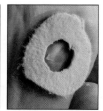

• **To continue a multi-day hike:** Remove the skin over blister. Cover the exposed blister with a hydrogel dressing or petroleum jelly and gauze. Secure the dressing in place with cloth tape or with flexible medical tape. Use tincture of benzoin. Add an ENGO® blister patch to footwear or socks.

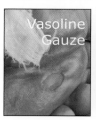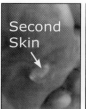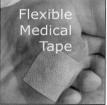

Treatment for Blood Blisters

- **Beneath skin:** Treat as per friction blister. Blood blisters, because they extend more deeply into the skin, are at higher risk of infection. Keep the affected area clean.
- **Beneath nail bed:** If large and painful, heat a small piece of metal (a paperclip works well…) over the blue flame of your cook stove until it's red hot and melt nail to release blood, pressure, and pain.

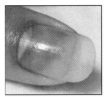 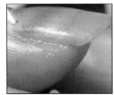 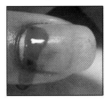

Full-Thickness Wounds

Physiology of Healing

Refer to the diagram at the bottom of this page. Full-thickness wounds pierce both the epidermis and the dermis, causing bleeding. The damaged blood vessels immediately constrict and within 5-15 minutes, specialized proteins (fibrin) form a clot that holds the wound edges together and stops further bleeding. Inflammation leads to local vasodilation and increased vascular permeability that, in turn, permit phagocytes and other supplies to seep into the tissue. Together with the clotting proteins, these form an internal barrier and scab that help protect the wound against invading bacteria. Excess fluid and debris not picked up by the lymphatic system or ingested by phagocytes drains through the scab as pus. The internal protective barrier and scab continue to thicken and, over time, the clot is replaced by pink granulation tissue composed of new capillaries and fibroblasts that secrete collagen. New skin cells are constructed from the collagen and migrate over the granulation tissue, building from the inside out. Collagen forms faster in a moist environment. The new capillaries are extremely fragile and bleed easily when disturbed. The granulation tissue gradually contracts and pulls the wound edges closer together. Eventually the scab falls off. Finally, weeks later, the epidermis is completely regenerated leaving fibrous scar tissue beneath.

Field Treatment for Full-Thickness Wounds

General Treatment for Full-Thickness Wounds

- Clean all wounds within two hours of the incident.
- Cover wound with a dry dressing and bandage. Monitor, reclean and rebandage when the dressing becomes wet through wound drainage or environmental factors.

Treatment for Low-to-Moderate Full-Thickness Wounds

- **Begin the cleansing process after bleeding has stopped. Do not clean a wound that is associated with severe life-threatening bleeding.**
- Wash the skin surrounding the wound with soap and clean water or using a 10% solution of povidone-iodine (PI); do not wash inside the wound itself.
- Use your fingers to distract the wound, then pressure flush numerous times with copious amounts

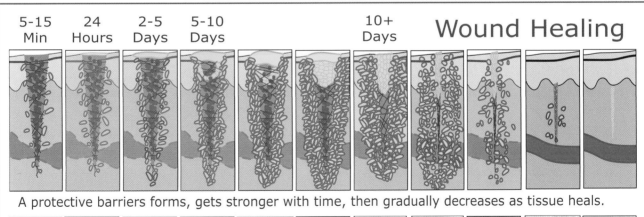

| 5-15 Min | 24 Hours | 2-5 Days | 5-10 Days | | 10+ Days | Wound Healing |

A protective barriers forms, gets stronger with time, then gradually decreases as tissue heals.

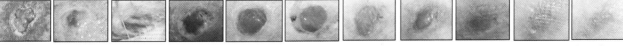

Inflammation (local redness, warmth, pain, tenderness and swelling) increases over the first 24 hours, stabilizes, then slowly decreases as the protective barriers get stronger.

Low-to-Moderate Risk Full-Thickness Wounds

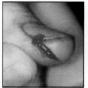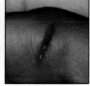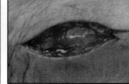

Clean edges
Not deep
Minimal or no damage to underlying tissue

High-Risk Full Thickness

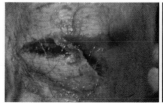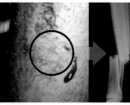

Deep   Ragged edges
Dirty   Damage to underlying tissue
Puncture   Animal bites

of clean water. A 30 cc or 60 cc irrigation syringe is ideal, but other delivery methods can also work well, such as a bicycle water bottle or a strong plastic bag with a corner removed. Flush using intense short bursts, rather than one long stream. Avoid forcing material into tissue pockets by flushing along the axis of the wound. Pat or air dry.

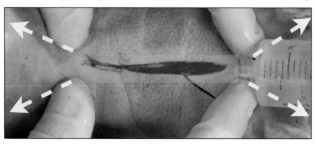

Distracting the wound and pressure flushing.

• *Avoid vigorous scrubbing; it may cause minor bleeding.* In the unlikely event of more severe bleeding, STOP the cleansing process and apply direct pressure until the wound has reclotted. Do not resume cleaning the wound until the bleeding has stopped; then, gently flush.

• Cover the wound with a thick

Wound Closure

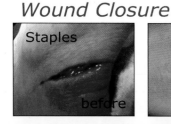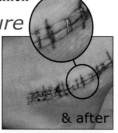

Staples
before   & after

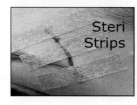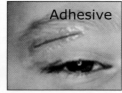

Steri Strips   Adhesive

gauze dressing and bandage.

• Monitor, reclean and rebandage the wound when

the dressing becomes wet from wound drainage, sweat, or environmental conditions.

• While wound closure often speeds the healing process, it also increases the chance of infection by preventing drainage. *Only attempt to close clean, shallow lacerations.* To close a shallow laceration, approximate edges with adhesive strips (Steri-strips®, tape strips, butterfly® closures), tissue adhesive (Dermabond®), or skin staples. NOTE that staples require a special stapler and tool for removal.

*Treatment for
High-Risk Full-Thickness Wounds*

• *Follow the wound cleaning process for low-to-moderate full-thickness wounds and include the following steps:*

• Remove any skin or tissue from the edges of the wound that is poorly attached or turning blue or black. Use a clean sharp scissors or scalpel. *Do not cut or remove deep tissue or structures.*

• Remove any remaining foreign material using clean tweezers or forceps following the initial flushing process. Gentle probing may be necessary. A large magnifying glass is often helpful.

• *Vigorous scrubbing, extensive probing, and excessive cutting may restart minor bleeding and should be avoided.* In the unlikely event of more severe bleeding, STOP the cleansing process and apply direct pressure until the wound has reclotted. Do not resume cleaning the wound until the bleeding has stopped; then, gently flush.

• Finish the cleansing process with multiple flushes of a 1% povidone-iodine solution (diluted from a 10% povidone-iodine solution or ointment), saline solution, or fresh echinacea tea.

• *Do not close high-risk wounds in the field* because of the increased chance for infection.

- Impregnate the gauze dressing with a 10% povidone-iodine ointment (or solution), white/light petroleum jelly or a petroleum-based antibiotic ointment. Do not apply directly onto or into the wound, since petroleum-based ointments are difficult to remove and 10% PI solution will damage healthy cells. Secure the dressing with a conforming bandage.

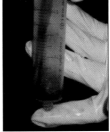
Measuring 1% PI solution for diluting

- Immobilize the limb or site using a splint to prevent mechanical disruption of the protective barrier if the wound is over a joint. All wounds associated with an unstable injury require splinting. If the limb is angulated or deformed, it may also require realignment. Refer to the previous discussions of unstable injuries and splinting earlier in this Section.
- Consider packing deep wounds with narrow gauze strips soaked in 1% PI solution to prevent premature closure and to encourage drainage. Remove, reclean and replace the packing four times a day (breakfast, lunch, dinner and before bed).
- Begin a Level 2 Evacuation for all patients who have wounds associated with an unstable injury.
- All patients with high-risk wounds are at high risk for contracting tetanus. If they have not had a tetanus vaccination or booster within the past five years, they MUST receive shots containing the antitoxin (tetanus immune globulin) and vaccine within 24 hours of the incident.

Treatment for Animal Bites

- All animal bites are high-risk wounds and at risk for contracting rabies. Thorough and aggressive wound cleaning is EXTREMELY important. Flushing is not enough to kill the rabies virus and all wounds should be physically swabbed; use a 2% solution of benzalkonium chloride (CureChrome®) or a 20% soap solution. Thoroughly flush all chemical agents after a few minutes of contact time.
- All mammals are susceptible to rabies and are potential carriers; however, only certain animals commonly transmit the virus to humans. Rabies reservoirs in the United States include skunks, raccoons, foxes and bats. Rodents, rabbits and hares, and urban cats and dogs are considered low risk.

- Contact local health officials for advice before beginning your trip; consider pre-exposure immunization. At-risk patients will need a 5-dose vaccine series and additional immune globulin. The first shot in the vaccine series should be given as early as possible and the site infiltrated with immune globulin. People who have been vaccinated against rabies do not need the immune globulin, but will require a booster dose of the vaccine. ***All people infected and presenting with the signs and symptoms of rabies die.*** The CDC recommends that all persons bitten by a wild animal receive post-exposure treatment UNLESS the animal has been captured and examined for rabies; begin a Level 2 Evacuation. See Rabies under Section VIII, Medical Illnesses, for more information.

Impaled Objects

Assessment

- In general, because of the high risk of infection and difficulty of transport, all objects impaled in skin and muscle tissue should be removed if they are easy to remove (splinters, nails, cactus spines, fishhooks, etc.) and do no additional damage to the underlying structures as they are being removed. ***Do not attempt to remove objects impaled in a patient's skull, eye, chest or abdomen.***

Field Treatment

- Many small impaled objects, such as splinters or nails, may be easily removed with fingers, tweezers, or forceps; occasionally you may need to make a small incision through the skin along the axis of the object, in order to cleanly remove the entire object. Use a clean sharp knife or scalpel.

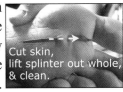
Cut skin, lift splinter out whole, & clean.

Do not cut underlying structures in an attempt to loosen any impaled object. Tiny hair-like spines from cactus or nettles can be removed with any type of sticky tape (duct tape works well).

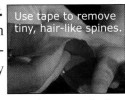
Use tape to remove tiny, hair-like spines.

- Once the object has been removed, any existing puncture wounds are at a high risk for infection; treat accordingly. ***If the impaled object cannot be removed easily and safely, it must be stabilized in position and the patient carefully evacuated.***

Push down
on the eye
as you pull
sharply on
the line.

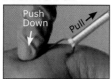
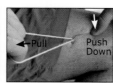

Wound Infection

Bacteria may be delivered with the same object that damaged the tissue or may migrate into the wound from the patient's skin. While arterial bleeding will flush some bacteria, it rarely completely cleans the wound. Bacteria take approximately two hours to become established in the tissue, where they are significantly more difficult to remove. If the protective barrier is overwhelmed by invading bacteria, a local infection will develop, increasing, rather than decreasing, the inflammatory response. The protective barrier may become overwhelmed by the presence of too many bacteria or suffer a mechanical breakdown secondary to local movement. The chance for developing an infection is higher immediately after the injury and lowers as the protective barrier becomes well established. Once established, a local infection may progress through the lymphatic system into the bloodstream and become systemic, eliciting a low-grade fever as the immune system responds. Fevers below 102° F stimulate the immune system and create a hostile environment for the invading bacteria. As the fight continues and toxins build, the patient feels tired and sick.

Cellulitis is an infection of the skin and underlying tissue typically caused by streptococci or staphylococci bacteria that enter via a minor insult to the patient's skin: insect bite, fungal infection, dry chafed skin, etc.; the break may not be obvious. Cellulitis often spreads rapidly and may develop into a life-threatening systemic infection.

Assessment

Local Wound Infection

• A local infection will present with increased redness, tenderness, and pain at both the wound site and in the surrounding tissue.

• Swelling increases and may pull the wound edges apart.

• The wound continually drains large amounts of pus OR the skin heals, seals the wound, and pre-

vents drainage. If this occurs, a pus pocket will form underneath the skin at the wound site.

Systemic Wound Infection

• In a systemic wound infection, pain, tenderness, and swelling continue to increase as more of the tissue surrounding the wound becomes infected.

• Redness continues to increase and red streaks may appear radiating along the affected limb, towards the trunk of the body.

• The patient complains of general soreness and fatigue.

• Fever and chills are common.

Cellulitis

• Cellulitis may occur with or without a wound and is more prevalent in the lower leg and feet.

• The rapidly spreading skin rash has the associated signs and symptoms of inflammation: increasing tenderness, swelling, redness, and warmth.

• Fever, chills, and red streaks indicate a systemic infection.

• The presence of blisters, crepitus, and dead tissue indicate a severe infection.

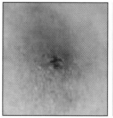
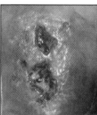
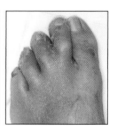

Local   Systemic   Cellulitis

Field Treatment

Treatment for Local Wound Infection

• The treatment goal is to contain and reduce the infection through aggressive cleaning.

• The wound site and the affected tissue are either immersed in hot water or covered with hot compresses 105°-112° F (or as hot as the patient can bear) for 30 minutes, until the wound opens. In the case of an abscess, a pustule head develops and a small incision can be made through the skin to expose the pocket and permit drainage.

• The wound edges are pulled apart and aggressively cleaned in the same manner as any high risk wound. The wound should never be squeezed to remove pus pockets; squeezing may force invading bacteria into healthy tissue and increase the infection.

- 10 % povidone-iodine ointment should be applied to the first few layers of the dressing. The wound should then be bandaged and splinted to help establish a new protective barrier.
- The wound should be soaked and recleaned on a regular basis, four to six times a day. The patient should be closely monitored for a developing systemic infection.
- Maintaining a clean wound and dressing helps speed healing and prevent the spread of any drug-resistant bacteria.
- Consider a Level 3 Evacuation if oral antibiotic therapy for a systemic infection is not available.

Treatment for Systemic Wound Infection

- The treatment goal is to contain and reduce the infection through aggressive cleaning and anti-biotic therapy.
- The wound should be treated in the manner out-lined for a local infection (see above) AND:
- Administer fever-reducing medications, such as OTC aspirin, ibuprofen, naproxen sodium, or ac-etaminophen if the patient's temperature is 102° F or greater. The body's immune system functions ef-ficiently in the temperature range between 99°-101° F; therefore, patients with a low-grade fever should not be given fever-reducing medications.
- The patient should rest and avoid exercise in order to decrease the production of metabolic waste.
- Administer fluids to increase the elimination of waste. Monitor the patient's urine color and output.
- Start an oral course of systemic antibiotics and monitor the patient's condition. Begin a Level 2 Evacuation if there is no improvement in 48 hours or if the infection worsens. Resistant strains of staphylococcus aureus (MRSA) are becom-ing increasingly prevalent and may not respond to penicillin-based or traditional antibiotics. Doxycycline provides good coverage against mild infections from many gram-negative and gram-positive organisms, including most CA-MRSA. Administer 100 mg by mouth every 12 hours until inflammation has resolved. Avoid sun during ther-apy and 5 days after the course is complete; sun blocks are typically ineffective. IV vancomycin is the treatment of choice for resistant infections.

- Begin a Level 2 Evacuation if antibiotic therapy is not an option.

Treatment for Cellulitis

- If associated with an obvious wound, clean and soak as per local wound infection.
- If no wound appears to be present, soak as per local wound infection.
- Start an oral course of systemic antibiotics and the patient's condition.
- Begin a Level 3 Evacuation if antibiotics are not available and signs and symptoms are mild.
- Begin a Level 2 Evacuation if S/Sx are systemic and/or severe, including the presence of red streaking emanating from the infection site, fever, chills, crepitus, blisters, and/or the presence of dead tissue.

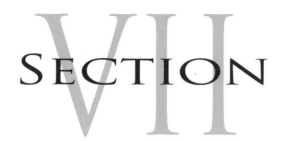

SECTION VII

Environmental
Injuries & Illnesses

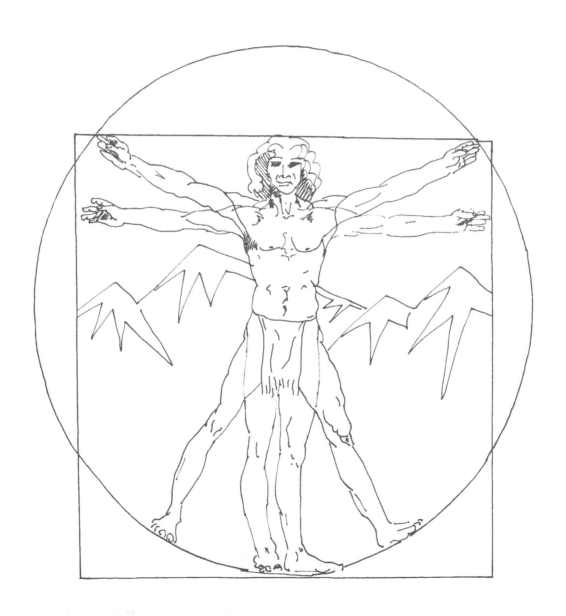

Environmental Injuries & Illnesses

Assessing Environmental Mechanisms

Possible environmental problems are related to the current weather conditions, such as hot, cold, wind, rain, sun, or lightning; or to a specific environmental mechanism, such as a bite, sting, toxin exposure; or exposure to changes in pressure and oxygen level either at altitude or during SCUBA or free diving. Each weather condition or mechanism will yield a finite set of possible environmental problems that may be ruled out depending upon the patient's S/Sx.

Environmental Conditions or MOI	Possible Problems	Page
Being Outdoors	Dehydration	112
Cool to Cold Weather typically below 70° F (44.5° C)	Hypothermia	117
	Chilblains	124
	Raynaud's Phenomenon	125
	Frostbite	122
Hot Weather typically above 85° F (30° C)	Heat Stroke	127
	Heat Exhaustion	127
	Heat Syncope (fainting)	127
	Heat Cramps	127
	Heat Rash	127
	Hyponatremia (low sodium)	130
Sun Exposure	Sunburn	113
	Photokeratitis (Snow Blindness)	114, 197
	Phototoxic Reaction	115
	Photoallergic Reaction	115
Lightning Storm	Cardiac Arrest & Dysrhythmias	64, 135
	Respiratory Arrest	64, 135
	Thermal Burns	132, 135
	Ruptured Eardrum	195, 135
	Nervous System Insults (confusion, amnesia, paralysis, blindness, etc.)	135
Prolonged Cold Water Immersion	Cold Water Immersion Injury	126
Water Submersion	Drowning	139
	Near-drowning	139
Topical Exposure to Plant or Animal Material	Absorbed Toxin	140
	Local / Systemic Allergic Reaction	149
Ingested Plant or Animal Material	Ingested Toxin	140
	Local / Systemic Allergic Reaction	149
Inhaled Smoke, Hot Air, or Stove Exhaust	Respiratory Burn	134
	Carbon Monoxide Poisoning	135
Bite or Sting	Injected Venom	142
	Local / Systemic Allergic Reaction	149
Hot Water, Objects, etc.	Thermal Burn	132

Environmental Conditions or MOI	Possible Problems	Page
Altitude	Mild AMS	153
	Moderate AMS	153
	Severe AMS: HAPE / HACE	153
SCUBA Diving	Pulmonary Over Pressure Syndrome	159
	Nitrogen Narcosis & Oxygen Toxicity	160
	Decompression Sickness (Bends)	161
	Barotrauma (Squeeze)	164
Free Diving	Shallow Water Blackout	165
	Barotrauma (Squeeze)	164
Abrupt Changes in Direction or Speed	Sea & Motion Sickness	165

Dehydration

Pathophysiology

Dehydration occurs when water loss is greater than water intake. It typically occurs during exercise, a heat challenge, or as a result of nausea, vomiting, and diarrhea from a medical MOI; it may occur under any environmental condition. Water imbalances directly affect cellular metabolism. The body responds to water loss by vasoconstricting peripheral vessels to maintain perfusion pressure and by decreasing urine output to conserve its existing water supply. As perfusion decreases, cellular function, mental acuity, and physical performance also decrease. The concentration of waste products in the patient's urine increases proportionally with decreasing urine output and their urine color becomes dark yellow or brown. If the loss continues, the patient will show the clinical pattern for volume shock: progressively increasing pulse and respiratory rates, followed by decreased blood pressure and decreased AVPU levels. Urine output and concentration are the primary evaluative tools; thirst is an unreliable indicator of hydration status.

Prevention

- Maintain fluid and electrolyte balances. Replace fluid loss by drinking water; cool water is tolerated better than lukewarm water. Drink slowly, with small sips, to prevent vomiting.
- Monitor urine output and concentration. Normal urine color for a well hydrated person is clear or pale yellow.
- Thirst is an unreliable indicator of hydration status; drink before you are thirsty.

Assessment

- The patient presents with a history of fluid loss and insufficient replacement. Possible causes include heavy exercise, exposure to a hot environment, severe vomiting, or diarrhea.
- Urine output is decreased; urine is concentrated and dark yellow or orange-brown in color.
- The patient may complain of headache or nausea. Vomiting is possible in severe cases due to electrolyte loss.
- Mental and physical performance is significantly impaired. The patient may be irritable, or lethargic.

Field Treatment

- The treatment goal is to replace fluids and electrolytes.
- Replace water and electrolyte loss slowly at 1 liter per hour to prevent vomiting, using a commercial or improvised Oral Rehydration Solution. Cool water is tolerated better than lukewarm or cold water.
- To improvise an Oral Rehydration Solution, mix 1/2 tsp salt (sodium chloride), 1/4 tsp salt substitute (potassium chloride), 1/2 tsp baking soda (bicarbonate), 2-3 tbsp of table sugar, honey, or Karo® syrup in 1 L water. The ratio of salts to sugar should be at least 1 part salt to 2 parts sugar for absorption.
- Electrolytes may also be replaced using foods high in simple sugars, potassium, and sodium, such as bananas, raisins, pretzels, or salted crackers.
- Monitor urine output and concentration.
- Severe fluid loss may require IV replacement. Begin a Level 1 Evacuation if you cannot reverse and maintain the patient's hydration status.

Sun Exposure

The sun bombards the earth with a constant stream of electromagnetic radiation in the form of waves. Electromagnetic radiation is measured in nanometers (nm), where 1 nm is equal to one millionth of a millimeter. The shorter the wavelength, the higher the energy. Visible light falls between ultraviolet (UV) radiation on one side and infrared radiation (IR) on the other.

Ultraviolet radiation (UVR) is responsible for tanning, sunburn, photosensitivity reactions, many skin cancers, and skin aging; it is divided into three components: UVA, UVB, and UVC. The overwhelming majority of the shorter and more dangerous UVC waves are absorbed by the ozone layer. The longer UVA (95%) and UVB (5%) waves penetrate the atmosphere and scatter when they reach the ground. UVR is strongest when your shadow is shorter than you are, typically 10 a.m. to 4 p.m. Reflective surfaces, such as snow, water, and white sand increase exposure. Some UVR exposure per day is necessary for skin cells to synthesize Vitamin D. The human body requires vitamin D to maintain normal blood levels of calcium and phosphorous, to maintain a healthy immune system, and to regulate cell growth. How much depends on your age, body weight, skin pigmentation, and where you live. UVB radiation has higher energy and is responsible for sunburn. UVA has lower energy, penetrates much deeper, and is responsible for tanning, for aging of the skin, and for many photosensitive reactions. Infrared radiation (IR) is felt as heat.

Sunburn
Pathophysiology

Sunburn is the most common burn seen in the backcountry. To avoid serious problems, it is vital to protect the skin from overexposure to UVR. UVB radiation from the sun damages and kills healthy cells that in turn, stimulates a local inflammatory response. The resulting vasodilation and increased vascular permeability are responsible for the familiar pain,

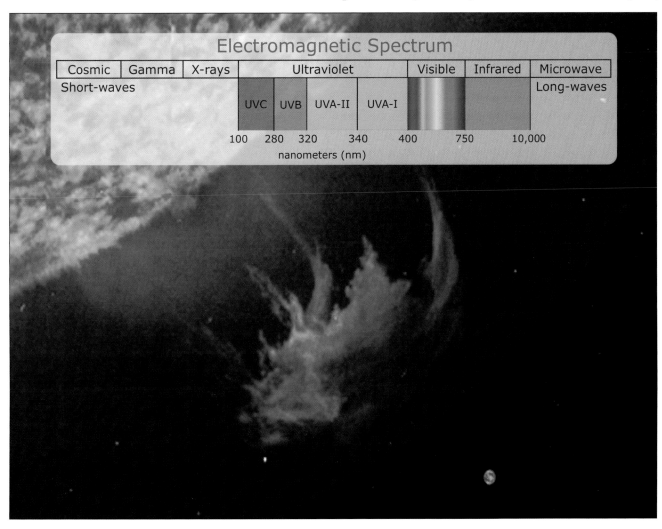

Electromagnetic Spectrum

Cosmic	Gamma	X-rays	Ultraviolet	Visible	Infrared	Microwave

Short-waves

UVC	UVB	UVA-II	UVA-I

Long-waves

100 280 320 340 400 750 10,000

nanometers (nm)

redness, heat, and swelling associated with sunburn. As fluid shifts from the blood vessels into the tissue spaces, it causes swelling and a corresponding drop in fluid volume. If the fluid that has shifted into the tissue is not balanced by increased water intake, general dehydration ensues. The dehydration resulting from superficial and partial-thickness sunburns directly predisposes patients to hypothermia, heat exhaustion, heat stroke, altitude sickness, and indirectly, to hyponatremia. Excessive UVB rays can also damage the eyes, causing a reversible sunburn of the cornea known as Ultraviolet Photokeratitis.

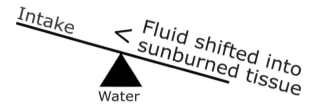

Prevention

Prevention of Sunburn

- Seek shade during the peak exposure hours. UVR is strongest when your shadow is shorter than you, typically from 10 a.m. to 4 p.m. High altitude, snow, water, and white sand increase exposure.

- Clothing offers safer and more effective sun protection than sunscreen. Dark clothing provides more protection than light, dry clothing more than wet, and a tight weave gives more protection than a loose weave. Light-colored sunblock clothing is commercially available and works extremely well.

- Use waterproof sunscreens with minimum SPF 30 that contain helioplex® as adjunct protection to augment clothing for broad spectrum UVA-UVB protection. Opaque zinc oxide offers the most complete and safest skin protection.

Prevention of Ultraviolet Photokeratitis

- Protective eye wear is mandatory in mountain, river, ocean, and desert environments, where sunlight and glare are unavoidable. All types, including prescription glasses, contact lenses, and intraocular lens implants, should absorb the entire UVR spectrum. Polarization or photosensitive darkening are additional sunglass features that are useful under specific circumstances, but these features do not, by themselves, provide UVR protection. Consider goggles, wraparound glasses, or glasses with side protection. Bring a back-up pair of glasses.

- An emergency pair of "slit glasses" can be made from duct tape and a piece of cord or cloth.

- A wide-brimmed hat blocks about 50% of UVR and significantly reduces the amount of light entering above or around glasses.

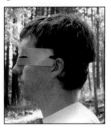

Assessment

Assessment of Sunburn

- The patient has a history of having the affected are exposed to direct sunlight without sun protection.

- Sunburn causes local redness and pain, with or without blistering, in sun-exposed areas. Sloughing of dead skin (peeling) often occurs as healing progresses.

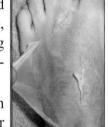

- Inflammation, redness, and pain increase during the 24 hours after exposure.

Sunburn

Redness and pain increase during the first 24 hours due to inflammation.

Assessment of Ultraviolet Photokeratitis

- Exposure greater than one hour in direct sunlight is generally required to develop UV photokeratitis. High altitude, snow, water, and white sand increase the potential for injury.

- S/Sx are usually delayed for 6-12 hours after exposure and often accompany a sunburned face.

- The patient complains of bilateral eye pain, grit or dirt in their eyes, headache, and light sensitivity.

- Due to extreme pain, assessment may require a SINGLE dose of a topical ophthalmic anesthetic. Use only once. Multiple doses significantly impair healing. Refer to Section VIII, Medical Illnesses, pages 197-201, for a discussion of eye assessment and for details on local ophthalmic anesthesia and eye exams.

- The affected eyes appear red; surrounding tissue may be swollen.
- A horizontal band may be seen across the eye, when a patient squints and their eye is stained with fluorescein dye. Refer to Section VIII, Medical Illnesses, for a discussion of eye assessment and for details on fluorescein use and eye exams.

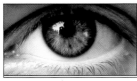
Normal Eye

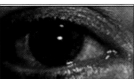
Red and Swollen Eye

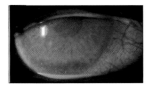
Eye stained with fluorescein

Treatment

Treatment of Sunburn

- Treat superficial burns with topical aloe vera and vitamin E.
- Administer ibuprofen or naproxen sodium for pain, to reduce inflammation, and promote healing.
- Flush partial-thickness burns with clean water. Open closed blisters and remove dead skin prior to cleansing. Pat or air dry. Keep the affected area moist. Use white/light petroleum jelly, silver sulfadiazine (Rx), Second Skin®, or cover the affected area with a micro-thin dressing. Re-clean twice a day. Leave micro-thin dressings in place unless an infection develops. Lance the dressing if leaking fluid creates a "blister" under it. Use caution when using silver sulfadiazine; in rare cases it may cause an allergic reaction.
- Replace fluid loss with water. Monitor urine color and output and adjust water intake as necessary.
- If a heat challenge exists, replace electrolytes with commercial Oral Rehydration Solution (ORS), slowly at one liter/hour to prevent vomiting, or give food containing sodium. Cool water is tolerated better than lukewarm or cold water.
- Begin a Level 1 Evacuation to a burn center if the patient has partial-thickness burns covering more

than 20% of their total body surface area (TBSA). Refer to Thermal Burns on page 132 for details.

Treatment of Ultraviolet Photokeratitis

- Remove from sunlight until the S/Sx subside (usually within 24-48 hours).
- Severe cases may require bandaging. Treat with bacitracin ophthalmic ointment four times a day until S/Sx are relieved. Monitor for corneal ulcer. Consider a Level 3 Evacuation.
- Treat headaches with NSAIDs: aspirin, ibuprofen, naproxen sodium, or acetaminophen.
- While cold compresses may offer some relief from the pain, consider using topical ophthalmic NSAIDs (Rx: ketorolac 0.5% ophthalmic solution) to control mild to moderate pain. Stronger pain medications (Rx: oxycodone with acetaminophen) may be required in severe cases.

Photosensitivity

Photosensitive reactions are caused by light-activated compounds. The most common types are phototoxic reactions, photoallergic reactions, and polymorphous light eruptions. While each has a different pathophysiology, their S/Sx are similar and may be difficult to tell apart. In *phototoxic* reactions, incoming light activates a compound that directly damages cell membranes and/or cellular DNA, resulting in a strong inflammatory response that looks like very severe, or exaggerated, sunburn. Phototoxic reactions tend to be limited to exposed areas and do NOT require previous exposure.

In *photoallergic* reactions, incoming light activates a compound, usually a drug that binds with skin proteins to create an allergen. The allergen activates the patient's immune system initiating a cellular response that produces cytotoxic (killer) T-cells. These T-cells, in turn, destroy healthy skin cells. The subsequent inflammation causes an itchy, bumpy dermatitis that may include the formation of small, clear blisters.

A *polymorphic light eruption* (PLME) is a type of photoallergic reaction that is common to light-sensitive, fair-skinned individuals, and women, typically those living in cold climates, during spring and early summer as sun exposure increases. Repeat episodes are less likely as the summer progresses; PLME often recurs each year after the first incident and is typically diagnosed based on the patient's history.

Assessment

While phototoxic reactions, photoallergic reactions, and PLME may be difficult to tell apart, in most cases photoallergic reactions and PLME produce an itchy, bumpy dermatitis, while phototoxic reactions appear as a severe sunburn.

Treatment

- Identify and discontinue the sensitizing agent.
- Resolution is variable once the offending agent is removed and depends solely upon the chemical composition of the compound.
- PLME resolves on its own in a few days.
- Cool compresses may offer symptomatic relief.

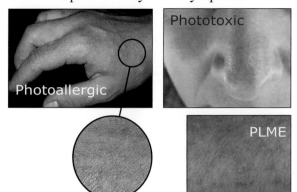

Distinguishing Between Phototoxic & Photoallergic Reactions

Distinguishing Feature		Phototoxic	Photoallergic
Frequency of occurrence		High	Low
Amount of agent required to elicit a reaction		Large	Small
Onset of S/Sx after exposure		Minutes to hours	24-72 hours
Multiple exposure to agent required to elicit a reaction		No	Yes
Distribution		Sun-exposed areas only	Sun-exposed areas; severe reactions may spread to include unexposed areas
Clinical characteristics		Exaggerated sunburn	Dermatitis
Immunologically mediated		No	Yes
Signs & Symptoms	Blisters	Severe reactions only	Severe reactions only
	Redness & Swelling	Yes	Yes
	Pigmentation changes	Possible	No
	Separation of nail bed	Possible	No
	Itching	Uncommon	Yes

Common Photosensitizing Drugs Encountered in the Outdoors

Drug Class	Drug	Phototoxic	Photoallergic	Other
Antibiotics	Tetracyclines (doxycycline, tetracycline)	Yes	No	Yes
	Fluoroquinolones (ciprofloxacin, gemifloxacin, levofloxacin)	Yes	No	No
	Sulfonamides (TMP/SMX)	Yes	No	No
NSAID	Ibuprofen	Yes	No	Yes
	Ketoprofen	Yes	Yes	No
	Naproxen	Yes	No	Yes
	Celecoxib	No	Yes	Yes
Antifungals	Terbinafine	No	No	Yes
	Itraconazol	Yes	Yes	No
	Voriconazole	Yes	No	Yes
Sun Screens	Para-aminobenzoic acid (PABA)	Yes	Yes	No
	Cinnamates	No	Yes	No
	Benzophenones	No	Yes	No
	Salicylates	No	Yes	No
Fragrances	Musk ambrette	No	Yes	No
	6-Methylcoumarin	No	Yes	No
Oral Contraceptives	All Estrogen-Progestin combinations	No	Yes	Yes
Diuretics	Acetazolamide	Yes	No	No

Hypothermia

Pathophysiology

Hypothermia occurs when a person cannot maintain their normal body temperature in the face of a cold challenge. The cold challenge increases as a person is exposed to progressively decreasing temperature, increasing wind, and increasing humidity. People respond to a cold challenge by increasing their heat production through shivering and maintaining their core temperature through peripheral vasoconstriction. Any type of heat production requires an efficient metabolism and the burning of ingested or stored calories. As the availability of calories decreases, so too does a person's ability to produce heat through shivering or exercise. Fitness, hydration status, health, and injury all affect a person's metabolism and their ability to produce heat. Effective vasoconstriction is dependent upon a healthy circulatory system.

The initial effects of vasoconstriction are readily apparent in a person exposed to a severe cold challenge. In a normal cold response, skin becomes pale and cool as peripheral circulation decreases. The frequency of urination increases with the vasoconstriction. The urine is clear unless dehydration is present. Eventually, as their core temperature drops, a normal response to cold becomes hypothermia and a cold person becomes a patient. Normal core temperatures range from 97°-99° F (36° to 37.2° C). As a patient's core temperature drops below 96° F (35.5° C), their mental status gradually becomes affected and they may become lethargic or irritable. Left untreated, their level of consciousness may decrease on a downward spiral from awake and lethargic or irritable to voice-responsive, pain-responsive, and finally unresponsive; their pulse rate, respiratory rate, and blood pressure drop respectively. Though still alive, the severely hypothermic patient often appears dead. They are unresponsive, having no visible respirations, no palpable pulse, and no measurable blood pressure. Patients with core temperatures below 90° F (32.2° C) may present as voice-responsive, pain-responsive, or unresponsive. At core temperatures below 90° F (32.2° C), the electrical conduction pathways in a hypothermic patient's heart become increasingly unstable and predisposed to arrest. For this reason, rescuers must prevent patients with core temperatures below 90° F (32.2° C) from exercising, which returns cold, acidic blood to the core; avoid peripheral rewarming in a hot tub or sauna, which initiates vasodilation in the extremities and a subsequent decrease in blood pressure; and prevent abrupt trauma, including chest compressions, which will initiate V-fib in patients with an undetectable, but functioning, cardiac rhythm. When assessing hypothermic patients without a hypothermia thermometer, all patients below an awake and alert status must be presumed to have a core temperature below 90° F (32.2° C) and moderate or severe hypothermia.

The onset of hypothermia is variable and depends on the severity of the cold challenge, the length of exposure, and the health of the patient. Acute hypothermia may occur in minutes to hours with cold water immersion, regardless of the victim's health. Subacute hypothermia may occur in hours to days in a mountain or river environment, where decreased caloric intake predisposes the climber, hiker, or paddler to hypothermia from a moderate cold challenge. Expedition members with predisposing factors, such as poor health, inadequate nutrition, or poor hydration, can develop a chronic cold response during prolonged exposure to cool environmental conditions, particularly if they have limited caloric intake and no glycogen or fat stores. They may easily become hypothermic when presented with a slight increase in the cold challenge.

Prevention

- Be prepared for environmental cold challenges with weather knowledge, good equipment, fitness, adequate nutrition, and good health.
- Balance intake and stored calories with the anticipated energy output. Provide rest days to resupply glycogen (sugar) and fat stores before a strenuous event involving a potential cold challenge.
- Keep hydrated.
- Avoid smoking; nicotine is a strong vasoconstrictor.

Assessment

Assessment of Cold Response

- The patient has a history of exposure to a mild, moderate, or severe cold challenge.
- The patient is alert and cooperative with a core temperature above 96° F (35.5° C). Judgement is intact.
- The patient's skin may appear pale or white, cool and moist.

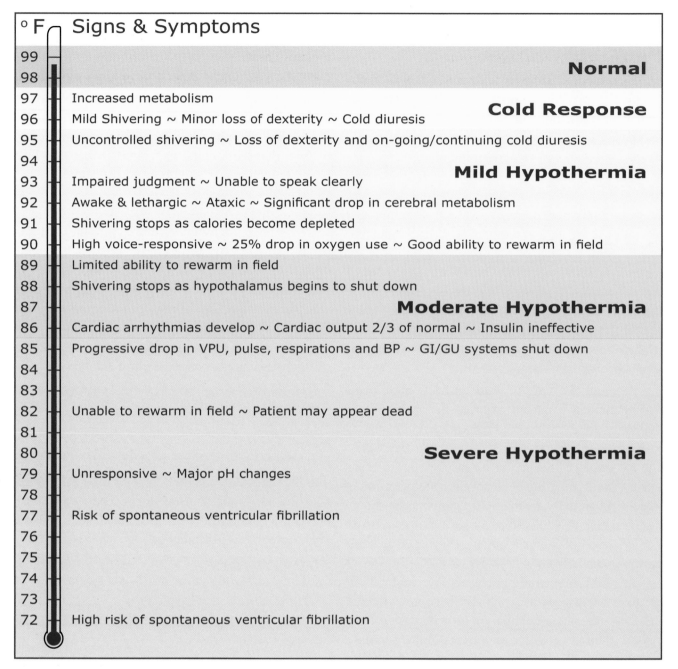

°F	Signs & Symptoms
99	**Normal**
98	
97	Increased metabolism
96	Mild Shivering ~ Minor loss of dexterity ~ Cold diuresis — **Cold Response**
95	Uncontrolled shivering ~ Loss of dexterity and on-going/continuing cold diuresis
94	**Mild Hypothermia**
93	Impaired judgment ~ Unable to speak clearly
92	Awake & lethargic ~ Ataxic ~ Significant drop in cerebral metabolism
91	Shivering stops as calories become depleted
90	High voice-responsive ~ 25% drop in oxygen use ~ Good ability to rewarm in field
89	Limited ability to rewarm in field
88	Shivering stops as hypothalamus begins to shut down
87	**Moderate Hypothermia**
86	Cardiac arrhythmias develop ~ Cardiac output 2/3 of normal ~ Insulin ineffective
85	Progressive drop in VPU, pulse, respirations and BP ~ GI/GU systems shut down
84	
83	
82	Unable to rewarm in field ~ Patient may appear dead
81	
80	**Severe Hypothermia**
79	Unresponsive ~ Major pH changes
78	
77	Risk of spontaneous ventricular fibrillation
76	
75	
74	
73	
72	High risk of spontaneous ventricular fibrillation

- Frequency of urination increases; urine color is clear to pale yellow unless dehydration is present.
- The patient may be mildly shivering.

Assessment of Mild Hypothermia

- The patient has a history of exposure to a mild, moderate, or severe cold challenge.
- The patient is awake and lethargic, awake and irritable, or high voice-responsive. "Remember the "rule of umbles": The patient is mumbling, fumbling, grumbling, tumbling, etc.
- The patient's core temperature is between 90° F (32.2°) and 96° F (35.5° C). Judgment may be impaired.

- The patient's skin is typically pale, cool, and moist. In temperatures below freezing, frostbite may be present.
- Frequency of urination increases; urine color is clear to pale yellow unless dehydration is present.
- The patient may be shivering uncontrollably.

Assessment of Moderate Hypothermia

- The patient has a history of exposure to a mild, moderate, or severe cold challenge.
- The patient is voice-responsive with a decreased pulse rate, respiratory rate, and blood pressure.
- Their core temperature is between 86° F (30° C) and 90° F (32.2° C). When assessing hypothermic

118 Environmental Injuries & Illnesses

patients without a hypothermia thermometer, assume all patients below an awake status to have moderate or severe hypothermia.

- The patient's skin may appear white or cyanotic (blue) and cold. In temperatures below freezing, frostbite is usually present.

- The patient may no longer be shivering and urination has decreased or stopped.

Assessment of Severe Hypothermia

- The patient has a history of exposure to a mild, moderate, or severe cold challenge.

- The patient's skin may appear white or cyanotic (blue) and cold. In temperatures below freezing, frostbite is usually present.

- The patient is no longer shivering and urination has decreased or stopped.

- Patient is low voice-responsive, pain-responsive or unresponsive with a significantly decreased pulse rate, respiratory rate, and blood pressure. The patient may be unresponsive and appear dead with no visible respirations, palpable pulse, or blood pressure. Check for a pulse for 60 seconds; if not present, recheck after three minutes of rescue breathing; oxygen helps to stabilize cardiac rhythms.

- The patient's core temperature is below 86° F (30° C). When assessing hypothermic patients without a hypothermia thermometer, assume all patients below an awake status to have moderate or severe hypothermia.

Field Treatment

Treatment of Cold Response

- Examine your resources and question your decision to continue in the face of the present cold challenge.

- Replace lost calories with simple sugars and carbohydrates. Consider providing rest days to resupply glycogen (sugar) and fat stores before re-exposure. Consider exercise if calories are in place.

- Replace lost fluids with hot liquids. Avoid caffeinated drinks.

- Consider adding external heat.

- Consider decreasing the cold challenge by providing dry insulation and shelter.

- Avoid smoking; nicotine is a strong vasoconstrictor.

Treatment of Mild Hypothermia

- Field rewarming is usually effective.

- The treatment goal is to reduce the cold challenge and increase the patient's ability to produce and retain heat.

- Reduce the cold challenge by creating a dry wind-proof shelter and add heat in any feasible manner, such as fire, hot tub, sauna, heat packs, hot water bottles, or exposure to another person's body heat. Increase the patient's ability to retain heat by removing any wet clothing and adding layers of dry insulation.

- One effective method of field rewarming is to place the mildly hypothermic patient into a sleeping bag, seal it completely around their face, and then place them (bag and all) inside two sleeping bags joined together with a warm person on each side. The bags should be well insulated from the ground and inside an effective shelter.

- Replace lost fluids with hot liquids. Avoid caffeinated drinks.

- Replace lost calories with simple sugars and carbohydrates.

- Maintain treatment until the patient's body temperature returns to normal and they have replaced their caloric stores and fluids. This usually requires a few days.

- Avoid smoking; nicotine is a strong vasoconstrictor.

Treatment of Moderate Hypothermia

- There is a limited ability to rewarm the patient in the field; attempt passive rewarming only.

- The treatment goal is to reduce the cold challenge and begin a Level 1 Evacuation with ALS to a major trauma center.

- Reduce the cold challenge using the methods described below for Severe Hypothermia.

Treatment of Severe Hypothermia

- The goal is to carefully reduce the cold challenge and begin a Level 1 Evacuation with ALS to a major trauma center.

- Reduce the cold challenge by creating a dry, wind-proof shelter. Add external heat reluctantly, carefully, and slowly to the patient's hypothermia package by using hot packs or hot water bottles outside an insulation layer. An effective method of packaging a severely hypothermic patient for litter transport or for preventing hypothermia for litter patients in a cold challenge is shown in the photographs on page 121. An effective hypothermia package has five critical components: ground insulation, an external vapor barrier, two insulation layers, hot packs between the insulation layers, and an internal vapor barrier. Each component is discussed in more detail at the bottom of the page. Lay out all the components, as shown in the photographs on page 121 and roll them into a compact package prior to loading the patient. Then, roll or axially lift the patient to load them into the hypothermia package; the process is similar to loading a backboard or litter. Once loaded, seal each layer, beginning with the innermost layer first and moving outward. Make sure to create a removable cover to protect the patient's face. During long transports, the entire package may be placed into additional sleeping bags joined together and next to two warm bodies while in camp.

• At core temperatures below 86º F (30º C), the patient's heart is extremely fragile and predisposed to arrest. AVOID dropping the patient or rapid peripheral rewarming.

• Begin rescue breathing. In addition to adding internal heat, positive pressure ventilations increase the delivery of oxygen to the heart and help electrically stabilize it.

Treatment of Cardiac Arrest in Hypothermia

• If a cardiac monitor is not available and definitive care is within three hours, continue rescue breathing (PPV) and do not start chest compressions. Place the patient in a hypothermia package and gently begin a Level 1 Evacuation.

• If a cardiac monitor is not available and definitive care is NOT within three hours, continue rescue breathing (PPV), start chest compressions and place the patient in a hypothermia package. If spontaneous pulse and respirations do not start within 30 minutes and communication is available, consult a physician. If communication with a physician is not available, continue CPR and rewarming efforts for 60 minutes. If unsuccessful, consider stopping resuscitation efforts.

• If an AED is available and states that shocks are indicated, give one shock. If the core temperature of the patient cannot be determined or is above 86° F, treat the patient as if normothermic. If the patient's core temperature is below 86° F, discontinue use of the AED after the initial shock until the patient's core temperature has reached 86° F and continue as if normothermic. Defibrillation and drugs are generally not effective when the patient's core temperature is below 86º F (30º C).

Improvised Hypothermia Package

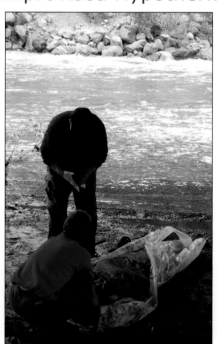

Ground Insulation
• Preferred: one closed-cell foam sleeping pad on bottom; one 1.5+ inch-thick inflated sleeping pad on top.
• Alternate: two sleeping pads of any type.
External Vapor Barrier
• Preferred: full-zippered bivy sack.
• Alternate: large plastic tarp.
Two Insulation Layers
• Preferred: mummy-style synthetic sleeping bags with full zippers.
• Alternate: any kind of sleeping bag.
Hot Packs Between Insulation Layers
• Preferred: mylar hydration packs filled with boiling water, sealed with improvised plastic bag "gasket" and pressure tested before use.
• Alternate: any filled, sealed, and tested water bottle.
Internal Vapor Barrier
• Preferred: mylar "space bag."
• Alternate: mylar space blanket, garbage bags.

Improvised Hypothermia Packaging

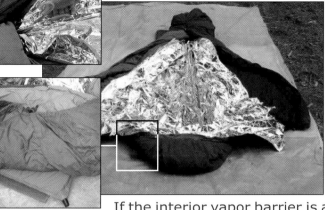
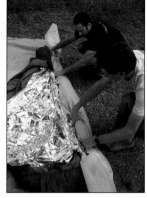
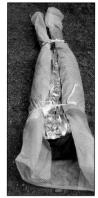

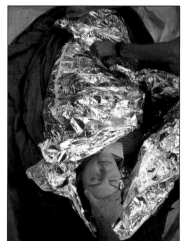
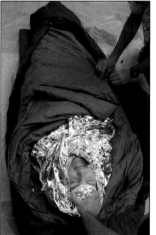
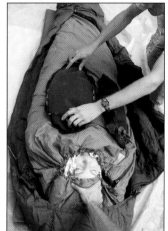

If the interior vapor barrier is a space bag and your patient is spine injured, you'll need to cut the bag down the center in order to safely roll them into the package. Once the hypothermia package is fully assembled, lift the patient and axially slide the hypo-pack under them in a manner similar to loading a backboard or litter. If there are only a few rescuers and lifting is not a safe option, roll the patient into the hypo-pack. Before rolling, fold one side of the package underneath to eliminate any bumps. Once the patient is in the bag, carefully cover them one layer at a time. Remember to maintain spine stability if they are spine injured and to lay hot water bags over their chest and between the two sleeping bags.

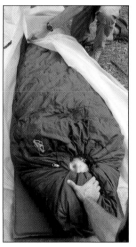
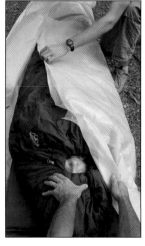
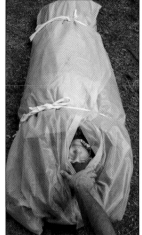

To prevent people from becoming cold while sleeping when the temperature unexpectedly drops or to treat mild hypothermia, zip two sleeping bags together and place the cold person in their own sleeping bag between two other people. While a bit tight, it is quite warm. Use hot water bags or bottles protected with socks or sweaters if more heat is required; if necessary, a vapor barrier may also be added.

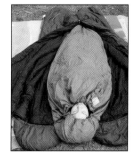
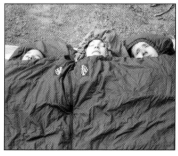

Frostbite
Pathophysiology

At rest, humans are thermoneutral at outside temperatures of about 82° F (28° C). Frostbite occurs with exposure to temperatures below 32° F (0° C). Hypothermia, traumatic injury, circulatory diseases, fatigue, illness, and high altitude may compromise peripheral circulation and predispose patients to frostbite. Average skin temperature is 91° F (33° C). As the skin temperature drops below 91° F (33° C), peripheral blood vessels begin to constrict. Maximum constriction is reached at 59° F (15° C) and sensation is lost around 50° F (10° C). At 50° F (10° C) the blood vessels in the dermis briefly vasodilate every 10-15 minutes to maintain cellular perfusion. The cycles are stronger and faster in acclimated people. Due primarily to vasoconstriction, the areas most commonly frostbitten are the face, including the nose, cheeks, and ears; the hands; the feet; and the penis. Water crystals form in the intracellular fluid at 28° F (-2° C). Crystals form in the epidermis and interstitial fluids first. As the water crystals grow in the interstitial fluid, the concentration of solutes increases, disturbing the electrolyte balance. In an effort to maintain the normal concentration level of solutes, water is pulled from the cells via osmosis into the interstitial fluid. Cellular function decreases as water is removed. As crystals continue to form and grow, the cells become so dehydrated that they stop producing energy and eventually freeze. Vasoconstriction coupled with increased blood viscosity leads to small blood clots. As the process continues, crystals eventually form in the blood and sub-dermal tissue. Damage increases with both increasing crystal size and the duration of freezing and is apparent only after rewarming.

As perfusion decreases, the extremity becomes cold and painful. With the freezing of surface tissue (frostnip), the skin takes on a white, waxy appearance and feels numb; the affected area has a soft, doughy texture. As deeper tissue is frozen, ice crystals become visible within the skin layers, all sensation disappears, and the frostbitten area is hard and "wooden" to the touch. The longer an area remains frozen, the greater the eventual damage. Rapid and controlled rewarming in "warm" water is essential to minimize the damage caused by the formation of ice crystals. Ultimately, tissue damage due to frostbite may require

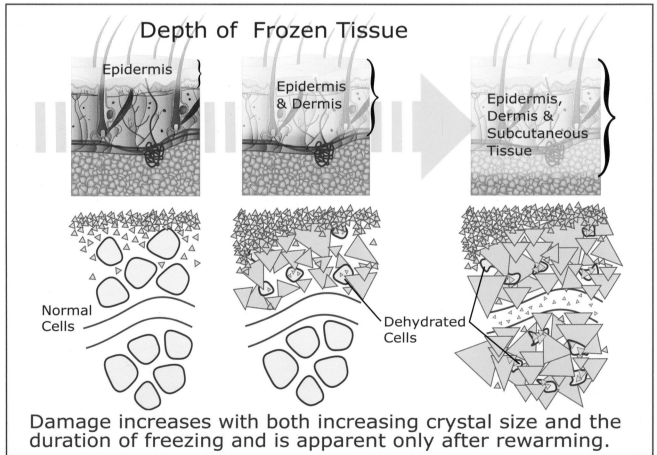

Depth of Frozen Tissue

Epidermis

Epidermis & Dermis

Epidermis, Dermis & Subcutaneous Tissue

Normal Cells

Dehydrated Cells

Damage increases with both increasing crystal size and the duration of freezing and is apparent only after rewarming.

amputation; however, the depth and severity of the damage is not apparent until hours or days after the rewarming process has been completed. Although tissue damage is exacerbated after rewarming by subsequent refreezing and use, walking on frozen feet prior to rewarming does no additional harm. There is extreme pain associated with the return of perfusion; the pain medication of choice is morphine. Within a few hours after rewarming, the skin appears swollen and red, cyanotic, or mottled in color. It is usually accompanied by an intense itching and burning pain. Blisters commonly develop within a 12-24 hour period. The appearance of clear or pink distal blisters indicates less damage than the formation of dark proximal blood blisters. Early numbness is a poor sign that may be replaced later with a deep throbbing pain. In severe cases where tissue damage is extensive, early numbness will be followed by severe proximal swelling, leaving the distal frostbitten area cold, severely discolored, and without perfusion or blisters. Mummification usually begins within a few days. The healing tissue is predisposed to a secondary bacterial infection and must be treated as a high-risk wound until the swelling subsides. It must not be refrozen or used.

Prevention

- Prevent hypothermia.
- People having diseases of the circulatory system, such as diabetes and Raynaud's phenomenon, are predisposed to frostbite.
- Avoid alcohol; over one third of all frostbite cases involve alcohol.
- In mountaineering situations, subjectively monitor protected extremities, such as the hands and feet, for numbness or lack of sensation while traveling. Only inspect feet visually when in camp.
- Avoid local constriction, such as tight boots and gloves, too many socks or glove liners, rings, etc.
- Consider setting up camp or changing route as environmental conditions deteriorate.
- Avoid smoking; nicotine is a strong vasoconstrictor.

Field Assessment

- The patient has a history of exposure to temperatures below 32° F (0° C).

Assessment of Frostnip

- The patient complains of numbness and lack of motor skills, especially in their extremities.

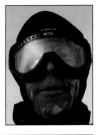
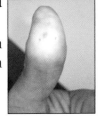

- The affected area feels soft and dough-like upon palpation.
- The skin appears white and waxy.

Assessment of Frostbite

- There is a complete loss of sensation with no movement.
- The affected tissue feels solid and "wooden" to the touch.
- On exam, the skin is white with ice crystals visible within the skin layers.

Field Treatment

Treatment of Frostnip

- The treatment goal is rapid and early field rewarming.
- Treat any existing hypothermia first.
- Consider spontaneous rewarming by increasing exercise and local perfusion.
- Consider rewarming skin-to-skin. For example, warm noses, cheeks, and ears using warm hands; warm hands in the groin area or under the arms; and, warm feet on a friend's stomach while in camp.
- Consider rewarming by immersing the extremity in "warm" (104°-108° F or 40°-42.2° C) water for 30-40 minutes. Monitor the temperature constantly. Remove the limb when adding additional hot water to prevent thermal burns.
- Administer OTC ibuprofen to promote healing.
- Avoid smoking; nicotine is a strong vasoconstrictor.
- If no blisters have appeared after 24 hours, the limb may be used. Although the damage is minimal, the limb is predisposed to refreezing and care should be taken to keep it warm.
- If blisters appear, the damage is significant and the limb should not be used or refrozen.

Treatment of Frostbite

- Consider walking the patient out on frozen feet, if less than 24 hours from a major hospital. Consider field rewarming only if the patient is more than 24 hours from medical care and subsequent use and refreezing can be avoided.
- Treat any existing hypothermia first.
- For controlled field rewarming, rewarm the limb in "warm" (104°-108° F or 40°-42.2° C) water for 30-40 minutes. Monitor the temperature constantly.

Remove the limb from the water when adding additional hot water to prevent thermal burns. An improvised "pot" can be made from a folded, rolled and tied ensolite pad covered with a heavy pack liner.

- Administer pain medications prior to rewarming. Rx: opium derivatives, such as morphine.
- Treat the affected area as a high-risk wound. Apply cotton between digits during the healing phase.
- Avoid smoking; nicotine is a strong vasoconstrictor.
- Avoid using or refreezing the affected area.

Post Re-warming Prognostic Signs

Favorable

- Normal sensation, color and warmth.
- Swelling within three hours.
- Early formation of clear blisters that extend to the tips of the digits.

Unfavorable

- No Swelling.
- Late formation of small, blood-filled blisters.
- Black tissue.

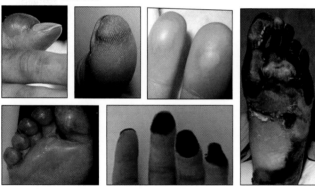

Chilblains

Pathophysiology

Chilblains is believed to be caused by a pre-existing vascular abnormality in the extremities. It occurs with repeated exposure of bare skin to a cold (32º-60º F or 0º-15.5º C), wet, and often windy environment. During exposure, the peripheral vessels constrict, denying perfusion to skin layers. After prolonged vasoconstriction, during the rewarming process, patients complain of burning and itching in affected areas. The inflammatory response is activated and 12-24 hours after rewarming, the affected area becomes swollen and red with patches of cyanotic (blue) tissue or nodules. In severe cases, small blisters may appear. Symptoms usually last 12-14 days with the affected area prone to a secondary bacterial infection. Continued exposure may lead to scarring and changes in skin pigmentation. Chronic chilblains is often seasonal with complete healing during the summer months.

Prevention

- Wear protective clothing.
- People with Raynaud's disease are predisposed to chilblains.
- People with chronic and severe chilblains may need to avoid cold, wet, and windy environments.
- Herbs that help to prevent chilblains include teas made from fresh ginger, angelica, or prickly ash that stimulate circulation, or teas made from yarrow, hawthorn, or horse chestnut that promote vasodilation.
- Massage the hands and feet regularly to increase local circulation.
- Avoid smoking; nicotine is a strong vasoconstrictor.

Assessment

- The patient has a history of skin exposure to cold (30º-60º F or 0º-15.5º C), wet, and windy conditions.
- The patient experiences localized burning and itching in affected areas upon rewarming.
- Localized blotchy patches, swelling, redness, tender blue nodules, and, in severe cases, small blisters or pustules, appear 12-24 hours after rewarming.
- Signs and symptoms persist for 10-14 days.

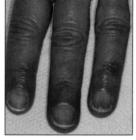
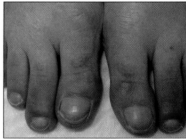

Field Treatment

- Avoid continued exposure to cold, wet, and windy conditions.
- Apply topical ointments containing the herbs aloe vera and rue to the affected areas.
- Elevate the affected areas to reduce swelling.
- Keep the affected area clean, warm, and dry. Monitor for secondary bacterial infection.
- Avoid smoking; nicotine is a strong vasoconstrictor.

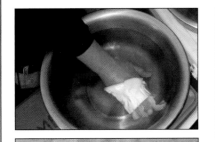
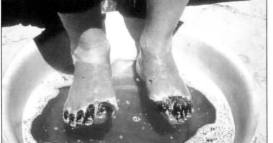
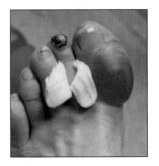

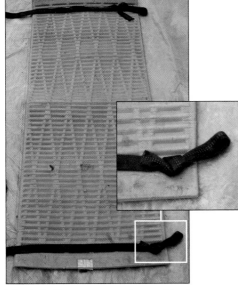

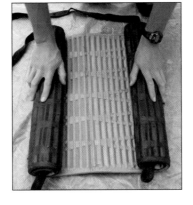
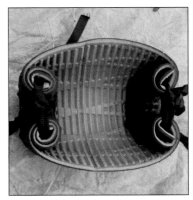

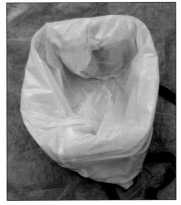
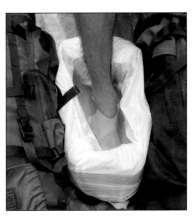

Field Rewarming Pot

Leave a small part of the over-hand knot exposed and roll pad from each end, fold, tie, cover with a trash bag, and fill with hot water. If the pad is a bit flimsy, you will need to support it on either side during use.

Raynaud's Phenomenon

Pathophysiology

As previously discussed (see Hypothermia and Frostbite) humans respond to cold by constricting peripheral blood vessels and shunting warm blood to the core. In people with Raynaud's phenomenon, normal vasoconstriction is exacerbated by abrupt spasmodic contractions of arterioles. The vasospasm may last minutes to hours, but is seldom severe enough to cause tissue loss.

An attack is characterized by repeated episodes of color changes of the skin during cold exposure or emotional stress. Raynauds usually strikes the patient's fingers or toes; on rare occasions, it may affect the tips of the ears, nose and tongue. During an attack, the affected area typically feels cold and numb, as blood flow is interrupted. The skin initially turns white as oxygenated blood is withdrawn. In response, veins and capillaries dilate and the skin color changes to blue as the tissue is flooded with unoxygenated blood. Finally, as the attack ends and blood flow returns, the skin area may flush bright red, throb and tingle. In most cases, the blood flow to the skin will remain low until the area is rewarmed. After warming, it generally takes 15 minutes for the tissue to completely recover. Interestingly, not all people experience all of the color changes.

Recurrent cases of Raynaud's phenomenon can result in atrophy of the skin, subcutaneous tissues and muscle. In extreme cases it may cause ulceration and ischemic gangrene. Females are five to seven times more likely to develop Raynaud's than men. Cause is unknown; there is no complete treatment or cure beyond minimizing cold exposure. Trigger temperatures vary with the individual. Smoking, repetitive trauma or prior vascular injury predispose people to Raynaud's.

Prevention

• Prevent hypothermia.

• Keep extremities warm. Wear loose-fitting protective clothing: insulated boots, heavy socks, gloves, etc. Avoid local constriction, such as tight boots and gloves, too many socks or glove liners, rings, watches, etc.

• Avoid smoking; nicotine is a strong vasoconstrictor and may provoke and/or worsen an attack.

• Avoid use of vasoconstrictors, such as beta-blocker medications, cold preparations that contain pseudoephedrine, caffeine, narcotics, some migraine headache medications, some chemotherapeutic drugs, and the blood pressure medication, clonidine.

• Herbal teas that stimulate circulation may help: fresh ginger, angelica, and prickly ash.

• Herbal teas made from yarrow, hawthorn, and horse chestnut promote vasodilation and may help.

• Control stress; it may trigger an attack.

Assessment

• The patient rapidly develops white, cyanotic, or flushed skin upon exposure to cold or to stressful situations.

• Numbness, pain, and/or throbbing is common in the affected area.

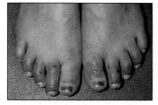

Field Treatment

• Rewarm the affected area; soaking in warm water works well.

• In situations where the environment cannot be modified, consider a vasodilating calcium channel blocker, such as extended-release nifedipine.

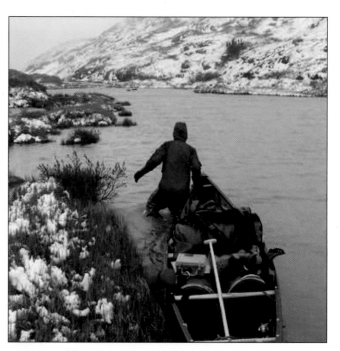

Cold Water Immersion Injury
Pathophysiology

Cold water immersion injuries, also known as "immersion foot" or "trench foot," develop after prolonged immersion, usually greater than 10-12 hours, in cold water (32°-50° F or 0°-10° C). The constant immersion causes prolonged vasoconstriction and decreased local perfusion. Lack of oxygen to the local tissue causes increased permeability in the capillary beds resulting in local edema and swelling. The skin may be red, whitish, or cyanotic (blue). Initial symptoms include tingling and numbness. The extent of the injury is significantly increased when the limb is kept immobile below the heart for example while sitting in a raft with the feet immersed in cold water. Rewarming causes extreme pain and the extremity appears hot, red, and dry; small red blisters are common. This phase may last 4-10 days. In appearance, damage to the limb may be indistinguishable from frostbite and treatment is similar. Severe or repeated immersion can result in gangrene and extensive tissue loss. Complete healing takes place over a period of months to years; there is a high risk of infection during the healing process. There is also a prolonged decrease or loss of sensation as the tissue heals and the patient remains predisposed to all forms of cold injury.

Prevention

- Prevent hypothermia.
- Wear protective clothing, such as dry suit boots, waders, and gloves. Keep feet warm and dry; change socks daily. Using foot powder that contains aluminum hydroxide may help. Don't sleep in wet socks.
- Massage the feet regularly to increase local circulation. Avoid local constriction.
- Herbal teas made from fresh ginger, angelica, or prickly ash stimulate circulation and may help.
- Herbal teas made from yarrow, hawthorn, and horse chestnut promote vasodilation and may help.
- People with diseases of the circulatory system, such as diabetes and Raynaud's phenomenon, are predisposed to cold water immersion injury.
- Consider setting up camp or changing route as environmental conditions deteriorate.
- Avoid smoking, dipping, and patches; nicotine is a strong vasoconstrictor.

Assessment

- History of prolonged immersion (typically greater than 10-12 hours) in very cold water (32°-50° F or 0°-10° C).
- The patient's feet are cold, numb, and swollen.
- The skin color may be red, white, or cyanotic (blue) before rewarming; tissue may die and turn black after rewarming.
- CSM is decreased in the affected extremity.

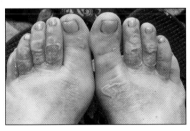 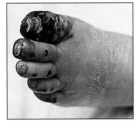

Field Treatment

- The treatment goal is rapid field rewarming. Begin a Level 2 Evacuation to a major trauma center.
- Treat any existing hypothermia first.
- Warm the affected area gently. Pat or air dry. ***Do not rub.*** Elevate feet.
- Administer 400-600 mg ibuprofen four times a day.
- Treat the affected area as a high-risk wound. Gently wash the limb and apply cotton between digits. Pad all blisters; do not break. Re-clean and pad

as necessary during the healing phase. If blisters break, debride and treat as a high-risk wound, applying topical aloe vera every six hours; consider oral antibiotics. If possible, elevate the affected limb and eliminate or minimize all pressure on damaged tissues.

- Encourage the patient to actively move their affected limb(s), but don't manipulate or massage them. Damaged tissues are highly susceptible to infection. Gangrene is possible and leads to amputation.
- Avoid using the affected limb and avoid repeated immersion.
- Avoid smoking; nicotine is a strong vasoconstrictor.

Heat Illnesses
Pathophysiology

Most serious illnesses and heat-related problems occur as the heat challenge overwhelms the ability of the body to cool itself. The heat challenge is a combination of metabolic and environmental conditions; it increases as temperature increases, wind speed decreases, humidity increases, and exercise levels increase. Fever, shivering, tremors, convulsions, hyperthyroidism, sepsis, stimulants, and other drugs and conditions can increase heat production, increase body temperature, and predispose people to heat illnesses.

The body responds to an increasing heat challenge through systemic vasodilation to increase radiant, conductive, and convective cooling and by sweating to increase evaporative cooling. The ability to effectively dissipate heat is variable and dependent upon the health of an individual and their level of acclimatization. In fit, healthy individuals, initial heat acclimatization occurs within 3-5 days, with greater than 80% occurring within 2-3 weeks, and 100% weeks-to-months later. Heat acclimatization is slower in persons with poor health. During acclimatization, major changes occur in the thermoregulatory centers of the brain, within peripheral vessels, and within the heart. Sweating, and therefore evaporative cooling, is increased and begins at a lower core temperature, while electrolyte loss from both sweat and urine is minimized. Metabolic efficiency is significantly increased; essentially, more usable energy is produced with less heat. Peripheral blood flow increases and starts earlier, increasing radiant, conductive and convective cooling. The redistribution of blood flow to the peripheral vessels combined with the high loss of fluids and electrolytes places a tremendous burden on the heart. Patients having preexisting cardiac problems are more likely to arrest. Once acclimated, the combination of increased stroke volume and decreased pulse effectively reduces the workload on the heart and the chance of arrest. Maintaining hydration and electrolyte balances are critical to the body's ability to dump excess heat. Urine, not the amount of fluid intake, is the primary evaluative tool when assessing water balance; it should be clear or pale yellow. Mental status is the primary evaluative tool when assessing severe heat injuries. Any change in the patient's mental status, from alert and cooperative to irritable, anxious, dizzy, or lethargic, is a significant finding. If vasodilation and sweating do not serve to maintain a normal mental status, heat injury has occurred; and, if left untreated, death will rapidly follow.

When the body's core temperatue reaches 108° F (42.2° C), proteins, including the enzymes responsible for all chemical reactions within the human body, break down. This rapidly leads to irreversible multiple organ failure and death. Water stores heat; the body is roughly 65% water. Death, secondary to heat stroke, tends to occur during the second day of exposure in unacclimated people, as stored heat from the previous day carries over into the present. Exertional heat stroke occurs when the heat challenge is too great and overwhelms the cooling ability of the body. Classical heat stroke occurs when dehydration leads to a loss of cooling mechanisms. With a 3% loss of water during an exercise-related heat challenge, vasodilatation decreases by more than 50%. With a 7% loss, the rate of sweating decreases by 25% and the onset is delayed. Most deaths due to heat stroke are combinations of the classical and exertional heat stroke. Heat exhaustion is often a precursor to heat stroke. It occurs when a person becomes dehydrated during a heat challenge and their core temperature rises, but remains below 105° F (40.5° C).

Prevention

- Allow time for heat acclimatization to occur before engaging in activities that require exertion.
- Maintain water and electrolyte balances. Cool oral fluids are more easily absorbed than warm or very cold ones.

- With unacclimated persons, confine exercise to early morning and evening in a heat challenge situation until fully acclimated.
- Avoid sunburn; sunburn causes dehydration and predisposes people to all heat-related problems.
- Avoid standing with locked knees; regular movement, even if slight, maintains venous pressure and helps eliminate fainting.

Assessment

- The patient has a history of exposure to a moderate or severe heat challenge. The heat challenge increases with increased temperature, decreased wind, increased humidity, and increased exercise.

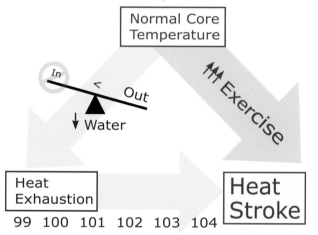

Assessment of Heat Rash

- Heat rash usually occurs in a humid environment following a prolonged period of sweating. The sweat ducts become blocked with sweat and skin cells activating the inflammatory response.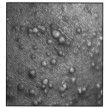
- The patient shows red, swollen skin with small pustules.

Assessment of Heat Cramps

- Heat cramps are the result of electrolyte imbalance and are common in the large muscle groups of the thigh and abdomen.

Assessment of Heat Syncope (Fainting)

- Heat syncope usually occurs when a person is standing with their knees locked, with minimal or no movement, and is exacerbated by dehydration.

Assessment of Heat Exhaustion

- The patient presents with a history of moderate to severe heat challenge and limited or no fluid replacement.

Cooling Mechanisms

Heat Challenge
Environmental
- ↑ Temperature
- ↑ Humidity
- ↓ Wind

Metabolic
- ↑ Exercise

Passive Heat Loss
- ↑ Vasodilation

Active Heat Loss
- ↑ Sweating

In = Out

Water

Core Temperature

Normal
The heat challenge is balanced by active and passive cooling mechanisms.

Exertional Heat Stroke
The active and passive cooling mechanisms are functioning; however, the heat challenge is so large that it overwhelms both.

Heat Challenge
Environmental
- ↑ Temperature
- ↑ Humidity
- ↓ Wind

Metabolic
- ↑ Exercise

Intact Cooling Mechanisms
Passive Heat Loss
- ↑ Vasodilation

Active Heat Loss
- ↑ Sweating

In = Out

Water

Core Temperature ≥ 105º F

Classical Heat Stroke
The active and passive cooling mechanisms have failed due to dehydration and are overwhelmed by the heat challenge.

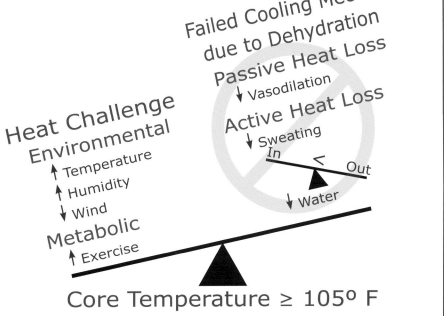

Heat Challenge
Environmental
- ↑ Temperature
- ↑ Humidity
- ↓ Wind

Metabolic
- ↑ Exercise

Failed Cooling Mechanisms due to Dehydration
Passive Heat Loss
- ↓ Vasodilation

Active Heat Loss
- ↓ Sweating

In < Out

↓ Water

Core Temperature ≥ 105º F

- Water loss is greater than intake and the patient is dehydrated. The patient complains of headache and occasionally nausea. Vomiting is possible in more severe cases. Chills are common.
- Urine output is decreased and the urine is concentrated and dark.
- The patient's skin will usually be pale, cool, and moist from the water loss and subsequent vasoconstriction.
- The patient's core temperature is usually elevated, but below 104° F (40° C).
- The patient looks and feels "sick."
- The patient's mental status may be normal, irritable, or lethargic.

Assessment of Heat Stroke

- The patient presents with an altered mental status in the presence of a moderate to severe heat challenge. Heat stroke should be suspected with minor AVPU changes. If patient is anxious, irritable, lethargic, dizzy, or exhibiting bizarre behavior in the presence of a heat challenge, immediately begin treatment for heat stroke. Severe changes in the patient's level of consciousness (VPU) are later signs and indicate more severe injury.
- The patient's core temperature is usually greater than 105° F (40.5° C), but may be significantly lower in some individuals.
- Seizures are common.
- Coma and death are possible.

Field Treatment

Treatment of Heat Cramps

- Replace fluids and electrolytes. Cool oral fluids are more easily absorbed than warm or very cold ones.
- Rest. Massaging the affected muscles is often helpful.

Treatment of Heat Syncope (Fainting)

- Consciousness returns quickly and spontaneously.
- Cool the patient and replace fluids and electrolytes.

Treatment of Heat Rash

- Lightly scrub the affected area with soap and water to clear blocked sweat ducts.
- Monitor the affected area for infection.
- Note that decreased sweating may predispose the patient to heat stroke.
- Limit exercise and heat exposure.

Treatment of Heat Exhaustion

- Stop exercise and cool the patient. Cold water immersion is very effective in humid environments, while evaporative cooling of the bare skin on the entire body is up to four times faster in arid climates. Use a combination of spray misting and fanning for effective evaporative cooling. Avoid overcooling and shivering; shivering increases body temperature and is counterproductive.
- Replace lost fluids and electrolytes slowly to avoid vomiting. Cool oral fluids are more easily absorbed than warm or very cold ones.
- The patient is at risk for further heat injuries and should be closely monitored. If their environment cannot be modified, for example, by changing the hiking route or decreasing the level of exercise to permit acclimatization, begin a Level 3 Evacuation.

Treatment of Heat Stroke

- Stop exercise and cool the patient. Cold water immersion is very effective in humid environments, while evaporative cooling of the bare skin on the entire body is up to four times faster in arid climates. Use a combination of spray misting and fanning for effective evaporative cooling. Avoid over cooling and shivering; shivering increases body temperature and is counter productive.
- If the patient is alert, replace lost fluids and electrolytes slowly to avoid vomiting. Cool oral fluids are more easily absorbed than warm or very cold ones.
- Alert patients, who have not undergone a significant level of consciousness change (VPU), may remain in the field, but should be considered at high risk for further heat injuries and closely monitored. If their environment cannot be modified, for example, by changing the hiking route or decreasing the level of exercise to permit acclimatization, begin a Level 2 Evacuation.
- Begin a Level 1 Evacuation for all VPU patients to a major trauma center after cooling; maintain their critical systems en route.

Hyponatremia
Pathophysiology

Body cells require uninterrupted communication with the brain in order to function normally.

This communication is electrochemical in nature and exists because electrolytes are capable of carrying an electrical current when in solution. All mineral salts are electrolytes. Sodium is the primary electrolyte in the extracellular fluid, while potassium is the primary electrolyte in the intracellular fluid. Both are crucial to maintaining water balance and neurological function. Changes in the concentration of electrolytes will disrupt all body functions and, if severe, will lead to death.

Potassium and sodium are normally excreted in urine and sweat; stores are limited and balance is maintained through oral intake. Normal consumption of food containing electrolytes is usually all that is necessary; however, sodium loss in an un-acclimated person during a significant heat challenge is typically thirty-to-fifty times greater than normal. If the lost sodium is not replaced and an extremely large amount of water is consumed, the water effectively "dilutes" the sodium remaining in the blood and plasma. As the sodium level within the blood drops, sodium diffuses from muscle tissue into general circulation. If the consumption of plain water, or any liquid not containing sodium, continues without the addition of food or salt, sodium will continue to be lost in urine. When enough sodium is lost, normal electrical communication in the affected muscles is also lost, causing muscle spasms and cramps. At the same time, and because the blood/brain barrier prevents sodium from leaving the brain, water from the cerebral blood vessels moves into brain tissue similar to the way a sponge swells and enlarges when soaking up water. The resulting cerebral edema causes significant mental status changes, nausea and vomiting, and eventually a decrease in level of consciousness (VPU), seizures, and coma. Death is possible due to brainstem herniation and the subsequent mechanical compression of the brainstem's vital functions. These progressive signs and symptoms are known as hyponatremia (low sodium), electrolyte sickness, or water toxicity. Unfortunately the S/Sx of hyponatremia mimic, in its early stages, heat exhaustion and later, heat stroke. Treatment of these heat-related illnesses with large volumes of water without replacing electrolytes is the primary cause of hyponatremia. Regardless of the cause, replace electrolytes whenever replacing fluids.

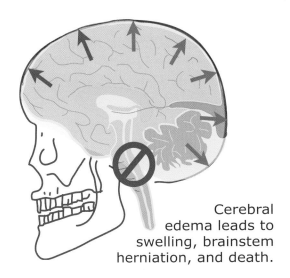

Cerebral edema leads to swelling, brainstem herniation, and death.

Prevention

- Replace electrolytes by eating foods containing salts (sodium and potassium) and sugar (to help facilitate the absorption of the electrolytes from the digestive system); the ratio is two parts sugar to one part salt. Commercial Oral Rehydration Salt solutions (ORS) may be used to treat mild cases of hyponatremia and to treat or prevent dehydration, but are less effective than foods high in sodium for treating more severe cases of hyponatremia. Fruit juices, soda, and beer contain little sodium and are not effective replacement drinks. In the absence of electrolyte replacement solutions, a pinch of salt and two pinches of sugar per 8 oz. glass of water are usually all that is necessary. Salt tablets are too concentrated and often cause nausea and vomiting.

- Persons exercising in a hot environment, especially if unacclimated, should increase their dietary sodium intake.

Assessment

Early S/Sx

- The patient presents with a history of drinking large amounts of plain water, or other drinks lacking in sodium, and not eating foods high in sodium.

- Their urine is clear and copious. Most patients suffering from hyponatremia have urinated within the past two hours.

- General weakness, dizziness, and fatigue, followed by nausea and vomiting is common. Diarrhea is possible.

- The patient looks and feels sick; bizarre or irrational behavior is common.

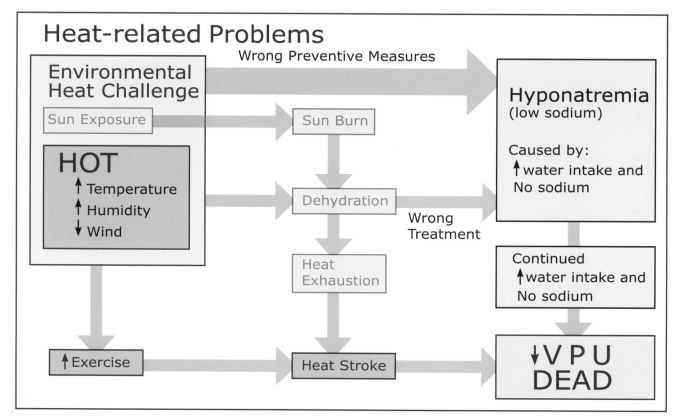

Heat-related Problems

Environmental Heat Challenge

Sun Exposure

HOT
↑ Temperature
↑ Humidity
↓ Wind

↑ Exercise

Wrong Preventive Measures

Sun Burn

Dehydration

Heat Exhaustion

Heat Stroke

Wrong Treatment

Hyponatremia
(low sodium)

Caused by:
↑ water intake and
No sodium

Continued
↑ water intake and
No sodium

↓ V P U
DEAD

Late S/Sx

• The patient exhibits an ongoing decrease in AVPU; the likelihood of seizures and death increases as AVPU drops.

Field Treatment

BLS Treatment

• If a significant heat challenge is present and the patient is unacclimated and complaining of the heat, assume and treat for heat stroke.

Follow-up Treatment

• Confirm the diagnosis based on the patient's history of water intake and urine output/frequency.

• Most cases of hyponatremia are mild and may be treated in the field by severely restricting water intake and adding sodium to the patient's diet until S/Sx resolve.

• For mild cases, add sodium via food. VERY mild cases may often be successfully treated with an Oral Rehydration Salt solution.

• Awake patients, who have not undergone a significant AVPU change and have responded to treatment, may remain in the field IF you can modify their diet to maintain a balance between water and sodium intake, modify their environment, change the route, and significantly decrease exercise to provide further time for acclimatization.

• If field treatment is unsuccessful or NOT possible, begin a Level 2 Evacuation.

• Begin a Level 1 Evacuation with ALS for all V, P, or U patients.

Distinguishing between Heat Exhaustion, Heat Stroke & Hyponatremia

• During a heat challenge, ALWAYS assume heat stroke, STOP exercise and COOL the patient. When the patient is comfortable with a normal core temperature and no longer complaining of the heat, confirm their hydration status based on their history and treat them accordingly.

• A history of NOT drinking water combined with dark urine and a decreased urine output indicates heat exhaustion.

• A history of drinking a lot of water combined with clear urine and significantly increased urine output indicates hyponatremia.

Thermal Burns
Pathophysiology

Superficial and partial-thickness sun and thermal burns activate the body's normal inflammatory response causing vasodilation and an increase in the permeability of the local blood vessels and capillary beds. Vasodilation causes local redness and heat while increased permeability allows fluid to leak into the surrounding tissue causing swelling and blisters. Swelling follows the generic swelling curve. It may begin immediately and continue to develop over the next 24 hours. Insensible fluid loss is increased as much as fifteen times greater than normal. Fluid lost within the surrounding tissue due to swelling is not available for general perfusion until the burn heals and it is reabsorbed. Fluid loss in patients who have superficial burns greater than 50% of their total body surface area (TBSA), as is common with severe sunburn, and those who have partial-thickness burns on greater than 20% of their total body surface area, may lead to volume shock; the patient may require IV therapy to maintain their fluid balance. Patients with large surface area burns in the backcountry often die from volume shock. Those with less serious superficial and partial-thickness burns are predisposed to dehydration, heat exhaustion, heat stroke, hypothermia, and altitude sickness because of the lost fluid.

Since the vessels in the burn area are vasodilated due to the inflammatory response, they cannot constrict in the presence of cold; thermoregluation is severely compromised or lost. Patients, who have superficial and partial-thickness thermal or sunburns greater than 10% of their TBSA, are predisposed to hypothermia and should not be immersed in cool or cold water for more than a few minutes, if at all. Because of the high degree of efficiency of evaporative cooling, they should also be careful when repeatedly soaking and wearing wet cotton clothing in a desert environment. Patients with thermal burns covering less than 10% of their total body surface area should immediately immerse the burned area in cold water to cool the burn and relieve pain.

Full-thickness burns destroy the entire skin layer including capillaries, blood vessels, and nerves; therefore, there is no surface perfusion. Often, underlying tissue is also affected. Full-thickness burns may appear less severe than superficial or partial-thickness burns because the destroyed nerves do not transmit pain and the lack of perfusion eliminates swelling. The skin appears white or grey. Because there is no perfusion, healing occurs slowly and is limited. All dead tissue must be removed to prevent infection. Full-thickness burns are at high risk for infection.

Prevention
- Be extremely careful when lighting and cooking on portable stoves or fires. Avoid grease fires!
- Avoid using flammable liquids to start campfires.
- Be extremely careful when pouring hot liquids or when walking near stoves or campfires with boiling water.

Assessment
- Superficial burns are characterized by redness, pain, and tenderness in the affected area.
- Partial-thickness burns are initially characterized by redness, pain, and tenderness in the affected area. Later, within 24 hours, clear, fluid-filled blisters appear.
- Full-thickness burns are characterized by no redness, pain, or tenderness in the affected area. The patient's skin appears unnaturally white, grey, or black. The burned area may extend deeply into the body and involve underlying structures, which may also appear black. There will be little or no bleeding.

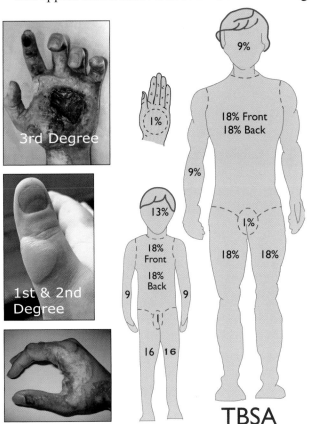

Field Treatment
- Immerse thermal burns in cool water to cool damaged tissue and reduce pain. Exercise extreme care in immersing patients in water, if the burned

area is greater than 10% of their TBSA they are susceptible to hypothermia.

- If the patient is alert, give oral fluids and electrolytes to help prevent dehydration. Monitor the patient's urine; it should be clear or pale yellow in color. Dark-colored, concentrated urine indicates a fluid imbalance and additional fluids and electrolytes are required.

- Aloe vera may be applied to all superficial burns to help ease pain and promote healing.

- For partial-thickness burns, remove all dead tissue, apply silver sulfadiazine ointment to the affected area, and cover with a breathable gauze dressing to reduce pain and fluid losses; reclean and replace twice a day. Silver sulfadiazine ointment is a Rx sulfa drug that may cause an allergic reaction in some patients with a history of sulfa allergies. Occlusive dressings promote infection; do not cover a burn with occlusive dressings. Spenco 2nd Skin® may be used on small partial-thickness burns. Since burns remain sterile for 24-48 hours burn treatment should not delay an evacuation.

- If ointment or dressings are unavailable, a protective scab will develop if the burn is left open to the air.

- Large TBSA superficial and partial-thickness burn patients have a limited ability to thermoregulate and are predisposed to hypothermia, heat exhaustion, and heat stroke.

- Full-thickness burns are at high risk of infection. Treat as a full-thickness wound. Consider evacuation. If medical care is within 24 hours, cleansing should not delay the patient's evacuation.

- Burn patients are also at risk for contracting tetanus. Check the patient's immunization history.

- Administer pain and anti-inflammatory medications, such as aspirin, ibuprofen, or naproxen sodium.

- Begin a Level 1 Evacuation with ALS to a major burn center for partial-thickness burns over 20% of the patient's TBSA, all burns totaling over 30% of the patient's TBSA, all respiratory and full-thickness burns, and burns to the head, hands, or groin.

Respiratory Burns

Inhalation of steam or hot gases may directly damage lung tissue. Swelling of the upper airway can happen within minutes or hours after inhaling hot gases and, if severe enough, can completely obstruct the airway causing respiratory arrest. Toxins present in the inhaled gases may cause immediate muscular contraction of the smooth muscle lining of the lower airway and subsequent bronchial constriction. They may also activate the inflammatory response within the lining of the lower airway causing vasodilation, fluid leaks, delayed swelling, and bronchial constriction. In addition, fluid may accumulate in the alveoli causing severe respiratory distress and arrest. Respiratory distress may appear at any time within the 24 hours following inhalation. Patients who develop severe respiratory distress from the inhalation of steam or hot gases in the backcountry, often die. The cause of a respiratory burn or smoke inhalation in a wilderness environment is usually a forest fire.

Assessment

All patients who report having inhaled gases, especially hot gasses, are at risk for delayed respiratory swelling and constriction even if they do not present with the early clinical pattern for respiratory distress. If respiratory distress does not develop within 24 hours, respiratory problems associated with inhalation may be ruled out. All patients, who have been exposed to gas inhalation who develop the clinical pattern for respiratory distress, will need an immediate Level 1 Evacuation and hospital care.

Early Clinical Pattern for Respiratory Distress

- The patient exhibits a change in normal mental status to alert and anxious.

- The patient assumes the tripod position and complains of difficulty breathing.

- Wheezing sounds are present in both lungs.

- The respiratory rate increases and the patient exhibits a broken speech pattern, known medically as word or phrase apnea.

- The patient's pulse rate increases.

Late Clinical Pattern for Respiratory Distress

- The patient's level of consciousness decreases (VPU).

- In severe cases, wet lung sounds, such as rales or gurgling, are present.

- The patient has a productive cough, having clear or, in rare cases, blood-tinged mucous.

- Cyanosis (blue color) may develop in mucous membranes.

- The patient's pulse and respiratory rates continue to increase; respiratory arrest is possible.

Field Treatment

- The field treatment for respiratory burns and smoke inhalation is extremely limited and the fatality rate is high. Focus your attention on early recognition and fast evacuation.
- All patients in respiratory distress should be supported in a sitting position.
- Administer supplemental oxygen.
- The effect of positive pressure ventilations may be limited due to the constriction of the patient's lower airway and developing pulmonary edema.
- Begin a Level 1 Evacuation with ALS to a major burn center for all patients exposed to hot gases, even if S/Sx of respiratory distress are not present.

Carbon Monoxide Poisoning

Carbon monoxide (CO) is colorless, odorless, tasteless, and initially non-irritating; S/Sx are delayed and often accumulative. In a wilderness environment, CO is typically generated as a by-product of incomplete fuel combustion in a stove or lantern. CO may also be encountered in SCUBA diving when a faulty diving air compressor generates "bad" air. S/Sx vary widely based on exposure level, duration, and the general health and age of an individual. Even minimal CO exposure at high altitude is potentially fatal.

Assessment

- The patient has a history of using a combustible stove or lantern inside an enclosed space.
- Exposure to a low concentration of CO yields lightheadedness, confusion, headaches, vertigo, and flu-like S/Sx.
- Exposure to higher concentrations of CO or exposure for longer times, causes the patient to develop pink, flushed mucous membranes, an increased pulse rate, decreased BP, cardiac arrhythmia, delirium, hallucinations, dizziness, unsteady gait, confusion, seizures, CNS depression, unresponsiveness, respiratory arrest, and death.
- Long-term neuropsychiatric sequelae are common.
- Oxygen saturation via a pulse oximeter is an unreliable indicator of CO poisoning.

Field Treatment

- Remove the patient from the toxic environment and place them in a sitting or semi-reclined position in clean air.
- If available, administer oxygen ASAP using a non-rebreather mask.
- Administer rescue breathing (PPV) and CPR as necessary. Respiratory arrest may occur if you are unable to maintain effective blood oxygen levels.
- Begin a Level 2 Evacuation for all awake patients.
- Begin a Level 1 Evacuation for all V P U patients to a hyperbaric center.

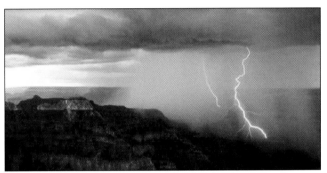

Lightning Injuries
Pathophysiology

Lightning, like all electrical current, travels the path of least resistance. Patients, who are "struck" by lightning, may come in contact with the electrical current through a direct hit, a splash, or ground conduction. The severity of lightning injuries is associated with the type of "strike" and its subsequent pathway. Splash and ground current are the most common forms of injurious strikes and patients struck in either manner are more likely to survive than those struck by a direct hit. Pathways through the head and chest commonly cause respiratory and cardiac arrest. Even with successful resuscitation, permanent damage to the central nervous system is possible. General confusion and amnesia are common, and may persist for several days. Heart dysrhythmias may occur immediately or may be delayed for several days. Current following muscular pathways may cause immediate muscular contractions and subsequent unstable injuries to tendons or bones; temporary paralysis is common. Entrance and exit wounds are rare and are associated with direct contact with a metal fence or shroud. The most common pathway is peripheral, causing temporary fernlike or star-burst burn patterns on the patient's skin. A peripheral pathway or "flashover" may also cause minor thermal burns as water is converted into steam. The patient's clothes may literally be "blown off" by expanding steam. Deeper thermal burns are possible if the patient is in direct contact with metal objects. Over 50% of lightning victims rupture one or both eardrums from the rapidly heated and expanding air (thunder) associated with all lightning strikes. The expanding air may throw a victim multiple feet; therefore, all lightning victims should be treated as trauma patients.

Lightning Physics

Thunderstorms and lightning are created when rapidly rising warm, moist air collides with the cold air of the upper atmosphere. Water molecules within the rising warm air become ionized (negatively charged) as they enter the cooler air in the upper atmosphere. Between 5 and 10 kilometers above the surface of the earth the negatively charged water vapor condenses and turns to water droplets and ice crystals. When heavy enough to overcome the updraft, the droplets or crystals fall as rain or hail, bringing the cooler air and their negative charges with them. As negative charges accumulate at the bottom of the cloud, a step leader shoots at 150-foot intervals toward the ground. Because like charges repel each other, the negative charges at the bottom of the cloud force electrons in the ground and all objects below the cloud to the periphery of the storm away leaving positive charges to accumulate directly below the cloud. As the positive charges increase in strength, they create electron streams that move upward towards the cloud and connect with the negative step leader moving down. The initial upward stroke is followed by a massive return stroke. Thunder is the result of the superheated air abruptly expanding outward from the completed circuit. The process continues until the charges are equalized between the cloud and ground. A "single" lightning bolt is really a series of sequential strokes, one immediately after the other. The multiple strokes are responsible for the characteristic flickering and branching of lightning.

Common Thunderstorm Formation Scenarios:

There are three common scenarios in which thunderstorms are generated: mountainous regions with cool nights and hot days, a cold front moving in under an existing warm air mass, and dark land masses surrounded, or partially surrounded, by cooler water. All are briefly discussed below; refer to the illustrations on page 137.

1. During the hottest part of the summer, mountainous regions with cool nights and hot days produce daily thunderstorms that tend to develop in the mid-afternoon or early evening. Falling cool air from the high mountains feeds the developing storms, as it dives under the warm air at lower elevations pushing it upward. Local lakes increase the moisture content of the system and increase the severity of the thunderstorms.

2. When a cold front moves in under an existing warm air mass, the warm air is forced rapidly upward producing waves of thunderstorms along the leading edge of the cold front.

3. Dark land masses surrounded, or partially surrounded, by cooler water give rise to daily midsummer thunderstorms. Water retains its relative coolness from the winter due to its tremendous volume and heat capacity. When the darker land masses heat up in the hot summer sun, the strong thermal gradient produces daily thunderstorms in the afternoon or evening. This is an annual phenomenon in Florida, the Gulf states, the Atlantic region states, and all lake regions.

Prevention

• Know the local weather patterns (both frontal and diurnal).

• Seek shelter when you hear thunder.

• Stay away from high, exposed places such as ridges and peaks, and open areas, such as fields and open water, during a thunderstorm.

• Do not take shelter directly under isolated trees.

• During a thunderstorm, remove all metal, such as watches, necklaces, earrings, belt buckles, rings, MP3 players, iPods, climbing racks, and ice axes, from contact with your body.

• Seek shelter in dry areas not exposed to the storm's rain shadow and insulate yourself from the ground. Consider crouching with your feet together to reduce step conduction and lower your positive streamer.

• If awakened by thunder at night while in a tent, get up and squat on your sleeping pad until the storm passes.

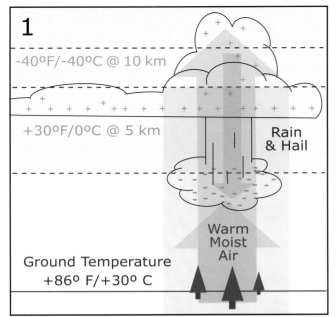

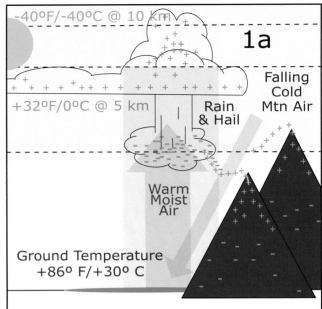

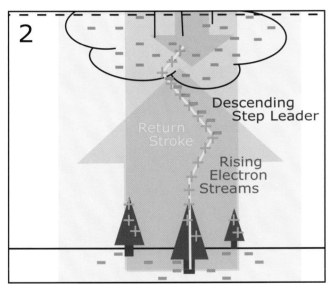

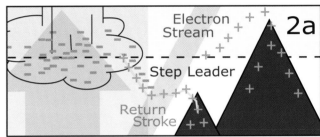

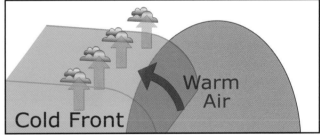

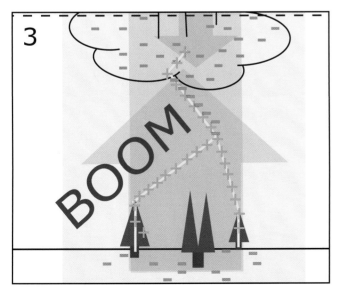

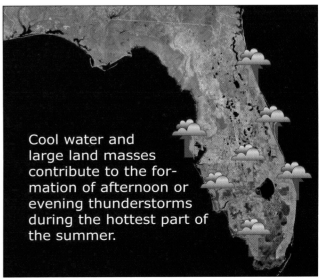

Cool water and large land masses contribute to the formation of afternoon or evening thunderstorms during the hottest part of the summer.

- Avoid shallow caves, gullies and overhangs. Caves should be dry and at least two-to-four times your height in length.
- Avoid holding onto metal fences, wires, or shrouds during a thunderstorm.
- Move if your hair stands on end, you see or hear static electricity, or you see a blue ring around objects; a lightning strike is imminent.
- If caught in a strike zone, move in an organized fashion toward a safer area; keep a minimum distance of 30 feet between people.

Assessment

- Both respiratory and cardiac arrest are possible.
- If a lightning victim is awake, they will usually remain awake.
- Assume that any person with a severely altered mental status in the vicinity of a thunderstorm has been struck by lightning.

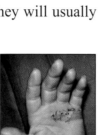
Entrance Wound

- Traumatic injuries are likely. Assume that all lightning victims have an unstable spine; spinal cord damage is possible. Assess and rule out traumatic injuries using the procedures described in Section VI, Traumatic Injuries. Temporary paralysis, numbness, and weakness are common.

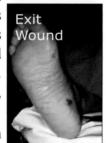
Exit Wound

- If patient's clothes have been blown off, check for superficial linear burns.
- Small entry/exit wounds are possible at conduction/contact points with metal fences or shrouds.
- The patient may have thermal burns from contact with metal or plastics.

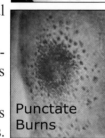
Punctate Burns

- Patients may be temporarily blinded with corneal damage and/or develop cataracts at a later date.
- The patient may present with punctate burns along the current pathway.
- Ruptured eardrums are common due to the sound and pressure wave created by rapidly expanding air (thunder); patients may be disoriented and temporarily deaf. They may have tinnitus or vertigo.
- Fern-like patterns on patient's skin indicate a positive lightning strike.

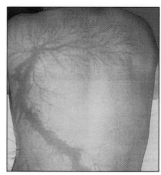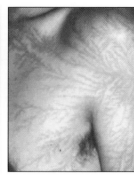

- General confusion, headaches, amnesia, and exhaustion are common and may persist for several days or weeks. Permanent personality changes, including irritability and depression, may occur.
- Patients may present with cardiac dysfunction and arrhythmias or they may develop these over time.
- Pulmonary edema is possible, but rare.

Field Treatment

- Immediately begin CPR if the patient is in cardiac arrest. Recovery with CPR is possible. Continue rescue breathing (PPV) if respirations are absent and pulse is present. It's common for lightning patients to require ventilations for hours before resuming breathing on their own.
- Immobilize the patient's spine and rule out traumatic injury as the situation warrants. Any associated paralysis is usually temporary.
- Treat all linear and punctate burns as partial or full-thickness (rare) thermal burns.
- Ruptured eardrums tend to heal on their own within 2-3 weeks. Avoid getting water in the ear. DO NOT FLUSH the patient's ears. Have their eardrum visually inspected before permitting them to swim or shower. Refer to Section VIII, Ear Infections & Problems, pages 193-197, for more assessment and treatment information.
- Fern-like patterns on the patient's skin are temporary and will disappear in 24-48 hours.
- Begin a Level 3 Evacuation for all lightning-struck patients who are awake, have had no loss of consciousness, and are asymptomatic.
- Begin a Level 2 Evacuation for all lightning-struck patients who are awake with an altered mental status and minor S/Sx.

Begin a Level 1 Evacuation to a major trauma center with ALS for all lightning-struck patients who are currently V, P, or U.

Drowning & Near-drowning

Pathophysiology

Pre-Resuscitation Pathophysiology

Drowning is the cause of numerous deaths in the outdoors each year. Upon submersion in water, 85% of drowning victims involuntarily inhale, flooding their lungs with water; 15% experience an immediate spasm of their larynx that prevents water from entering their lungs. In both cases, due to a systemic loss of oxygen, the victims will quickly become unresponsive; after a few minutes their hearts will stop, and, in most cases, after roughly five additional minutes they will suffer permanent brain damage. If not rescued, all drowning victims will die. If rescued, the unresponsive patient who still has a pulse has an excellent chance for recovery if positive pressure ventilations are started immediately. A patient who has no pulse and no respirations may completely recover with immediate CPR.

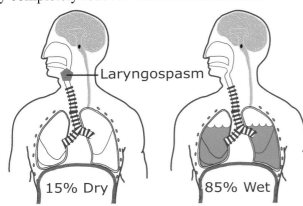

Mammalian Diving Response

In rare cases, usually associated with cold water and young children, a few victims may also have a complete recovery if rescued within one hour and if CPR is started immediately. These "lucky" few will have experienced both a laryngospasm and an immediate shell/core response known as the "Mammalian Diving Response" (MDR). An MDR immediately slows their metabolic processes while preventing water from entering their lungs, thus giving protection for up to one hour. Therefore, ***CPR should be initiated immediately with all drowning victims recovered within one hour of immersion who have no pulse and no respirations.*** If a recovery occurs during CPR, it will usually happen within the first few minutes. If pulse and respirations are not forthcoming, continue resuscitation efforts for a full 30 minutes.

The Mammalian Diving Response:

- Requires immersion in water colder than 68° F (20° C).
- Initiates a laryngospasm that prevents water from entering the victim's lungs.
- Temporarily stops breathing.
- Slows pulse.
- Vasoconstricts nonessential vascular beds and shunts blood to coronary and cerebral circulation.
- Lowers the patient's metabolic rate.
- Is more prevalent in the very young.
- Provides resuscitative protection for up to one hour.

Post-Resuscitation Pathophysiology

If CPR or rescue breathing (PPV) is successful, a patient may still die from delayed pulmonary edema within 72 hours of the near-drowning incident. Most near-drowning patients aspirate greater than 4 ml of water per kg of body weight; aspirating 1-3 ml of water per kg of body weight leads to significantly impaired gas exchange. During resuscitation aspirated water is absorbed into the microvascular bed surrounding the alveoli where it may wash out the surfactant and stimulate mast cell degranulation. If the mast cells degranulate, inflammation will occur within 24 hours and plasma will leak into the alveoli, causing pulmonary edema, respiratory distress, and potentially arrest within 72 hours of the event. The amount of central nervous system damage, caused by the lack of O_2 and corresponding acidosis, will determine the patient's ultimate outcome. If the period of ischemia is limited or the victim rapidly develops core hypothermia or a MDR, the damage may be limited, and the patient may recover with only minor neurologic sequelae. The incidence of pulmonary edema increases with the amount of particulate matter, such as salt, dirt, sand, and chemicals, dissolved or suspended in the water. Delayed infection is also a potential respiratory complication that may result in the patient's death from bacteria in the aspirated water.

Prevention

- Wear a life-jacket.
- Know how to swim in rapids and surf, as well as open water. For organizations, this means training both your guides *and* your clients.

- Prevent hypothermia through judgement, equipment choice, and caloric intake.
- Wear protective equipment, such as helmets, knee pads, and elbow pads to prevent traumatic injuries that might compromise swimming ability.
- Be trained in rescue.
- Avoid the use of alcohol and drugs, as these may impair judgment.

Assessment
Basic Life Support

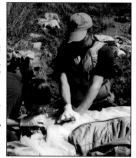

- If a traumatic MOI is present, the patient's spine should be stabilized during both rescue and treatment.
- If the patient is in respiratory arrest and has a pulse, their chances of recovery are good.
- If the patient is in both respiratory and cardiac arrest, recovery with CPR is possible.
- Decreased water quality increases the chance for delayed pulmonary edema over the next 24 hours and subsequent respiratory infections.

Post-Rescue/Resuscitation Assessment of Pulmonary Edema

- The patient complains of difficulty breathing.
- The patient may present or develop rales or wet lung sounds, a persistent cough, or increasing anxiety. They may assume a sitting or standing tripod position and have difficulty speaking in full sentences.

Field Treatment
Basic Life Support Treatment

- Begin immediate BLS resuscitation efforts if immersion time is less than one hour; begin rescue breathing (PPV) if respirations are absent. Begin CPR if a pulse is absent, regardless of core temperature. Consider stopping CPR after 30 minutes.
- If trauma is a potential MOI, immobilize the patient's spine.
- Treat the patient for hypothermia, as necessary.
- Anticipate vomiting during resuscitation.

Post-Rescue/Resuscitation Treatment

- Continue to treat for hypothermia as necessary.
- Be prepared for additional episodes of vomiting.
- Rule out traumatic injuries, using the procedures discussed in Section VI, Traumatic Injuries.

- Unless the water quality is extremely poor, patients who self-rescue are not at risk of developing delayed pulmonary edema. In heavily contaminated or muddy water, consider a Level 3 Evacuation in the case of self rescue. Monitor the patient for at least 6 hours and begin a Level 1 Evacuation if S/Sx of respiratory distress appear.
- Begin a Level 2 Evacuation for all patients who are awake after a successful resuscitation with no S/Sx of respiratory distress; the chance of a complete recovery is good.
- Begin a Level 1 Evacuation for all patients who become awake after a successful resuscitation and present or develop respiratory distress.
- Begin a Level 1 Evacuation for all patients who remain V, P or U after a successful resuscitation; they have an increased chance of a poor outcome.
- As the water quality decreases, the probability of delayed pulmonary edema and subsequent respiratory infections increase.
- Continue to monitor survivors for a secondary respiratory infection for 3-7 days.

Wilderness Toxins
General Pathophysiology

Toxins are proteins released in the body through one of four mechanisms: injection, ingestion, inhalation, and absorption. The common mechanism for most wilderness toxins is a venomous bite or sting. Bites and stings may be further broken down according to the individual type: insects, mammals, aquatic life, and reptiles. Ingested toxins may be either plant or animal in nature. The most common inhaled toxin is smoke. Plant saps and "hairs" may produce skin irritations and a local dermatitis.

Toxins may affect any, or all, of the body's systems. Toxic reactions may roughly be broken down into proteolytic, hemotoxic, and neurotoxic effects. Proteolytic (protein destroying) effects are primarily associated with bites or stings and may be cytotoxic (cell-destroying), hemotoxic (blood-destroying), myotoxic (muscle-destroying), or hemorrhagic (bleeding) in nature. Dead tissue predisposes the injury site to infection. Hemotoxins target the circulatory system and may cause: increased swelling by interfering with the clotting mechanism and by destroying microvascular beds (anticoagulants, hemorrhagic factors); cardiac dysrhythmias or arrest by damaging the heart directly (cardiotoxic); or, vascular shock, by damaging the intravascular control mechanism (vasotoxic). Neurotoxins target the nervous system and may cause muscle spasms, tingling or paralysis, respiratory arrest, seizures, coma, headache, hypertension leading to stroke or cardiac arrest, anxiety, hallucinations, altered mental status, fever, and generalized weakness.

The S/Sx and treatment of any toxic reaction depends on the chemical composition of the specific toxin; reactions may be local, systemic, or both. In most cases, unless you have studied both the MOI and the specific toxin, you will NOT be able to prevent, assess or treat that toxin. Do your research prior to leaving for a trip. Prevention is avoidance. Research the habitat and natural history of all potential toxic flora and fauna, prior to leaving for a trip. Antivenin and/ or antidotes are often available for severe reactions; however, field administration is rarely recommended. The general treatment regime for a toxic reaction is to remove or dilute the toxin, to administer or evacuate the patient to an antidote or antivenin, to provide basic life support as necessary, and to treat the patient's S/Sx until the toxin is metabolized. If the type, time, and amount of toxin are unknown, assessment and treatment are difficult. Many toxins also cause an immediate or delayed allergic reaction. ALWAYS monitor for an allergic reaction and be prepared to treat anaphylaxis. In addition, many insect bites or animal bites transmit serious infections or diseases.

General Prevention

- Most insect bites and stings may be prevented by wearing protective clothing, by shaking out all clothing and bedding before wearing or sleeping, by using a repellent, and by avoiding confrontation through habitat awareness. Insect repellents containing DEET are the most effective; however, the CDC considers concentrations of DEET greater than 35% to be toxic. Clothing and nets may be soaked in or sprayed with permethrin, a non-toxic insecticide specifically designed for that purpose; a single application is good for several weeks.

- The bites and stings of most animals may be prevented by avoiding confrontation through habitat awareness.

- Avoid ingesting unknown substances.

General Assessment

General Assessment

- A detailed history of the toxin spelling out what, where, when, how much, and the size/weight of the patient is required in order to treat with an antidote or antivenin. When dealing with an incomplete history, follow the general treatment guidelines outlined below.

- All wounds associated with any bite or sting have a high potential for infection.

- Monitor the patient and prepare to treat for anaphylaxis.

- Depending upon the method of delivery, contracting an infectious disease is possible. Refer to Section IX, Infectious Diseases.

- Severe S/Sx indicate a serious envenomation, which is often life threatening.

Proteolytic Toxins

- Proteolytic toxins typically cause: rapid edema and swelling, intense pain, interstitial bleeding, and the death of local tissue.

Neurotoxins

- Neurotoxins may cause limb weakness, numbness and/or paralysis; loss of memory, vision and/ or intellect; headache; respiratory depression; eyelid droop, increased sweating and salivation; double vision, reduced reflexes, and/or difficulty swallowing.

- S/Sx are often delayed.

General Field Treatment

All Toxins:

- Monitor the patient for anaphylaxis and treat if present.

- Support critical systems.

- Remove and dilute all toxins by limiting their absorption (e.g.: washing or flushing with water, administering activated charcoal, etc.) and enhancing elimination (e.g.: forcing fluids, administering oxygen, etc.).

- Treat S/Sx as they develop.

- Treat wounds associated with envenomations as high-risk wounds.

- Begin a Level 1 Evacuation with ALS to a major hospital for patients who exhibit serious, or potentially serious reactions.

North American Bites & Stings

Bees, Wasps & Hornets

Bee, wasp, and hornet encounters are common in all wilderness environments in warm weather. Stings are unpleasant, but rarely life threatening unless accompanied by a systemic allergic reaction. Be prepared to treat anaphylaxis.

Assessment

• Pain, redness and mild swelling at the site are common to all stings.

• Bees leave their stinger and venom sac in place. Wasps do not and often sting multiple times.

Treatment

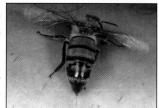

• Remove bee stingers at their base or the site will become infected.

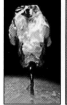 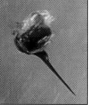

• Weak bases or unspiced papain-based meat tenderizer paste may break down the toxin if applied immediately after the sting; remove within 15 minutes.

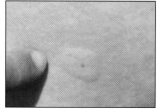

• Cool compresses relieve pain.

• Use oral or topical antihistamine.

• Monitor for a local or systemic allergic reaction. Be prepared to treat anaphylaxis.

Fire Ants

A fire ant grasps its victim with its mandibles, arches its body to drive an abdominal stinger into the skin, and releases its venom. The ant then pivots around its mandibles and continues to sting in a circular pattern. Skin lesions occur in clusters.

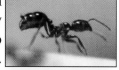

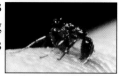

Assessment

• Following a fire ant sting, the patient feels an im-

mediate burning pain at the site that quickly moves up the lymphatic system and into the lymph gland.

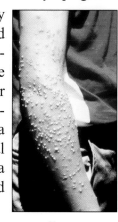

• Within seconds a tiny, itchy welt appears and is followed within 24 hours by a small blister or blisters. The fluid in the blister becomes cloudy after 8-10 hours. The blister eventually ruptures and forms a crust. The wound heals several days later, sometimes leaving a small scar. Scratching may lead to a secondary infection.

• The ant's mandibles leave two small puncture marks.

Treatment

• Administer an oral antihistamine for mild reactions. Evacuate patients with severe reactions.

• Cool compresses relieve pain. Keep the bite site clean and monitor for a secondary infection.

• Monitor the patient for a local or systemic allergic reaction. Be prepared to treat anaphylaxis.

Widow Spiders

Widow spiders build an irregular, rather messy, web and tend to hang upside down near its center awaiting prey. Widow spiders have very poor eyesight and are not aggressive. If the spider feels threatened, it immediately lowers itself to the ground and runs away. While both male and female widow spiders are venomous, males rarely bite humans. Most bites to humans are defensive and are delivered when the spider is accidentally squeezed or pinched by clothing or bedding. Not all widow spiders are black. Not all ventral abdominal (belly) markings appear as the classic red hour glass.

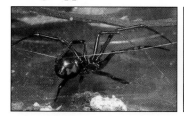 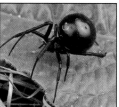

Assessment

• The initial bite may be painless and go unnoticed, may feel like a pin prick, or may be very painful. The worst pain occurs within first 8-12 hours and may continue for several days.

- Bite marks may or may not be present. A small bleb may develop within an hour. The blister may become larger with a blanched center and eventually ulcerate.

- Numbness at the site and involuntary muscle spasms develop within 30-60 minutes in the large muscle groups of the abdomen, lower back, and limbs. The abdominal pain mimics a ruptured ovarian cyst or appendicitis. In pregnant females, it may cause premature labor by increasing the contraction of the uterus.
- Other systemic reactions include high blood pressure, nausea, light sensitivity, restlessness, difficulty breathing, sweating, diarrhea, and seizures.
- Characteristic facial swelling with drooping eyelids may develop hours after the bite.

Treatment
- Apply ice or cool compresses.
- Clean and irrigate any wound as necessary.
- Administer pain medication and muscle relaxants as necessary.
- All children, pregnant women (venom may initiate contractions), and individuals with hypertension should be evacuated at Level 1 and admitted to a hospital. Antivenin is available and reserved for severe cases.

Wolf, Hobo, Jumping, & Recluse Spiders

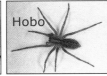
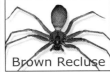

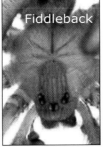

Spiders are difficult for lay people to identify accurately. If you are bitten or think that you have been bitten by a venomous spider, bring the spider or its parts with you for identification by a qualified arachnologist. Never throw away a spider that has definitely bitten a human. Positive species identification, size, sex, and age are important factors that can help to predict the severity of potential reaction and aid the attending physician in charting a course of treatment. Wolf and jumping spider bites tend to be less severe than hobo and brown recluse spider bites, however, the S/Sx of an envenomation present and develop in the same way.

Assessment
- Most spider bites develop a single small lesion, are not medically significant, and heal without advanced care.
- While some victims feel a sharp, stinging pain that gradually fades, in others the bite is painless and goes undetected.
- Venom is primarily a digestive toxin that destroys human tissue cells. Within a few hours, a red-to-purple halo may develop at the site, which is occasionally followed by a small blister. Over the next few days, the skin sloughs off the blister, leaving a raw area of exposed tissue generally a few millimeters to 1-2 centimeters wide; the affected site often takes weeks to heal.

- Larger ulcers—usually caused by skin-eating bacteria rather than the spider's toxin—may take months or even years to heal. Rarely, ulcers can become extensive, reach 30 cm in diameter, and require skin grafts.

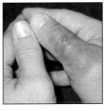
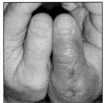
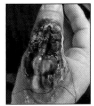

- Systemic symptoms are rare and indicate a more severe reaction.
- Secondary infection is possible and may be severe.

Treatment
- Antivenin is available to treat many spider bites, but it is only used to treat severe reactions.
- Apply cool to cold compresses intermittently to the site for the first four days; DO NOT USE HEAT.
- Aggressively clean blisters once the skin begins to slough. Monitor for infection and further tissue damage. Begin a Level 3 Evacuation for evaluation.
- If a secondary infection develops, re-clean as necessary, apply a topical antibiotic/antiseptic, administer oral antibiotics, and begin a Level 2 Evacuation.
- Begin a Level 1 Evacuation if systemic S/Sx develop.

Scorpions

Scorpions are nocturnal. They grasp their prey with pincers, arch their tails over their bodies, and deliver venom with their stinger. Venom glands are located lateral to the tip of the stinger.

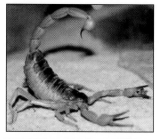
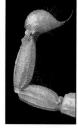

Giant Hairy Scorpion

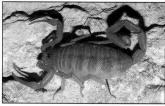

Centruoides (Bark Scorpion)

General Assessment

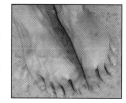

• All stings produce burning pain, minimal swelling, redness, occasional blisters, numbness, tingling, and local weakness in the affected limb.

Centruoides Assessment

• Centruoides venom is neurotoxic; death is possible but VERY rare.
• The site is hypersensitive to touch pressure, heat and cold; light tapping confirms the diagnosis.
• Neurological S/Sx may include anxiety, blurred vision, heavy sweating, increased salivation, difficulty swallowing, loss of bowel control, jerky muscular movements, and respiratory distress.

Treatment

• Apply cool-to-cold compresses to relieve pain and increase the patient's ability to break down the toxin.
• Evacuate patients with severe systemic S/Sx. The level of evacuation depends on their severity.
• Monitor for a local or systemic allergic reaction. Be prepared to treat anaphylaxis.

Centipedes

Centipedes are nocturnal hunters that prefer warm, temperate, and tropical regions. They spend most daylight hours underground or in rock piles and are capable of very fast movement when ex-

posed. Their venom is produced in a gland at the base of their fangs and is injected when they bite.

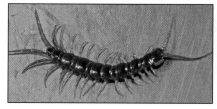

Assessment

• Small puncture wounds. Pain and tenderness vary from mild to severe.
• Local redness, swelling and itching are similar to Hymenoptera stings.

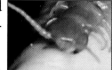

• Swollen, painful lymph nodes.
• Anxiety, palpitations, headache, nausea and/or vomiting.
• Most S/Sx last 4-8 hours; however, S/Sx from severe reactions may persist for days or weeks.

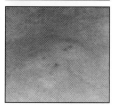

• Severe reactions may cause localized tissue death; bites are not fatal.

Treatment

• Administer an oral antihistamine and/or topical hydrocortisone for itching.
• Administer pain medications as necessary.
• Infiltrate the wound site with lidocaine to manage severe pain.
• Monitor the site for four hours for systemic S/Sx and for a secondary infection and/or tissue death.
• Begin a Level 3 Evacuation for patients with severe S/Sx.
• Monitor the patient for a local or systemic allergic reaction. Be prepared to treat anaphylaxis.

Pit Vipers (Crotalid)
Copperheads, Cottonmouths, & Rattlesnakes

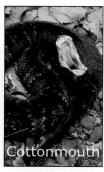
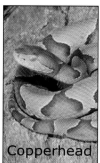
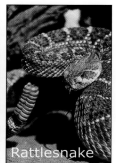

Copperhead   Cottonmouth   Rattlesnake

Vipers have a triangular-shaped head with an elliptical pupil and a heat-sensing pit located slightly below and behind their nostrils. Their venom is primarily proteolytic, although, some species' venom also contains neurotoxins. They have retractable fangs and generally opt to strike quickly and release; 20-30% of bites do not envenomate. Vipers can even strike and envenomate 20-60 minutes after they are dead. Rattlesnakes have a rattle at the end of their tail, although it may be absent, that vibrates with a tell-tale buzzing when the snake is threatened.

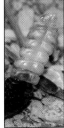

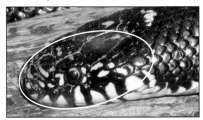
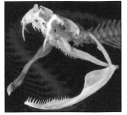

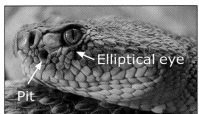
Elliptical eye
Pit
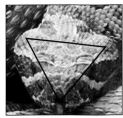

Assessment

- The patient may present with one, two, or more fang marks that may or may not be associated with minor bleeding.
- The patient experiences local burning pain, swelling, and bruising within 10-15 minutes. Local necrotic damage and secondary infection can be severe.
- Venous envenomation is extremely rare. If it occurs, it progresses rapidly to systemic S/Sx and death.
- Blood-filled blisters may develop locally within 6-36 hours following envenomation and progress up the limb. Tissue will blacken and slough as it dies.
- Moderate systemic S/Sx include general weakness, sweating, nausea/vomiting, lightheadedness, and low blood pressure.
- Severe hemotoxic systemic S/Sx include the appearance of small, purplish-red spots caused by bleeding into the skin (petechiae), coughing up blood, vomiting blood, tarry stools from intestinal bleeding, blindness, and pulmonary edema.

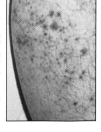

- Neurotoxic effects from envenomation from a Mojave rattlesnake may be delayed and include hoarseness, difficulty swallowing, eyelid droop and respiratory paralysis.

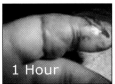
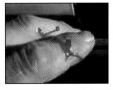
1 Hour

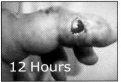
Day 14

12 Hours
Day 55

Treatment

- Immediately remove jewelry and constricting clothing from the vicinity of the bite.
- Antivenin is available for all North American pit vipers; it is best administered within 6 hours, and is primarily used to treat systemic reactions.
- Treat the bite as a high-risk wound; splint for transport.
- Begin a Level 1 Evacuation for all patients with systemic S/Sx to the nearest facility capable of administering antivenin. Begin a Level 2 Evacuation for patients with local S/Sx.

Coral Snakes (Elapid)

Coral snakes tend to be reclusive and spend most of their lives hidden in ground cover, emerging during rains or breeding season. Some species are almost entirely aquatic and spend most of their lives in slow-moving bodies of water that have dense vegetation. Coral snakes have a pair of short, hollow fangs fixed in the front of their upper jaw that release venom as they chew; the snake must hold on to successfully envenomate. Roughly 60% of bites do not envenomate. Venom is neurotoxic with minimal or no local effects. Coral snakes are not aggressive and most bites occur during handling. Without antivenom roughly 10% of victims die. Patients who survive the bite may require respiratory support for up to a week and may suffer persistent weakness for weeks to months.

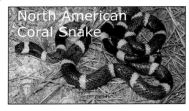
North American Coral Snake

Red on yellow, kill a fellow; Red on black, venom lack. (But only in North America.)

- Envenomation produces minimal or no local S/Sx; however, within 90 minutes the patient reports weakness or numbness in affected limb and, within 3-4 hours,

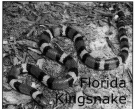
Florida Kingsnake

they experience tremors, drowsiness, or euphoria; increased salivation. Within 5-10 hours most patients exhibit slurred speech, double vision, difficulty swallowing, and respiratory distress. Complete flaccid (drooping) paralysis and respiratory arrest are possible. S/Sx may be delayed up for to 13 hours.

Treatment

- Splint and begin Level 2 Evacuation immediately; do not wait for S/Sx to appear.
- Upgrade to Level 1 if systemic S/Sx develop.
- Keep patient calm, quiet and still; DO NOT self evacuate.

Mexican Beaded Lizard & Gila Monster

Both the Mexican beaded lizard and gila monster are heavy, slow-moving venomous lizards that grow up to two feet in length and offer little threat to humans. They inhabit the scrubland, succulent desert, and oak woodland of the Southwestern United States and Mexico. They spend most of their lives underground in mammal burrows or rocks and emerge in mornings during spring and summer and after rain storms; sightings are rare. They have lots of loosely attached teeth and no fangs. Venom is released  into saliva from specialized glands in the jaw and enters the victim with chewing. The more irritated the lizard is, the more it salivates and the more venom is released. Irritated lizards may hang onto a limb and require physical removal. The longer a lizard remains attached, the worse the envenomation. That said, envenomation occurs in less than 70% of cases.

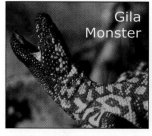
Gila Monster

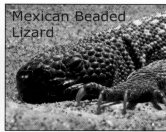
Mexican Beaded Lizard

- A bite from either lizard is presents with puncture wounds; the teeth may break off and remain in the tissue.
- The patient experiences severe burning pain at the site within five minutes that then progresses up limb; swelling follows.
- The pain generally lasts 3-5 hours and subsides after eight. Tenderness may last 3-5 weeks.
- Systemic S/Sx include weakness, sweating, and lightheadedness.

Treatment

- Remove the lizard by submerging it in water, covering its eyes with cloth, or prying its jaws apart with a stick
- Treat the bite as a high-risk wound. Probe for and remove any broken teeth.
- Administer pain medications as necessary.
- Begin a Level 3 Evacuation.

Venomous Aquatic Life

Venomous aquatic life may be divided into three treatment-dependent categories: acid-based for most venomous stings, heat-based for most puncture-related envenomations, and supportive care for specific life-threatening envenomations. Antivenin is available for many species; systemic allergic reactions are possible. Be prepared to treat anaphylaxis.

Venomous Aquatic Stings

Envenomation by the following aquatic organisms is treated by neutralizing it with a weak acid, a weak base, or a papin-based meat tenderizer: all jellyfish, fire coral, hydroids, anemones, sponges, sea lice, and bristleworm.

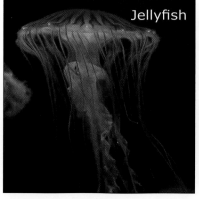
Jellyfish

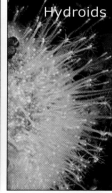
Hydroids

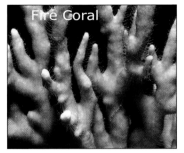
Fire Coral

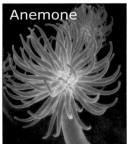
Anemone

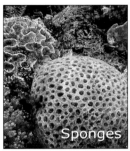

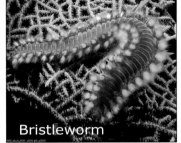
Sponges

Bristleworm

- Administer a systemic corticosteroid in a tapering dose for all severe reactions (60-100 mg prednisone over 14 days).
- Begin a Level 2 Evacuation for all patients with systemic S/Sx.
- Monitor the site for secondary infection.
- Monitor the patient for a local or systemic allergic reaction; be prepared to treat anaphylaxis.

Venomous Aquatic Punctures

Envenomation by the following aquatic organisms is treated by aggressive cleaning and soaking the site in hot water: starfish, urchins, stingrays, scorpionfish, lionfish, stonefish, catfish, and weeverfish.

Assessment

- Skin irritation develops in seconds to hours following a sting and is characterized by stinging, burning, redness, blistering, impression patterns, swelling, and itching.
- Systemic S/Sx include weakness, nausea, vomiting, diarrhea, headache, increased salivation, chills, and fever.

Treatment

- Flush the site with clean seawater. **Caution:** fresh water or pressure will trigger any stored nematocysts.
- Soak the site in vinegar (preferred) or other weak acid (40% isopropyl alcohol) or base (dilute ammonia) until the pain is relieved. A papain-based meat tenderizer—remove within 15 minutes—or baking-soda paste may also be effective.
- Nematocysts are coiled venomous stinging cells that release a thread-like stinger when triggered by contact with prey or fresh water. Remove any nematocysts from fire coral, jellyfish, anemones, or hydroids by powder and scraping.

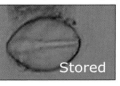
Stored

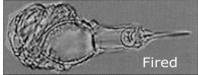
Fired

- Remove any embedded sponge spicules, bristles or spines using forceps and/or sticky tape.

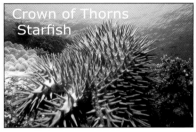
Crown of Thorns Starfish

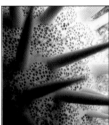

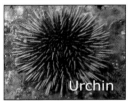
Urchin

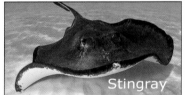
Stingray

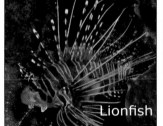
Lionfish

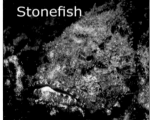
Stonefish

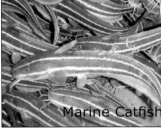
Marine Catfish

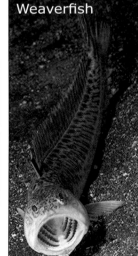
Weaverfish

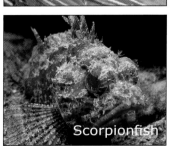
Scorpionfish

- The patient presents with an obvious wound with or with out bleeding.

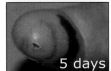

- The puncture site may exhibit mild to intense pain, redness, swelling, blisters, and sloughing.

- Systemic S/Sx include weakness, nausea, vomiting, diarrhea, headache, increased salivation, chills, fever, and delirium.

Treatment

- Soak the site in non-scalding hot water (45°C, 113°F) to tolerance until pain is relieved. Higher levels of heat tolerance may generally be reached by adding heat slowly versus sudden immersion.

- Remove any spine fragments embedded in muscle tissue and treat as a high-risk wound. Splint the limb if any fragments lie near joints.

- Administer pain medications as needed; consider infiltrating the site with lidocaine if the pain is severe.

- Monitor the patient for secondary infection.

- Consider administering prophylactic antibiotics.

- The evacuation level varies depending on the overall severity of the patient's S/Sx.

Other Aquatic Envenomations

Envenomation by the following aquatic organisms may be life threatening and treatment is supportive only: cone shell snails, blue-ringed octopuses, sea snakes, and box jellyfish.

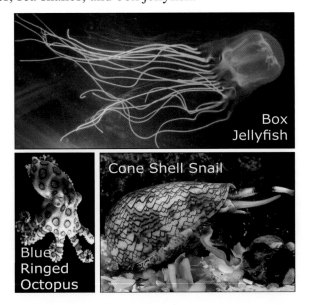

Box Jellyfish

Cone Shell Snail

Blue Ringed Octopus

Prevention

- The stinging cells on the tentacles of a box jellyfish are not triggered by touch, but by the chemicals found on skin. Wearing pantyhose—even under wetsuits—prevents envenomation.

Assessment

- Box jellyfish envenomation will initially present with characteristic local dermatitis.

- Cone shell snail envenomation will initially present like hymenoptera stings.

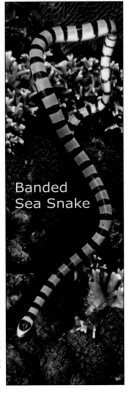

Banded Sea Snake

- Sea snake or blue-ringed octopus envenomation will initially present with little or no local S/Sx beyond bite marks; most Sea snake bites DO NOT result in envenomation.

- Following a bite or sting, local numbness may develop and spread to include the affected limb.

- Local redness, swelling, tenderness, and itching may develop.

- Systemic S/Sx are often delayed and include weakness, nausea, vomiting, diarrhea, headache, increased salivation, chills, fever, and delirium.

- Generalized paralysis often leads to respiratory and/or cardiac failure and death.

Treatment

- There is currently no antivenin available for cone shell snail stings or blue-ringed octopus bites; treatment is supportive only.

- Antivenin is available for box jellyfish and sea snakes and may be administered in the field; otherwise, begin a Level 1 Evacuation to a facility that can provide antivenin and supportive care.

- Soak box jellyfish stings in vinegar solution prior to removing tentacles and nematocysts and administering antivenin. The majority of box jellyfish envenomations do not result is death, especially when rapidly treated with vinegar. Small children are at higher risk than adults because of their smaller body size.

- Initiate rescue breathing (PPV) for all patients in

respiratory arrest from a box jellyfish envenomation. Continue PPV until the toxin is metabolized and the patient is breathing on their own. If the patient experiences cardiac arrest, initiate CPR.

Allergic Reactions

Pathophysiology

Allergies are a non-functional response of the patient's immune system to an ingested, inhaled, injected, or absorbed foreign protein (allergen). Prior exposure to an allergen is required to initiate an allergic hypersensitivity response. All allergic reactions involve the production of allergen-specific antibodies (IgE, IgA, or IgG) and/or cytotoxic (killer) T-cells. There are three common types of allergic reactions: acute IgE mediated allergies, subacute IgA or IgG mediated food allergies, and delayed contact allergies. Of the three types, two are of concern in a wilderness environment: IgE mediated allergies and contact allergies. Subacute food allergies are generally predictable, and therefore avoidable, based on an individual's medical history. It is important to note that allergies both develop and fade over time making the patient's history unreliable. Repeated contact with a specific allergen tends to sensitize people to that allergen and once sensitized, subsequent exposure to the same allergen tends to produce increasingly severe allergic reactions. People having a prior history of anaphylaxis should carry some form of injectable epinephrine and an oral antihistamine on or near their person when exposure is possible. People having known allergies should practice avoiding the responsible allergen. Immunotherapy may be helpful in eliminating serious allergies.

Contact Allergies

In the wilderness, contact allergies are usually caused by casual contact with the resin from the roots, stems, bark, berries and leaves of members of the Anacardiaceae family: "poison" ivy, oak, sumac, or mango skin (not juice). The resin contains urushiol that is released when the plant is injured. Urushiol is oily, spreads easily on contact, and may penetrate clothing and gloves. Depending on the thickness of the patient's skin, absorption may take hours. Once absorbed, the urushiol initiates an allergic response that mobilizes urushiol-specific killer T-cells to attack and destroy the affected skin cells.

The ensuing edema gives rise to the characteristic blebs associated with poison ivy, oak, and sumac.

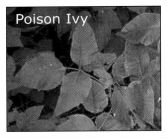
Poison Ivy

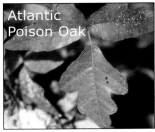
Atlantic Poison Oak

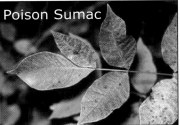
Poison Sumac

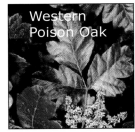
Western Poison Oak

Prevention

• Avoid the plants!

• Chemical skin protection is available.

• The resin chemically bonds with skin proteins about 30 minutes after contact. Wash with cold or cool water as soon as possible after suspected exposure. Hot water speeds absorption and worsens the rash. Use soap to emulsify the oil to make it easier to remove. Tech Lab's Oak & Ivy Cleanser® and Goop® are more effective than traditional soaps.

• The urushiol remains active for years. Recontamination by touching stored clothing and gear is common. Wash all clothing, gear, and pets that may have come in contact with the resin.

• Once the oil has been removed, the rash and serum from the blisters are not contagious.

• As long as the oil is no longer present, scratching does not spread the rash. However, scratching may cause secondary infections and increase the intensity of the itching.

Assessment

• Contact allergens often cause localized dermatitis with itching, burning, and occasional blisters. The itching, burning, and blisters from poison ivy, poison oak, or poison sumac may appear within a few hours of exposure, or may be delayed for up to 72 hours.

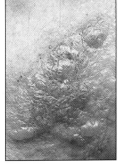

- In sensitized individuals, respiratory arrest may result from inhaling smoke from the burned plant.
- Ingested plants do not cause mucous lesions, but can lead to gastrointestinal S/Sx including perianal itching.

Treatment

- The resin chemically bonds with skin proteins about 30 minutes after contact. Wash with cold or cool water as soon as possible after suspected exposure. Hot water speeds absorption and worsens the rash. Use soap to emulsify the oil to make it easier to remove. Tech Lab's Oak & Ivy Cleanser® and Goop® are more effective than traditional soaps.
- Urushiol remains active for years. Recontamination by touching stored clothing and gear is common. Wash all clothing, gear, and pets that may

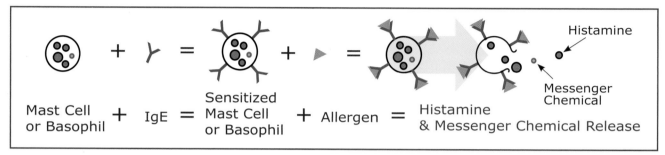

Acute Local Allergic Reaction

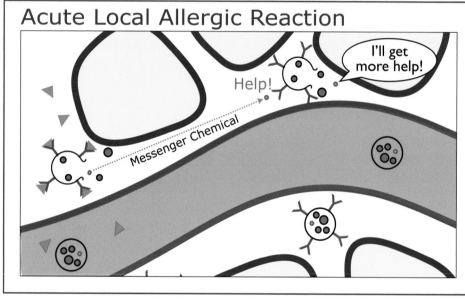

IgE is produced after prior exposure to an allergen.

IgE binds to mast cells in local tissue.

There is no IgE on the circulating basophils.

Allergens crosslink with the IgE.

Mast cells degranulate releasing histamine and chemical messengers into the tissue spaces.

Acute Systemic Allergic Reaction (Anaphylaxis)

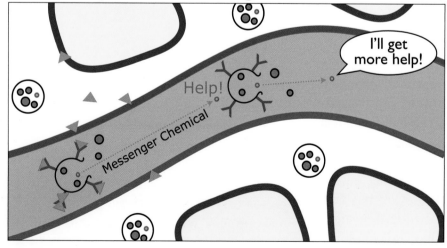

IgE is produced after prior exposure to an allergen.

IgE binds to the circulating basophils.

There is no IgE on the local mast cells.

Allergens crosslink with the IgE.

Basophils degranulate releasing histamine and chemical messengers into the blood.

have come in contact with the resin.

- Give an oral antihistamine, such as diphenhydramine (Benadryl®) dosed at 25-50 mg every 4-6 hours. Avoid topical antihistamines.

- Use drying agents or astringents on affected skin, such as Burrow's solution, oatmeal paste, calamine lotion. Open any blisters to release serum and to allow the topical agents to have contact with the underlying tissue. Tecnu Extreme® gel immediately relieves itching, dries blisters, and speeds healing.

- Severe skin reactions that cover more than 10% of the patient's body may require an oral Rx corticosteroid (prednisone).

- Monitor the affected areas for secondary infection; treat secondary infections with oral antibiotics.

- With severe reactions, monitor the patient for a systemic allergic reaction; be prepared to treat for anaphylaxis.

IgE Mediated Allergic Reactions

In the outdoors, IgE mediated allergic reactions tend to occur from bites, stings, ingested allergens, and medications. Once produced, IgE antibodies bind to local mast cells and/or circulating basophils. Both mast cells and basophils release histamine, prostaglandins, and cytokines when stimulated by an allergen/IgE antibody response. Histamine is a vasodilator and bronchial constrictor with receptor sites located in muscle, lung, brain, and GI/GU tissue. When the histamine receptors in muscle tissue are stimulated, they give rise to the S/Sx of local allergic reactions; when histamine receptors in the lungs, brain, and GI/GU systems are stimulated, the patient presents with the S/Sx of a systemic allergic reaction (anaphylaxis). Prostaglandins and cytokines act as messenger chemicals to recruit other mast cells and/or basophils and attract other inflammatory agents; they are responsible for spreading the initial IgE mediated allergic reaction and for late-phase inflammatory responses. A local allergic reaction is characterized by severe local swelling that may become progressively worse during the next few minutes or hours. A systemic allergic reaction (anaphylaxis) occurs when the allergen reaches the blood; the time between allergen uptake and the development of S/Sx varies with the delivery route (injection, ingestion, inhalation, absorption). Severe anaphylactic reactions produce a variety of signs and symptoms that are often life threatening. Hours after the initial allergic reaction, an inflammatory late-phase response may occur giving rise to similar S/Sx that may be more severe than the original.

Assessment

Local IgE Mediated Allergic Rhinitis (Hayfever)

- The stimulation of H-1 histamine receptors in the nasal mucosa increase nasal secretions, leading to a runny nose. Local swelling causes congestion. Neural stimulation from the swelling leads to sneezing. Swelling may spread to the eyes and cause itching and tears.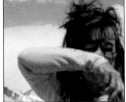

Assessment of Local IgE Mediated Allergic Reactions to Bites and Stings

- Toxic and local allergic reactions to bites and stings occur concurrently.

- H-1 histamine receptors in the local microvascular bed cause vasodilation and increased permeability leading to local redness and progressive swelling that eclipses the welt formed in response to the injected venom. Intradermal swelling stimulates sensory nerves and causes itching or burning sensations.

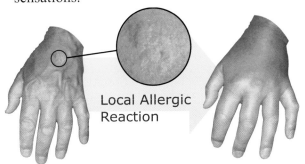

Local Allergic Reaction

Assessment of Systemic IgE Mediated Allergic Reactions (Anaphylaxis)

- No local allergic reaction occurs concurrently with most systemic allergic reactions. The more immediate the reaction, the greater its severity. The onset of the reaction depends on the MOI: typically within seconds to 20 minutes for bites and stings; within minutes to 4 hours for ingested allergens, and within seconds for inhaled allergens. Anaphylaxis is rare with contact allergens.

- Most systemic histamine releases cause itching, redness, and hives to appear usually on the groin, armpits, belly, flanks, or back. The reaction is away from the site of the bite or sting and may follow the ingestion or inhalation of an allergen.

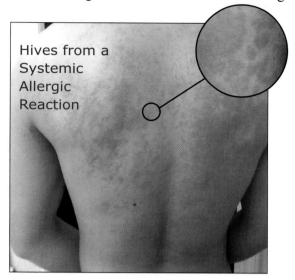

Hives from a Systemic Allergic Reaction

- The stimulation of H-1 histamine receptors in the brain releases neurotransmitters that cause anxiety.
- The stimulation of H-1 histamine receptors located in the small intestine causes muscular contractions that lead to increased peristalsis and abdominal cramps. The stimulation of H-2 histamine receptors in the stomach lining increases gastric secretions that lead to nausea, vomiting, and diarrhea.
- The stimulation of H-1 histamine receptors in bronchial muscle causes muscular contractions that lead to bronchial constriction and respiratory distress or arrest.
- The stimulation of H-2 histamine receptors in the heart increases the pulse and cardiac output.
- A systemic histamine release may cause flushing, vascular shock, and death as the entire circulatory system vasodilates.

Field Treatment

Treatment of Allergic Rhinitis (Hayfever)

- Treat intermittent symptoms with oral antihistamines and decongestants.
- Chronic symptoms may be treated with a Rx nasal corticosteroid spray taken alone, or in combination with an antihistamine and/or decongestant.
- Treat eye symptoms with antihistamine eye drops.

Treatment of Local IgE Mediated Allergic Reactions to Bites and Stings

- Give an oral antihistamine and follow standard dosing regimes. Adult dose of diphenhydramine is 25-50 mg every 4-6 hours; do not exceed 400 mg per day. Child dose is 1 mg per kg.
- Severe local reactions may require an oral Rx corticosteroid (prednisone) in a tapered dose for 14-28 days.
- Monitor the site for secondary infection; secondary infections are treated with oral antibiotics.
- Treat the concurrent toxic reaction separately.

Treatment of Systemic IgE Mediated Allergic Reactions (Anaphylaxis)

- When the mechanism is a bite, sting, or inhalation, epinephrine may be safely administered at the first S/Sx of a systemic allergic reaction, which is usually with the development of hives or red, itchy skin.
- When the suspected MOI is ingestion, give an oral antihistamine and monitor the patient. Administer epinephrine at the first S/Sx of respiratory distress.
- The preferred administration for epinephrine is an intramuscular injection of 1:1000 epinephrine in anterior portion of the mid-thigh. The adult dose is 0.3 cc; pediatric dose for children weighing less than 75 pounds is 0.15 cc.
- Treat concurrently with an oral antihistamine for 24-72 hours. Adult dose of diphenhydramine is 25-50 mg every 4-6 hours; do not exceed 400 mg per day. Child dose is 1 mg per kg.
- Closely monitor the patient. Give a second dose of epinephrine if the S/Sx do not disappear within 5-15 minutes or if they re-appear at any time. In rare cases, additional doses may be required to reverse the S/Sx.
- Monitor for a late-phase response (rebound) for 72 hours; most late-phase responses occur 4-6 hours after the initial treatment. Late-phase responses are treated in the same manner as an acute-phase response. Begin a Level 2 Evacuation for patients with a late-phase reaction.
- A recovery period of 24-72 hours is usually required for patients treated with epinephrine. The patient will remain hypersensitive to the respon-

sible allergen for an undetermined period of time. Evacuate according to your protocols.

- Begin a Level 3 evacuation if a limited amount of epinephrine is available and the possibility of re-exposure to the allergen exists. The patient will remain hypersensitive to the responsible allergen for an undetermined period of time.

Adjunct Treatments (second line only)

- An aerosolized epinephrine MDI, such as Primatene Mist® or Medihaler-Epi®, may counteract the effects of bronchocon- 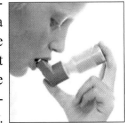 striction and laryngeal edema in some individuals. Rinse out the mouth and spit out immediately after using the inhaler to avoid gastrointestinal problems; don't swallow.

- Bronchospasm and wheezing may also be treated using an albuterol MDI 4-8 puffs every 15-20 minutes as needed.

Altitude Sickness

Pathophysiology

The term altitude sickness encompasses acute mountain sickness (AMS), high altitude cerebral edema (HACE), and high altitude pulmonary edema (HAPE); all pose a serious threat to climbers worldwide. As altitude increases the amount of available oxygen decreases. At 8,000 feet, there is 25% less oxygen than at sea level; at 18,000 feet there is 50% less oxygen than at sea level. Unless there is pre-existing respiratory damage, most altitude-related problems occur at elevations above 8,000 feet. The body initially responds to decreasing oxygen levels by increasing both respiratory and pulse rates in an effort to maintain oxygen perfusion to its tissues. One of the functions of the respiratory system is to facilitate pH balance; if respiratory rates remain abnormally high for a prolonged period of time (usually 24-48 hours), the normal blood pH (7.35-7.45) gradually becomes more basic, or alkalotic. The kidneys respond by excreting base (bicarbonate) into the urine. In most cases, the kidneys take one to three days to balance blood pH. In addition to pH changes, nitric oxide levels fall—steeply in some people—causing pulmonary vasoconstriction that raises pulmonary arterial pressure. Mild increases in pulmonary arterial

pressure increase lung perfusion and oxygenation and are adaptive. Full acclimatization takes 2-3 weeks, as red-blood-cell production and general metabolic efficiency increases.

If the attempt by the kidneys at balancing the blood pH fails, respirations cannot continue at a rate high enough to perfuse the body's tissue with oxygen (hypoxia). Hypoxia triggers increased cerebral blood flow in a failed attempt to oxygenate the brain. Water is retained by the kidneys to maintain blood pressure. In response to the increasing cellular hypoxia and changing blood pH, the permeability of the microvascular bed in tissues throughout the body increases. The ensuing system-wide leaks and edema are seen as visible swelling of the hands and feet. Combined with the increased cerebral blood flow, the patient presents with a headache, nausea, vomiting, and ataxia (HACE). If rising pulmonary pressure exceeds the capillary threshold in the lungs, plasma is forced into the alveoli damaging them and causing pulmonary edema and respiratory distress (HAPE). As such, the S/Sx of acute mountain sickness are progressive and identical to those of increasing respiratory distress and increasing intracranial pressure. With the development of severe AMS, death can occur within six hours.

There is an acclimatization zone between full acclimatization and the development of AMS. Resting pulse and respiratory rates increase above normal in the acclimatization zone secondary to altitude-driven hypoxia; however, there are no additional S/Sx of AMS because the kidneys are able to balance blood pH. As a climber acclimates to increasingly higher altitudes, their acclimatization level also increases. Complete acclimatization is limited to elevations less than 24,000 feet.

AMS Drugs

The same AMS prescription drugs are used for prophylaxis and treatment. Use prescription drug prophylaxis discriminately, NOT as common practice. Slow ascent is the preferred strategy for prophylaxis and descent is the preferred strategy for treatment. The drugs and dosages outlined below are for healthy individuals with no underlying medical conditions.

- Acetazolamide (Rx) is indicated for new climbers or for those with a history of AMS with a forced rapid ascent (greater than 5,000 ft/day) to camp at

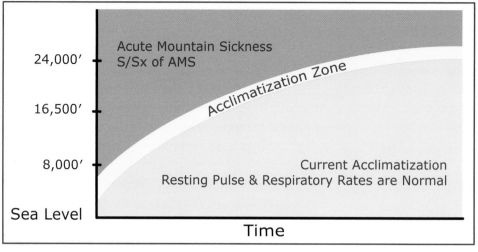

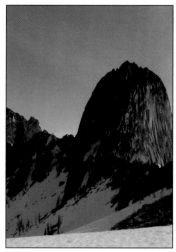

altitudes greater than 9,000 ft. Give 125 mg twice a day by mouth and continue for 3 days at fixed altitude; the dose is doubled to treat moderate and severe AMS. Use a potassium supplement. Acetazolamide is a sulfa drug and may cause anaphylaxis in sensitized individuals; if you carry acetazolamide, consider carrying epinephrine and an oral antihistamine. Side effects include frequent urination, numbness and tingling in the face, lips and occasionally hands, blurred vision and a general sense of weirdness. Beer and carbonated drinks lose their "fizz."

• Dexamethasone (Rx) is a corticosteroid that reduces the symptoms of AMS, but does not speed acclimatization; it may be used by climbers unable to take acetazolamide or in conjunction with acetazolamide for forced rapid ascents to altitudes greater than 14,000 feet (usually by flying to mountains and altitude for rescue purposes); it is also the gold standard for treating HACE. Give 4 mg four

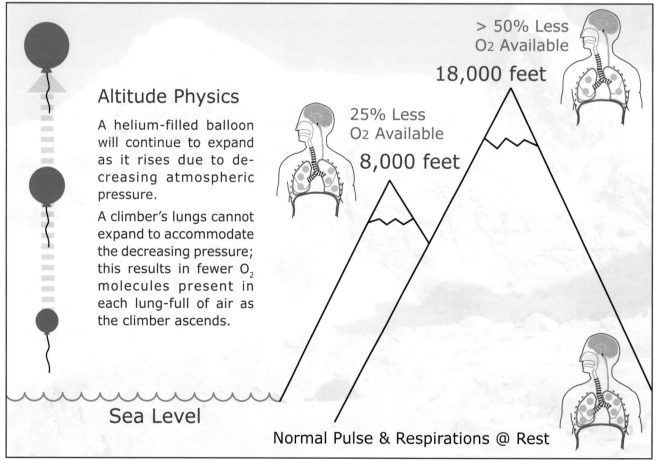

Altitude Physics

A helium-filled balloon will continue to expand as it rises due to decreasing atmospheric pressure.

A climber's lungs cannot expand to accommodate the decreasing pressure; this results in fewer O_2 molecules present in each lung-full of air as the climber ascends.

25% Less O2 Available
8,000 feet

> 50% Less O2 Available
18,000 feet

Sea Level

Normal Pulse & Respirations @ Rest

times a day by mouth or intramuscular injection. Continue until acclimatized or upon return to base altitude. Side effects include euphoria, upset stomach, difficulty sleeping, immunosuppression with prolonged use, ***and hyperglycemia in diabetics.***

- Nifedipine (Rx) is a calcium channel blocker that prevents pulmonary edema in susceptible individuals by relaxing smooth muscle that surrounds arteries, thereby reducing pulmonary arterial pressure. Give 30 mg by mouth two to four times a day during ascent using slow-release tablets; continue for 3 days at fixed altitude. Side effects include dizziness and mild tachycardia.

- Sildenafil citrate or tadalafil (both Rx) each prevent pulmonary edema in susceptible individuals by inhibiting the breakdown of nitric oxide and decreasing pulmonary arterial pressure; however, they have little effect on accumulated fluid in an already damaged lung. Give 50 milligrams of sindenafil citrate every eight hours or Tadalafil 10 mg every 12 hours. Sildenafil citrate may cause a systemic drop in blood pressure in some individuals; tadalafil has no significant side effects. DO NOT take either drug concurrently with nitrates. The ensuing drug interaction will cause a sudden and steep drop in blood pressure and potentially death. Nitrates are typically given to lower blood pressure in cardiac patients (nitroglycerin is one example; there are over 20 Rx forms of nitrates currently available).

- Salmeterol (Rx) is a beta-2 agonist; it increases activity of the membrane sodium channels largely responsible for clearing fluid from the alveoli. Given via an MDI or DPI inhaler (125 mcg) every 12 hours to treat HAPE. The main side effect is mild tachycardia.

Prevention

- Make a slow ascent. Allow the kidneys to maintain normal blood pH balance. Above 10,000 feet, ascend 1,000-to-2,000 feet per day with a rest day every 3,000-to-5,000 feet. This is a conservative pace that avoids high altitude pulmonary edema (HAPE) and high altitude cerebral edema (HACE) in most people by permitting the kidneys time to adapt to changing blood pH levels.

- Stay hydrated; avoid sunburn.

- Climb high and sleep low to avoid sleep hypoxia and a restless sleep.

- Avoid respiratory depressants, such as sleeping pills and alcohol.

- Restrict exercise levels during the first 24 hours at a new altitude to permit faster acclimation. Exercise increases oxygen demand.

- Eat a high-carbohydrate diet; avoid fats and proteins as they require more oxygen to digest and often lead to nausea. Avoid dehydration; closely monitor urine output and color. Normal hydration facilitates the kidneys' excretion of bicarbonate.

- Avoid all forms of nicotine.

- Consider taking Ginkgo biloba at 100 mg twice a day beginning 3-21 days before the climb and continuing throughout the climb. Ginkgo decreases the incidence and severity of AMS in some individuals and has no side effects.

Assessment

When assessing the severity of AMS, it is important to remember that not all S/Sx may be present. A pulse oximeter is useful to measure oxygen saturation, but is not predictive. Oxygen saturation at sea level is typically greater than 95% and drops at altitude; the amount of decrease depends on the individual, their level of acclimatization and the presence or absence of AMS.

Oxygen Saturation Levels

O_2 Sat	Symptom
95-100%	Normal
85-95%	Minimal sensory impairment
75-85%	Minimal mental impairment
65-75%	Increasing sensory & mental decrement
55-65%	Potential collapse

Assessment of Mild AMS

- Mild AMS usually occurs at elevations in excess of 8,000 feet. The onset of S/Sx is variable and includes a dull headache, abnormally high respiration rate, and shortness of breath during normal exercise.

- Other S/Sx include insomnia, Cheyne-Stokes breathing and/or anxiety attacks because of a depressed respiratory drive and associated hypoxia while sleeping. The parasympathetic and sympathetic systems are at war. The parasympathetic system wants to slow respirations to promote REM sleep; the sympathetic system wants to increase respirations to avoid hypoxia. The result is Cheyne-Stokes breathing. Cheyne-Stokes breathing begins with shallow panting breaths that gradually slow until breathing stops for a few seconds and then the cycle starts again. Climbers experiencing Cheyne-Stokes breathing may suddenly awaken with a feeling of suffocation when they stop breathing. Some suddenly sit up. This is disconcerting if you are sleeping next to them.

- Decreased appetite; often accompanied by nausea.
- Swelling of hands, feet, and occasionally face.

Assessment of Moderate AMS

- Moderate AMS usually occurs at new altitudes above 10,000 feet; the onset of S/Sx is variable and typically delayed 10-12 hours. They include a severe and increasingly debilitating headache, abnormally increased respirations and shortness of breath during mild exercise.
- Episodes of vomiting are possible.
- The victim is awake and irritable or lethargic with increasing fatigue.
- The development of rales or minor "crackling sounds" in the lungs is possible.

Assessment of Severe AMS (HACE/HAPE)

- Severe AMS (HAPE and/or HACE) usually occurs at new altitudes above 10,000 feet.
- The onset of S/Sx is variable; however, death may occur within 6 hours of presentation. S/Sx include a severe and increasingly debilitating migraine headache, abnormally increased respiration rate, and shortness-of-breath at rest, as well as persistent vomiting and decreased coordination (ataxia). Ataxia is often subtle and evaluation of a patient requires a specific test. The patient should walk in a heel-to-toe straight line. If their balance wavers, as if they are walking on a high wire, or if they stumble, they fail the test.
- Victims are initially awake and extremely lethargic or exhausted and quickly progress to V P U.
- The development of rales or minor "crackling sounds" in the lungs is possible, and if present, often progress to a productive cough and gurgling.

Field Treatment

Treatment of Mild AMS

- STOP the ascent and rest until the kidneys catch up, pH balance is restored, and S/Sx disappear, generally within 2-4 days.
- If S/Sx worsen, descend 1,000-2000 feet or until S/Sx resolve.
- Administer NSAIDs to reduce headache during rest days.
- Administer acetazolamide to speed acclimatization.
- Increase fluids and electrolytes to maintain hydration status; monitor urine output and color.
- To help avoid nausea, consume a diet high in carbohydrates; avoid proteins and fats.

Treatment of Moderate AMS

- STOP the ascent and DESCEND until S/Sx disappear, generally within 1,000-2,000 feet. The patient may or may not be able to self-evacuate. *Drug therapy is adjunctive in nature and does not substitute for descent.*
- Decrease and limit exercise.
- Use supplemental O_2 (1 L/min at rest) if available.
- Use a portable hyperbaric chamber to stabilize the patient prior to descent or if descent is not immediately possible.
- Administer acetazolamide (Rx) by mouth 250 mg twice a day *during* the descent.
- Administer dexamethasone (Rx) 4 mg four times a day by mouth or IM *during* the descent until S/Sx subside, usually within 12-24 hours.
- Administer nifedipine, sildenafil citrate or tadalafil for HAPE if crackling sounds are present in lungs.
- Administer salmeterol to reduce pulmonary edema if crackling sounds are present in lungs.
- Increase fluids and electrolytes; monitor the patient's urine output and color.
- Use promethazine (Rx) 25 or 50 mg suppositories three times a day for a maximum of 3 doses to control nausea and vomiting.

Treatment of Severe AMS (HACE/HAPE)

- STOP the ascent and DESCEND until S/Sx disappear, generally within 2,000-4,000 feet. A simple carry or litter evacuation is typically required. *Drug therapy is adjunctive in nature and does not substitute for descent.*
- Use supplemental O_2 (1 L/min at rest) if available.
- Use a portable hyperbaric chamber prior to descent or if descent is not immediately possible.
- Administer acetazolamide (Rx) 250 mg twice a

day by mouth during the descent.

- Administer dexamethasone (Rx) 4 mg four times a day for HACE by mouth or IM during the descent until S/Sx subside.
- Administer 20 mg sublingual nifedipine (Rx) for HAPE immediately and follow with 30 mg slow-release four times a day during the descent until S/Sx subside.
- Support HAPE patients in a seated or semi-reclined position to help facilitate their breathing.
- Positive pressure ventilations may be helpful, but difficult, during an evacuation.

Portable Hyperbaric Chambers

Because of their weight and expense, portable hyperbaric chambers tend to be found only in large expeditions to extreme altitudes that involve porters or at medical base camp facilities. Familiarize yourself with the specific chamber before use. Practice simulations are invaluable. There are three chambers in common use: the Gamow Bag®, the Certec Bag®, and the Portable Altitude Chamber® (PAC).

How to Use

- Portable hyperbaric chambers are NOT a substitute for descent or evacuation and are more effective if used in conjunction with AMS drugs and oxygen. ***Do not connect oxygen to the pump intake.***
- Insulate the chamber from the ground and place the patient's sleeping bag inside.
- Shade the chamber if in the sun.
- Patient should urinate and defecate before going inside the bag.
- Instruct the patient to breathe normally and to swallow as the bag is inflated to avoid overpressurizing their ears. If the bag should suddenly deflate, the subject should exhale.
- Give promethazine (Rx) 25 or 50 mg suppositories three times a day for a maximum of 3 doses to control nausea and vomiting in awake patients.
- Place V, P, and U patients on their side in case of vomiting.
- Put the patient into the bag, pump until the pop-off valve hisses, keep the patient at pressure for about one hour; remove patient and reassess. Additional cycles of inflation and reassessment are usually necessary until the patient is well enough to descend. HAPE typically requires 2-4 hours

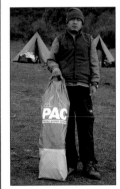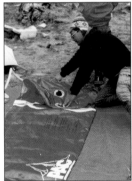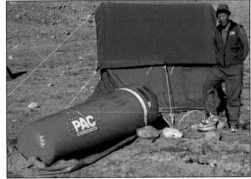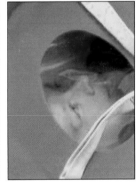

Chamber	Pros	Cons
Gamow Bag	• Foot pump.	• Zipper is prone to leak with extended use. • Reinforcement straps inhibit ease of patient entry.
Certec Bag	• Double envelope construction increases durability and pressure. • Easy to place patient inside.	• Hand pump strains lower back.
Portable Altitude Chamber (PAC)	• Foot pump. • Easiest bag to place patient inside. • Half the cost of the others.	

of treatment while HACE requires 4-6 hours. If successful, it generally provides a 10-12 hour evacuation window.

• Continue to pump fresh air into the chamber to flush the system and to prevent CO_2 build-up; constant pumping is a lot of work.

• Talk to and reassure patients while they are in the bag; claustrophobia and its associated anxiety are common.

• Tilt the bag if patient cannot tolerate lying flat.

AMS Summary

Prevention, as always, is preferable to treatment. Effective treatment requires early diagnosis. Until proven otherwise, all sickness at altitude should be treated as AMS; if in doubt: DESCEND. Four basic rules apply:

1. Stop ascent at first S/Sx.
2. Descend if S/Sx do not resolve within 2-4 days or if they get worse.
3. Descend immediately if patient exhibits pulmonary edema, ataxia or becomes voice-responsive, pain-responsive, or unresponsive.
4. Never leave an AMS patient alone; worsening S/Sx will affect their judgement.

Diving Injuries

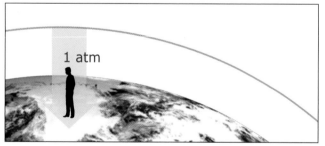

1 atm

Pressure is measured by pounds per square inch (psi), millimeters of mercury (mm Hg) or atmospheres (atm). Air has weight. The weight of a column of air at sea level is 14.7 pounds per square inch, 760 mm Hg, or one atmosphere. Water is heavier than air. The weight of a column of air at sea level—one atmosphere—is equivalent to 33 feet of water. Each additional 33 feet in depth increases the pressure by 1 atm. Our bodies are primarily comprised of water containing some dissolved gases. Liquids and body tissue do not compress under

pressure, gases do. Boyle's law states that at a constant temperature, the absolute pressure of a gas is inversely proportional to its volume; therefore, the volume of any gases trapped at the surface will decrease proportionally with the depth during descent.

As a diver descends, the increasing weight of the water above, increases the pressure on the diver's body and respectively decreases the volume of gas inside any enclosed space, such as the sinuses, ears, fillings, mask, and alveoli. Conversely, as a diver ascends, the water pressure is reduced and the gas inside any closed space expands.

SCUBA

SCUBA (Self Contained Underwater Breathing Apparatus) is necessary for a diver to breathe normally under water. SCUBA is compressed air contained within a steel or a aluminum tank. The regulator adjusts the pressure of the air delivered to a diver's lungs during each breath, permitting the diver to inflate their lungs normally regardless of the outside water pressure.

Decompression Chambers

Serious SCUBA diving injuries are pressure-related and treatment requires a Level 1 Evacuation to the nearest decompression chamber. Most successful at-sea evacuations are via helicopter. Patients should not be flown unless the cabin is pressurized to sea level; commercial aircraft are usually pressurized to 8,000 feet and should be avoided. Unpressurized aircraft—usually helicopters—must stay below 100 meters.

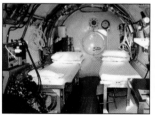 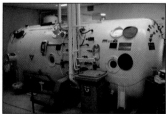

Multi-place decompression chambers are preferred to mono-place chambers in the treatment of serious diving injuries, so that medical personnel may directly work with the patient. Contact Diving Alert Network (DAN) for the location of the nearest decompression chamber. Be prepared. Know the location of the nearest decompression chamber and phone numbers of local rescue teams BEFORE leaving for a dive.

POPS
Pulmonary Over Pressure Syndrome

Pathophysiology

If a SCUBA diver holds their breath while ascending, they may rupture their alveoli as the air inside each sac expands. It takes very little pressure to rupture alveoli once the lungs are fully inflated; often only a few feet of ascent is all that is required.

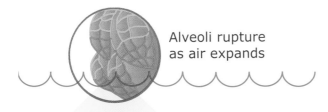

Alveoli rupture as air expands

Rapid ascent while holding breath

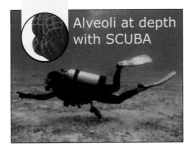

Alveoli at depth with SCUBA

Tiny air bubbles may leak into the pulmonary capillaries, travel back to the heart, and enter general circulation. The bubbles may become lodged in small arteries anywhere in the diver's body, subsequently blocking blood, and thus perfusion to that portion of the body. If the air bubble (arterial gas embolism or AGE) is in the brain, the diver will present with the S/Sx of a stroke. If the air bubble is in their heart, they will present with the S/Sx of a heart attack. If elsewhere in their body, they will present with localized pain and a subsequent loss of function. AGE is a major cause of death in sport diving. Escaping air may also leak into the middle compartment of the chest cavity (mediastinal emphysema). If it exerts undue pressure on the heart, the diver may present with the signs and symptoms of a mild heart attack. Usually, it continues to leak through the surrounding muscles and emerge as small bubbles beneath the skin of the diver's chest and neck (subcutaneous emphysema). While mediastinal and subcutaneous emphysema are the most common result of alveoli ruptures and often resolve without invasive medical treatment, the patient may, within a few hours, develop complications that do. Rarely, air may leak between the lung and the chest wall causing a delamination of the pleura (collapsed lung, pneumothorax) and respiratory distress leading to arrest. In a field setting, regardless of how the leaking air presents, the diver should be transported immediately with ALS for decompression in a hyperbaric chamber with adjunct medical care.

Prevention

- Ascend slowly and breathe normally; DO NOT hold your breath while ascending with SCUBA.

Assessment

- The MOI is a rapid ascent while breath holding.
- Onset occurs while the diver is surfacing, upon

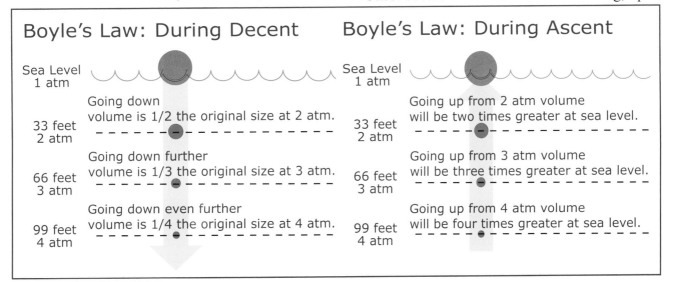

Boyle's Law: During Decent

Sea Level
1 atm

33 feet
2 atm

Going down volume is 1/2 the original size at 2 atm.

66 feet
3 atm

Going down further volume is 1/3 the original size at 3 atm.

99 feet
4 atm

Going down even further volume is 1/4 the original size at 4 atm.

Boyle's Law: During Ascent

Sea Level
1 atm

33 feet
2 atm

Going up from 2 atm volume will be two times greater at sea level.

66 feet
3 atm

Going up from 3 atm volume will be three times greater at sea level.

99 feet
4 atm

Going up from 4 atm volume will be four times greater at sea level.

surfacing, or within 10 minutes of surfacing. Drowning is a significant risk if the affected diver is in the water.

- Air often leaks into the middle compartment of the chest (mediastinal emphysema) and presents with the S/Sx of a heart attack. The escaping air usually continues to percolate through the mediastinum into the surrounding tissue to surface as small crackling bubbles under the skin (subcutaneous emphysema). Air bubbles in the neck often affect the patient's vocal chords and change the sound of their voice.
- Air bubbles that enter general circulation may lodge in small arteries and block blood supply to everything downstream (arterial gas embolism), causing

pain and loss of function in the affected tissue. S/Sx may present as a heart attack, stroke, respiratory distress, or joint pain, respectively. Bloody froth may issue from patient's mouth or nose.

- In rare cases, the diver's lung(s) may delaminate and collapse; patient presents with S/Sx of increasing respiratory distress and may arrest.
- Initially mild S/Sx often progress to life threatening in a few hours.

Field Treatment

- Support the patient's critical systems and evacuate with ALS to the closest decompression chamber; decompression is helpful even after long delays.

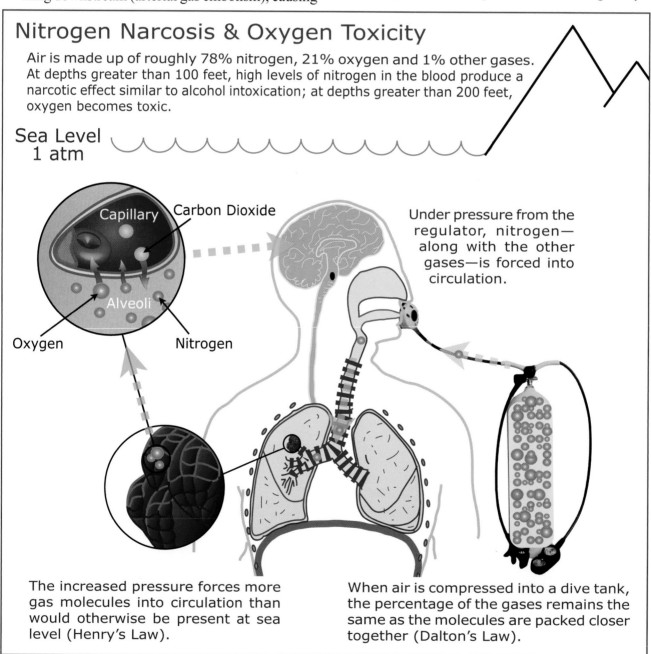

Nitrogen Narcosis & Oxygen Toxicity

Air is made up of roughly 78% nitrogen, 21% oxygen and 1% other gases. At depths greater than 100 feet, high levels of nitrogen in the blood produce a narcotic effect similar to alcohol intoxication; at depths greater than 200 feet, oxygen becomes toxic.

Sea Level
1 atm

Capillary

Carbon Dioxide

Alveoli

Oxygen

Nitrogen

Under pressure from the regulator, nitrogen—along with the other gases—is forced into circulation.

The increased pressure forces more gas molecules into circulation than would otherwise be present at sea level (Henry's Law).

When air is compressed into a dive tank, the percentage of the gases remains the same as the molecules are packed closer together (Dalton's Law).

- Place the patient in a neutral position on their back or on their left side. A head-down position will increase intracranial pressure, while a head up position encourages the movement of air bubbles to the brain.
- Administer supplemental O_2 at high liter flow.
- Reassure awake patients.
- Initiate rescue breathing and chest compressions as necessary. Consider stopping CPR after 30 minutes.

Nitrogen Narcosis & Oxygen Toxicity

Pathophysiology

Normal air is a mixture of gases containing 21% oxygen, 78% nitrogen, and 1% other gases, including carbon dioxide. Oxygen is required for normal metabolism; rising carbon dioxide levels in the blood stimulate the respiratory center to begin a new breathing cycle. Nitrogen, at normal or slightly increased pressures, remains inert. The percentage of gases in air remain the same while SCUBA diving (Dalton's Law), but the amount of gas dissolved in the blood increases as pressure increases (Henry's Law). When diving at depths near or greater than 100 feet using SCUBA with normal air, nitrogen accumulates in the blood. Large amounts of nitrogen alter the electrical properties of cerebral cellular membranes and produce a narcotic effect similar to alcohol intoxication. The sensation is generally pleasant; however, it may cause fatal lapses in judgement. In most cases, the afflicted diver fails to recognize the developing condition and recognition is dependent on an unimpaired diving partner. When diving at depths near or greater than 200 feet with compressed air, the ensuing high concentration of oxygen kills central nervous system cells.

Prevention

Prevention of Nitrogen Narcosis

- DO NOT dive at depths near or greater than 100 feet while using SCUBA with compressed air; 130 feet is usually considered the maximum safe limit for experienced divers.
- Dive with a friend. Unaffected divers can easily recognize those who become impaired.
- A helium/oxygen mixture is safer than compressed air for deep dives. Although expensive, it eliminates the problems associated with nitrogen.

Prevention of Oxygen Toxicity

- DO NOT dive at depths near or > 200 feet with compressed air. Use a helium/oxygen mixture and decrease the percent of oxygen according to dive depth.

Assessment

Assessment of Nitrogen Narcosis

- The MOI is SCUBA diving at depths near or greater than 100 feet. The results of nitrogen narcosis occur underwater.
- Onset is within minutes at depth, but varies with individuals.
- Diver's judgement becomes affected while using SCUBA with compressed air at depths near or greater than 100 feet. There is a change in normal mental status to awake and confused or lethargic; the diver may develop bizarre behavior. It is common for an affected diver to forget to check their air supply, depth gauge, bottom time, etc. and a secondary life-threatening problem may develop.
- The condition deteriorates as the depth increases.

Assessment of Oxygen Toxicity

- Oxygen toxicity causes tingling, focal seizures (facial or lip twitching), vertigo, nausea, vomiting, and constricted vision. About 10% of people experience seizures or fainting, which typically results in drowning.

Field Treatment

Treatment of Nitrogen Narcosis

- Reduce the pressure and the problem by ascending to shallow water; there are no aftereffects.

Treatment of Oxygen Toxicity

- Ascend to shallow water to reduce pressure; there is no treatment and damage may be permanent.

Decompression Sickness (the Bends)

Pathophysiology

When diving with SCUBA and compressed air, large amounts of nitrogen may become diffused into the diver's blood. Numerous factors increase the amount of nitrogen diffused into an individual diver's blood and tissue. Deep dives expose the diver to greater amounts of pressure and increase the nitrogen content proportionately. The longer the time a diver spends underwater, the greater the accumulation of nitrogen. Exercise increases perfusion and gas solubility in both blood and tissues. If the nitrogen remains in solution, it will diffuse back out of the blood and tissues through the diver's lungs as pressure is decreased "slowly." Nitrogen diffuses out of blood and tissue at roughly the same rate it enters; however, different tissues have different rates of absorption and the time required for nitrogen to come out of solution is dependent upon the specific type of tissue. More than 12 hours is required for nitrogen to diffuse out of fat. Residual nitrogen is the limiting factor for the number of deep dives that a diver may attempt within a 24-hour period; divers are predisposed to decompression sickness if too many deep dives are taken within that time frame. When a diver exercises at depth and then ascends without exercise, the rate of diffusion is slower during ascent than descent (because of the lack of exercise during ascent), and the diver is predisposed to decompression sickness. This is the reason for stage decompression. When an ascent is too rapid to permit the nitrogen to be diffused and expelled during normal exhalation, the diver's blood will become supersaturated with nitrogen and decompression sickness will occur. If a diver travels in an unpressurized aircraft within 24 hours after surfacing, nitrogen bubbles may also form.

Once a diver's blood becomes supersaturated, the nitrogen will come out of solution as small bubbles in the bloodstream. Since the bubbles are too big to move across the membranes into the alveoli and be removed during exhalation, they travel through the circulatory system until they become lodged in small arteries or capillaries. Once a vessel is blocked, perfusion is cut off to all the tissue supplied by that vessel. The presence of nitrogen bubbles within the microvascular bed may activate the clotting process, causing permanent obstruction. Minor cases of decompression sickness cause fatigue, itching or burning skin, local discomfort, and pain. Severe cases involving vessels in the brain, the spinal cord, and the lungs may cause death. Signs and symptoms of serious decompression sickness are those of stroke, spinal cord inju-

ries, and respiratory distress respectively. It may be impossible to tell the difference between severe decompression sickness and the problems associated with ruptured alveoli. The diver presenting with minor decompression sickness may, within a few hours, develop life-threatening problems. Regardless of how decompression sickness presents, the diver needs immediate decompression in a hyperbaric chamber to force the nitrogen bubbles back

Decompression Sickness

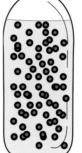

Similar to how soda is pressurized with carbon dioxide, nitrogen is forced into body fluids and tissue by the increased pressure from the dive tank.

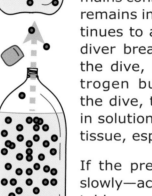

As long as the pressure remains constant, the nitrogen remains in solution and continues to accumulate as the diver breathes. The deeper the dive, the faster the nitrogen builds. The longer the dive, the more nitrogen in solution in the blood and tissue, especially fat cells.

If the pressure is released slowly—according to the dive tables—and followed by no exercise at sea level for 24-48 hours, the nitrogen comes out of solution slowly via the lungs, causing no harm.

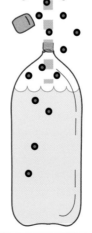

If the pressure is released quickly, by a rapid ascent and exercise, the nitrogen comes out of solution too quickly to off-gas normally via the lungs. Bubbles form in the blood and/or tissue, causing the S/Sx of decompression sickness.

into solution and reestablish perfusion to the affected areas before clotting problems develop. Adjunct medical care may be necessary before, during, and after decompression.

Prevention

- Stay hydrated to facilitate nitrogen off-gassing.
- Avoid dives that require stage decompression OR plan dives according to the U.S. Navy diving tables and be conservative.
- Know how to convert the dive tables for high-altitude diving.
- Avoid ascending at a rate greater than 60 feet per minute (1 foot per second).
- Avoid flying in unpressurized aircraft within 24 hours after a dive; allow surface time to fully decompress.
- Anyone with cardiovascular disease is predisposed to decompression sickness.
- Avoid nicotine products.
- Divers who have undergone minor decompression therapy should not dive for a minimum of 1-2 months following the therapy. Those who have undergone treatment for serious decompression sickness should not dive for 4-6 months. Divers should not dive again if they have undergone repeated treatments for serious decompression sickness.

Assessment

- The MOI is a rapid ascent.
- The onset of S/Sx is variable upon surfacing: 50% of cases occur immediately or within the first 30 minutes; 85% of cases occur within one hour; 95% of cases occur within three hours; and, 99% of cases occur within six hours. All abnormal S/Sx within 48 hours after a dive should be attributed to, and treated as, decompression sickness until proven otherwise.
- Early S/Sx may include unusual fatigue with itching, burning or mottled skin. Pitted edema indicates a more serious injury.

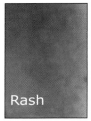
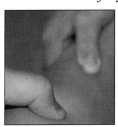
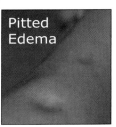

Rash

Pitted Edema

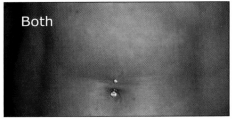
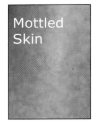

Mottled Skin

Both

- Deep aches, pain and tenderness in the joints of the shoulders, elbows or knees indicate the formation of nitrogen bubbles that may lead to life-threatening problems within a few hours.

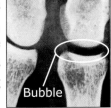

Bubble

- Serious S/Sx are variable and include: heart attack, stroke, and respiratory distress, often with a nonproductive cough.
- When the spinal cord is affected, the patient experiences girding abdominal and back pain, inability to urinate, numbness, tingling and weakness in the arms and/or legs that may progress to irreversible paralysis.

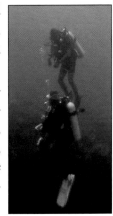

- Vertigo and ataxia indicate damage to the nerves of the inner ear.
- Headache, confusion, double vision, and difficulty speaking indicate brain involvement. Loss of consciousness is rare. Seizures are possible.

Field Treatment

- Support the patient's critical systems and immediately evacuate with ALS to the closest decompression chamber as per POPS treatment; decompression is helpful even after long delays.
- Place the patient in a neutral position on their back or on their left side.
- Administer 100% supplemental O_2 via a non-rebreathing face mask; this increases the gas gradient and the rate of nitrogen excretion.
- Reassure awake patients and administer oral fluids: one liter within the first hour. IV fluids are preferred and required with V, P, and U patients. Use isotonic sodium chloride solution or lactated Ringers and maintain urine output at 1-2 ml/kg/hr. Increasing the patient's fluid volume increases circulation, perfusion and the absorption of nitrogen bubbles.
- Place a urinary catheter in awake patients, who

are unable to urinate, and in all V, P, or U patients.

- Administer sublingual aspirin (650 mg) to decrease the formation of intravascular clots. Chewable baby aspirin is absorbed faster than regular aspirin.

- Rescue breathing and chest compressions as necessary. Consider stopping CPR after 30 minutes.

Barotrauma

(Squeeze)

Pathophysiology

Pressure increases as a diver descends; volume decreases. If the object surrounding the air is flexible, like a balloon (or alveoli), it shrinks as the air volume decreases. If the object is solid like a ping-pong ball (or sinus cavities, inner ear, etc.), it collapses as the air volume decreases. If pressure within the cavity can be equalized, the cavity will not collapse. Most of the body cavities that contain air are either flexible (alveoli) and do not require equalization or have connecting tubes (inner ear, sinuses) that, with training, permit the pressure to be equalized. One exception is the teeth; if a filling is poorly packed, there may be a small air cavity that causes pain and limits descent. Another unusual exception is when changing pressures cause temporary intestinal pain due to gas formation from partially digested or gas-producing foods, such as beans or tofu.

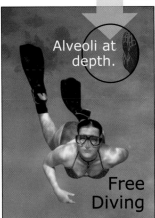

Alveoli at
Sea Level

Sea Level
1 atm

Alveoli at
depth.

Squeeze
Increasing water pressure during descent proportionally reduces the volume of any trapped gases. Gases trapped in a rigid container cause a pressure imbalance as the volume drops. If not equalized, the imbalance is painful and may damage the surrounding tissue.

Free
Diving

"Squeeze" problems are more common during descent. If the diver has a cold, allergy, flu, or sinus infection that causes swelling in the eustachian tubes or sinus passages, equalization may be difficult or impossible. Local decongestants—while offering short-term relief—may cause problems during ascent as they wear off. Eye squeeze is possible if the goggles worn do not permit equalization (exhaling through the nose into the air space).

Prevention

- Avoid diving (free diving and SCUBA) while congested from a cold, flu, allergy, sinus infection, or inner-ear infection.

- Descend and ascend slowly, allowing time for equalization.

- Avoid consumption of gas-producing foods prior to diving.

- Do not wear ear plugs or goggles without nose seals while diving; nose seals are necessary to equalize the pressure in the middle and inner ear.

Assessment

- The MOI is increased pressure on closed air spaces; onset is immediate.

- The diver experiences immediate pain in the affected area usually while descending.

- Severe pain in the ear, followed by a rush of cold water, a full feeling, and subsequent vertigo indicates a ruptured eardrum and may be accompanied by tinnitus (high-pitched whining or ringing) or hearing loss. The vertigo diminishes as the water in the ear reaches body temperature. Severe vertigo may be accompanied by nausea and vomiting that place the diver at risk for drowning.

- Severe pain behind the forehead, eyes or nose, accompanied by a nose bleed, indicates a rupture in the sinus lining.

- An unequalized face mask or goggles act like a suction cup applied to the eyes. The suction causes small blood vessels to dilate, leak and finally burst, leaving the eyes red and bloodshot. Vision is not affected.

- An increasing toothache indicates air pockets in or under a tooth or filling.

- Intestinal pain due to gas is usually self-limiting and of short duration.

Field Treatment

- Upon experiencing a "Squeeze," a diver should immediately stop their descent (or ascent) and attempt to equalize the pressure. If successful, they should continue at a slower pace; if unsuccessful, they should surface slowly.

- Tissue damage associated with pressure imbalances is treated according to the location and type of injury. Control pain with NSAIDs or Rx narcotic analgesics.

- If a ruptured eardrum is suspected, visually inspect the eardrum with an otoscope or cover and begin a Level 3 Evacuation for confirmation. If confirmed, administer systemic antibiotics to prevent an infection.

- Persistent dizziness or vertigo upon surfacing may be relieved by administering systemic decongestants.

Shallow Water Blackout

Pathophysiology

Rising levels of carbon dioxide within the blood stimulate the respiratory center in the brain to begin a breathing cycle. During the cycle, carbon dioxide is exhaled and oxygen is inhaled. This causes a decrease in blood levels of carbon dioxide, as oxygen levels rise. Oxygen is consumed during cellular metabolism and carbon dioxide is formed; rising carbon dioxide levels eventually stimulate the respiratory center and initiate another breathing cycle. Skin divers hold their breath to explore the underwater world when diving. Breath-holding interrupts the normal breathing cycle by limiting the oxygen uptake and permitting carbon dioxide levels to rise above normal. Eventually, before a diver runs out of oxygen, the respiratory center forces her to surface for a breath. If she hyperventilates before diving and succeeds in lowering her carbon dioxide level below normal, she will be able to hold her breath longer because her respiratory drive takes longer to stimulate. BUT she may run out of oxygen and lose consciousness before surfacing to breathe because of her depressed respiratory drive. If this happens and she is not quickly rescued, she will drown.

Prevention

- Avoid hyperventilation prior to free diving. A few deep breaths are acceptable to clear the lungs.

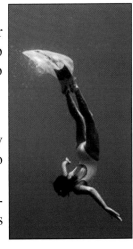

Assessment

- The patient has a history of hyperventilation prior to diving.

- A free diver loses consciousness while diving and needs to be rescued.

Field Treatment

- Administer positive pressure ventilations (rescue breathing) and chest compressions as needed. Consider stopping chest compressions after 30 minutes.

- Evacuate the patient per near-drowning.

Sea & Motion Sickness

Pathophysiology

Humans rely on input from musculoskeletal receptors, balance centers in the inner ear, and sight to orient themselves in space. Sea and motion sickness occur when the input from one or more of these senses is out of alignment.

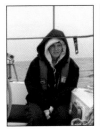 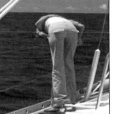 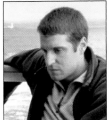

Prevention

- Avoid abrupt changes in direction and/or speed, which increase misalignment.

- Avoid all activities that involve focusing on near objects, such as reading or watching television.

- Avoid overeating, overheating, and foul odors. These exacerbate nausea and vomiting. Take slow, deep breaths of fresh, cool air.

- The bow, and sometimes the stern, of a vessel move up and down as the vessel passes through waves; depending on the size of the vessel, the stern drags through the water. Boats also rock from side to side. The further you are away from the central mass of the boat, the more movement you will encounter. Stay low, midline, and in the stern or middle of the boat, where there is the least motion.

- Focus on the horizon to help the brain reconcile conflicting input from the eyes, inner ear, and musculoskeletal receptors.
- If possible, have the patient steer the boat, as this makes them focus on the horizon and gets them thinking about something other than their own queasiness.
- If anchored and not throwing up, a swim often helps clear up seasickness.

Assessment

- Motion sickness is characterized by nausea and vomiting, pale skin, cold sweats, and hypersalivation.
- Prolonged seasickness leads to dehydration.

Field Treatment

Scopolamine

- Scopolamine reduces the CNS signals that initiate motion sickness; it is not effective once symptoms have begun. Start treatment 1-4 hours prior to exposure and continue throughout the trip. Common side effects of scopolamine are dry mouth, drowsiness and blurred vision. Scopolamine may be administered via a transdermal patch or oral tablet.
- The scopolamine patch is placed behind the ear, where it effectively prevents sea and motion sickness for up to three days; it may be cut into small, pie-shaped sections to reduce the dosage.
- Scopolamine tablets (1-2 tablets) may be taken orally on an empty stomach every 8 hours as needed.
- Use hard candy, ice chips, or gum to relieve dry mouth.

Ginger Root

- Ginger root is a highly effective antinausea remedy for sea and motion sickness and it avoids the drowsiness associated with OTC antihistamines.
- Give 1000 mg of powdered root or capsules one hour before exposure, with 250 mg four times a day thereafter.

Acupressure

- Acupressure has been used for centuries to treat sea and motion sickness.
- Apply pressure on the P6 point with your fingertip while concentrating on your breathing. The acupressure point is on the inside of your wrist. Measure three finger widths up your arm, from the wrist line. Use your thumb to locate the point in the hollow between the two bones and in the middle of the tendons. A slight soreness will let you know you have found the right location. Press the point firmly while you breathe out, and release pressure as you breathe in, repeating eight times on each wrist. Commercial wrist bands are available that apply continuous pressure.

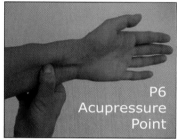 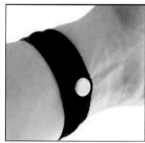

P6 Acupressure Point

Antihistamines

The brain contains histamine receptors in the hypothalamus, pons, and medulla oblongata, where the signals giving rise to sea and motion sickness originate. Sedating anti-histamines—those that cross the blood-brain barrier—block the signals and effectively prevent and treat motion sickness. Antihistamines cause drowsiness and should not be used by people operating vehicles or machinery.

- Cyclizine (OTC: Marezine®) 50 mg every 4-6 hours for patients 12 years old and over; 25 mg every 6-8 hours for children 6-11 years old. NOT RECOMMENDED for children under 6.
- Meclizine (OTC: Bonine®, Dramamine II®) 25-50 mg once a day for patients 12 and older. NOT RECOMMENDED for those under 12.
- Dimenhydrinate (OTC: Dramamine®) 50-100 mg every 4-6 hours for patients 12 years of age and over; 25-50 mg every 6-8 hours for patients 6-11 years old; 12.5-25 mg every 6-8 hours for children 2-5 years old.
- Promethazine (Rx) tablets or suppositories 25 mg every 8-12 hours for adults; 12.5 to 25 mg every 8-12 hours for children. The tablets may

Basic HDC Gravity System

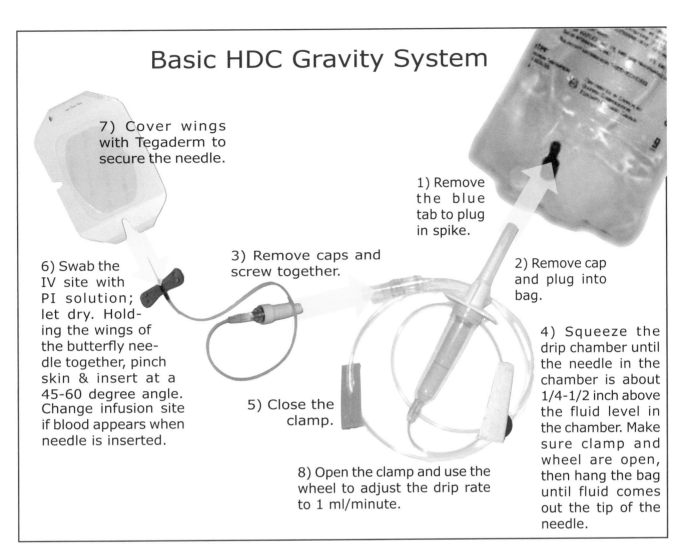

7) Cover wings with Tegaderm to secure the needle.

1) Remove the blue tab to plug in spike.

6) Swab the IV site with PI solution; let dry. Holding the wings of the butterfly needle together, pinch skin & insert at a 45-60 degree angle. Change infusion site if blood appears when needle is inserted.

3) Remove caps and screw together.

2) Remove cap and plug into bag.

4) Squeeze the drip chamber until the needle in the chamber is about 1/4-1/2 inch above the fluid level in the chamber. Make sure clamp and wheel are open, then hang the bag until fluid comes out the tip of the needle.

5) Close the clamp.

8) Open the clamp and use the wheel to adjust the drip rate to 1 ml/minute.

be combined with 25 mg of ephedrine or pseudoephedrine for better results in adults.

Dehydration and Hypodermoclysis (HDC)

Oral hydration is difficult in the presence of the vomiting and nausea caused by seasickness; subcutaneous infusion (hypodermoclysis) may be used to safely and easily treat mild-to-moderate dehydration.

- Isotonic infusion solutions containing sodium chloride—with or without glucose—may be used and given over a 24-hour period (or 500 ml given over 1-2 hours/3 times a day).
- Fluids are usually delivered by gravity at a rate of 1 ml per minute per infusion site. A maximum of two infusion sites may be used. About 1.5 L can be delivered continuously at one site and 3 L at two separate sites over 24 hours.
- Common infusion sites are the chest, abdomen (at least 2 inches from navel), thighs and upper arms. The infusion sites should have a minimum of one inch of fat and be spaced 1.5-2 inches

apart; if blood appears in the tubing, change sites. Once inserted, the needle should be able to move freely between the muscle and skin layers; muscle irritation will occur if the needle is placed too deeply and painful swelling will occur if it is placed within skin layers.

- Alternately, 500 ml may be given over 1-2 hours/3 times a day with hyaluronidase, an enzyme that temporarily breaks down the ground substance of connective tissue and enhances fluid absorption from subcutaneous tissue.
- The basic gravity-feed system consists of a normal saline solution (0.9 percent) bag, a tube with a drip chamber, a 21- or 23-gauge long-tube butterfly needle, povidone-iodine solution or alcohol skin preparation, and a sterile occlusive dressing (Tegaderm®).
- Document each infusion fluid amount, rate, site changes, adverse effects and start, stop, insertion and removal times, on the patient's SOAP

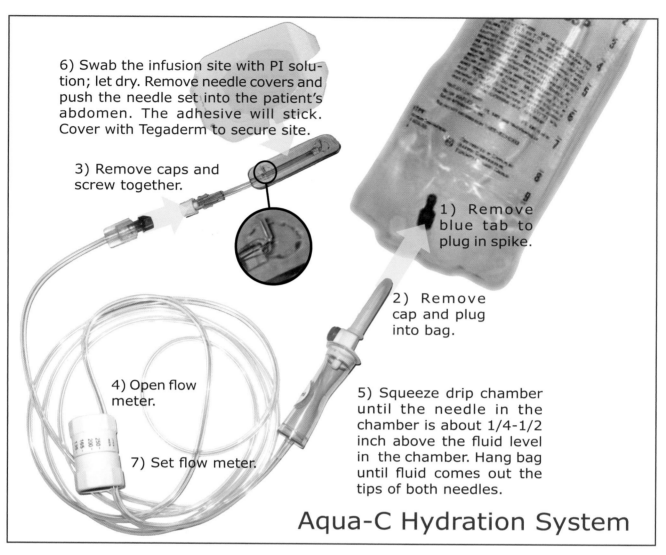

6) Swab the infusion site with PI solution; let dry. Remove needle covers and push the needle set into the patient's abdomen. The adhesive will stick. Cover with Tegaderm to secure site.

3) Remove caps and screw together.

1) Remove blue tab to plug in spike.

2) Remove cap and plug into bag.

4) Open flow meter.

7) Set flow meter.

5) Squeeze drip chamber until the needle in the chamber is about 1/4-1/2 inch above the fluid level in the chamber. Hang bag until fluid comes out the tips of both needles.

Aqua-C Hydration System

note. Label infusion sites, tubing and solution containers.

- Check patient and infusion site after one hour, and every two hours thereafter, for signs of edema, leakage or disconnection. Document.

- Local edema is the most common adverse effect. If edema is present, massage the tissue to enhance absorption. Document.

- The infusion can be started and stopped at any time by opening and closing the clamp on the tubing. There is no danger of clot formation.

- If using boluses (a large amount of fluid given over a short time), add a Y-connection between the needle and main tubing during assembly. Inject 150 U per L of hyaluronidase into the infusion bag and 75 U into each infusion site through the short injection port on the Y-connection near the needle.

- Change sites every 1500-2000 ml or if the patient experiences adverse effects; tubing and solution containers should be changed every 72 hours. Change dressings when the site is changed, or when loose, soiled or damp.

- Use the following formula to calculate drip rates (drops per minute), if a flow meter is not used:

$$\text{Drip Rate} = \frac{\text{Volume (ml)}}{\text{Time (min)}} \times \text{drops/ml}$$

- A special infusion set developed by Norfolk Medical, called the Aqua-C Hydration System, reduces the risk of needle insertion, greatly simplifies setting infusion rates using a flow meter, and permits two sites to be accessed with one administration set-up.

SECTION VIII

Medical Illnesses

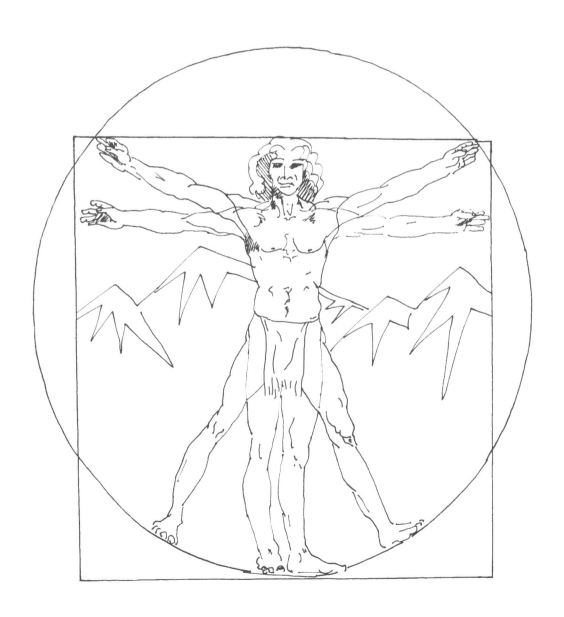

Assessing Medical Problems

There are tens of thousands of possible medical problems. Providing an accurate diagnosis and treatment plan requires years of training, access to a computer database, laboratory analysis, and sophisticated diagnostic tools, few of which are generally available in a wilderness setting. Prevention of common expedition-based medical problems typically requires an in-depth participant medical form and screening, attention to personal and camp hygiene, safe food preparation, water purification, and foreknowledge of any endemic infectious disease. Regardless of prior training and experience, it is more important to determine if the presenting medical problem is serious enough to require an evacuation and, if so, the urgency of that evacuation, than it is to accurately diagnose a specific problem. Follow the standard Patient Assessment System protocol described in Section IV, to rule out traumatic and environmental mechanisms before considering a medical mechanism.

SAMPLE History for Medical Problems

Non-traumatic pain is a common chief complaint for most medical patients. The majority of non-traumatic musculoskeletal pain is related to the activity and overuse and does not point to or mask a life-threatening condition. General muscle soreness that is not related to overuse, is typically caused by an infection. Note that non-traumatic, non-tender chest pain may indicate a serious heart or lung problem and abdominal pain, while often benign, can also be quite serious. To determine the potential cause of their pain, follow the standard SAMPLE history format on pages 51-52. Remember to ask all menstruating female patients if they are sexually active and, if so, what form of protection they use.

Physical Exam for Medical Problems

While there is no need to physically examine a medical patient head head to toe, you should explore all painful areas using gentle, firm pressure. Remember that pain and tenderness refer to different events; pain is a sign, tenderness is a symptom. When you ask a patient *What hurts?* and they tell you or point to a place on their body that hurts, that is "pain." When you *touch* them somewhere on their body and they say, *"Ouch!"* that's tenderness. While pain and tenderness frequently occur together with musculoskeletal injuries, it's not unusual for a patient with a medical problem to report an area as painful, yet find that the area does not hurt when it is palpated.

Abdominal Pain & Tenderness

Abdominal pain is a common complaint that is often difficult to diagnose. Abdominal pain is typically caused by a digestive, urinary, or reproductive system problem associated with the structure and function of its tubes.

Conceptually, the organs of the digestive system comprise a single, long tube, while the reproductive and urinary systems contain tubes, such as ureters, urethra, and fallopian tubes. Blocked tubes are accompanied by a loss of function, cramping, abdominal pain, and in more severe cases, guarding and tenderness. The pain is usually nonspecific, mild or severe, and does not necessarily relate to the severity of the problem.

Invading bacteria, viruses, parasites, and yeast commonly enter and travel via a tube (mouth, vagina, urethra, anus) and produce a variety of gastrointestinal infections that may have local or systemic consequences. Most intestinal infections usually produce diarrhea, vomiting, and abdominal cramps. More severe infections may cause fever, chills, severe pain, guarding, tenderness, and rupture.

Rupture of a tube causes fluids to leak into the abdominal cavity. The stuff sack lining the abdominal cavity, the peritoneum, is highly innervated and easily inflamed. Leaks quickly activate the inflammatory response and cause increasingly more fluid loss to edema; volume shock is possible. If the fluids contain invading bacteria, the subsequent infection may be fatal, even if the fluid loss is not. Patients who have a mechanism for abdominal fluid loss (infection, ulcers, etc.) and present with severe abdominal pain and tenderness often require surgery.

There are three basic types of abdominal pain: visceral, somatic, and referred; each is serviced by a set of different sensory nerves. Visceral nerves originate from different levels on both sides of the spinal cord and are unmyelinated. Their nerve end-

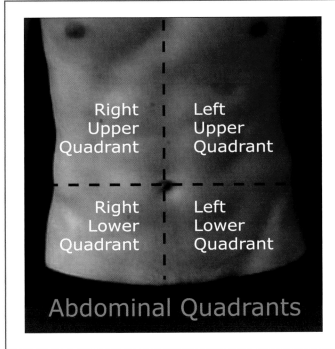

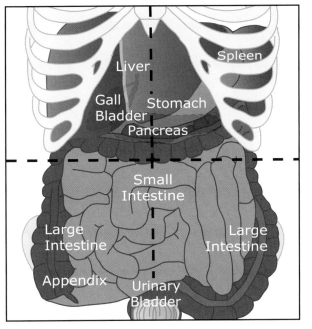

ings terminate in the walls of hollow organs and in the capsules of solid organs. They are stimulated by stretching, distension, and excessive contraction and produce a generalized dull pain or ache, which is usually described as crampy. In contrast, each somatic nerve originates at a specific level of the cord, is myelinated, and services a portion of the parietal peritoneum. Stimulation gives rise to a more specific, sharp, and intense type of pain that is seen as abdominal tenderness, guarding, or rebound pain. Finally, referred pain occurs when nerve pathways overlap, causing the pain to appear at a site away from its actual cause. Abdominal pain often begins as diffuse visceral pain, as an organ swells from inflammation, and then spreads to somatic pain, as the peritoneum becomes irritated. Patients suffering from severe abdominal pain typically present on their back or side with their legs drawn up and knees bent.

For assessment purposes, the abdomen is divided into four quadrants, as shown in the above diagram. Begin an abdominal exam in the quadrant farthest from the pain and palpate the painful quadrant last. Overlap your hands; use the top hand to push and the bottom hand to feel. Apply gentle, firm pressure to all quadrants; inflamed organs are tender. Look for rebound pain by gently pressing the patient's abdomen, then releasing the pressure suddenly. If patient complains of pain on release, the organ may be close to rupturing or recently rup-

tured. Likewise, if the patient "guards" their abdomen with their hands as you attempt to examine it and/or tightens their abdominal muscles (rigid abdomen) during an exam, an organ may be close to rupture or recently ruptured.

Vital Signs for Medical Problems

As with any patient, record multiple sets of vital signs; DO NOT skip any. A fever usually indicates an infection. Expect the patient's pulse and respirations to increase slightly in the presence of a fever.

Evaluating Medical Problems

A three-step process for evaluating patients suspected of having a medical illness is discussed below. If possible, consult with a physician. *When in doubt, take them out.*

1. Identify any urgent ***Red Flags*** ⚑ and, if found, begin a level 1 or 2 evacuation (Refer to the tables on the next page).

2. Identify any conditions, such as heart attack, asthma attack, diabetic reactions, or anaphylaxis that require emergency medications and, if possible, administer them.

3. If NO urgent ***Red Flags*** ⚑ exist, treat the patient's signs and symptoms and begin a level 3 evacuation. Alternately, refer to the ***Differential Diagnostic Chart for Common & Urgent Expedition Medical Problems*** on pages 174 & 175 and attempt to diagnose and treat the problem directly.

Evacuation Guidelines for Medical Problems

The urgency of a medical evacuation depends on the degree of involvement, or potential involvement, of any critical system. The greater the degree or potential, the more urgent the evacuation. Diagnostic patterns and guidelines for both non-urgent (level 3) and urgent (levels 1 & 2) evacuations are discussed in the following pages.

Level 1 Evacuation Red Flags ▶ : The patient's illness is immediately life threatening and the patient may die without rapid hospital intervention.

Begin a Level 1 Evacuation for:

• A patient exhibiting any abrupt change in mental status that does not spontaneously resolve within a few minutes or that reoccurs.
• A patient who is voice-responsive, pain-responsive, or unresponsive. Consider hypoglycemia and administration of glucose.
• Pain that is abrupt, new, and severe.
• A patient having chest pain or pressure that is not clearly attributable to heartburn. Consider heart attack (see page 178) and administration of aspirin and prescribed (Rx) nitroglycerin.
• A patient exhibiting acute respiratory distress from an unknown cause. Refer to Level 1 & 2 Evacuation guidelines for Asthma on pages 188-189.
• A patient excreting large amounts of bright red blood from the mouth or anus.
• A patient having vaginal bleeding, when the bleeding exceeds 5 soaked maxi-pads per day.
• A patient exhibiting severe abdominal pain with guarding. Bleeding into the abdominal cavity causes severe abdominal pain and tense (rigid) abdominal muscles. Patients typically present on their back or side with their knees bent. Movement increases the pain.
• A patient exhibiting abdominal pain that becomes specific or is accompanied by rebound pain. As perforation or rupture of an organ or tube becomes imminent, pain becomes specific to one or two quadrants and/or the patient shows pain on release of pressure during an abdominal exam.
• A patient exhibiting abdominal pain and tenderness with the clinical pattern of volume shock (i.e.: increasing pulse and respirations, pale skin, anxiety, hypotension, etc.).

Level 2 Evacuation Red Flags ▶ : The patient's illness may result in permanent disability OR the patient has the potential to develop a life-threatening problem that requires hospital intervention.

Begin a Level 2 Evacuation for:

• A patient exhibiting abdominal pain, loss-of-appetite and fever, with or without non-specific tenderness and chills that are NOT accompanied by diarrhea.
• A patient exhibiting abdominal pain and tenderness accompanied by stomach or intestinal bleeding (e.g.: coffee ground vomitus or black, tar-like stools).
• A patient having pain that begins slowly and gradually gets worse over a period of days.
• A patient having intracranial, thoracic, and abdominal pain—even mild pain—from an unknown medical mechanism in persons over 60 years of age.
• A patient having an open globe injury to the eye (see page 199).

Level 3 Evacuation (no Red Flags ▐): The patient's illness is NOT life threatening and has little or no potential to become life threatening; however, the patient is unable to continue with the trip OR needs advanced assessment and treatment beyond what is possible in a field setting.

Begin a Level 3 Evacuation for:

- A patient exhibiting minor problems that are persistent and uncomfortable, and do not respond to your field treatment.

- A patient having severe diarrhea and/or vomiting. Upgrade the evacuation level if the patient becomes dehydrated.

Consider a Level 3 Evacuation for:

- A patient exhibiting diffuse abdominal pain, with or without non-specific tenderness, that is accompanied by nausea, vomiting, and diarrhea. Minor abdominal problems tend to resolve within 24-48 hours. Treat the presenting signs and symptoms, maintain the patient's hydration status, and monitor for intestinal bleeding, perforation, or rupture. Refer to the Field Assessment of Abdominal Pain & Tenderness table on page 176 and the discussions on Intestinal Infections (Gastroenteritis) on page 206 and Appendicitis on page 209.

- A patient who has vomitus or a stool with small quantities of red blood that clearly originates from a local source—nose, mouth, or hemorrhoids. This is generally not serious.

General Supportive Treatment for Medical Problems

- *Rest:* Maintain the patient's core temperature, replace any lost fluids and electrolytes, and monitor their urine output and color.

- *Herbs:* Herbs that stimulate the immune system and have strong antimicrobial properties include: echinacea and golden seal in combination, ginseng and astragalus in combination, and hyssop.

- *Vomiting and diarrhea:* Vomiting and diarrhea are usually self-limiting; control only if the patient is in danger of becoming dehydrated. Control persistent vomiting (>12 hours) with Rx ondansetron oral disintegrating tablets (Zofran ODT®) 8 mg initial dose followed by 8 mg second dose eight hours later, then 8 mg every 12 hours for a maximum of three days; place the tablet on the patient's tongue and swallow when dissolved. Alternately use Rx promethazine 25 mg by mouth every 6-8 hours or suppository 12.5-25 mg every 12 hours; preload with diphenhydramine 25 mg by mouth 10 minutes prior to administration to avoid drug-induced side effects. Diphenhydramine (Benadryl®) may also be used if the other drugs are unavailable. Adult dose is 50 mg by mouth every 6 hours for 4 doses.

Mild diarrhea may be controlled with teas made from five finger grass or the inner bark of slippery elm. Control severe diarrhea with loperamide (Imodium®) by mouth 4-8 mg per day; DO NOT exceed 16 mg in 24 hours. Begin with the lowest dosage possible and repeat after each loose bowel movement. Constipation and abdominal cramps are possible side effects.

- *Itching:* Consider using diphenhydramine (Benadryl®) 50 mg by mouth every 6 hours to provide relief from the itching associated with rashes.

- *Fever:* Treat fevers greater than 102° F (39° C) with OTC acetaminophen, ibuprofen, or naproxen. Yarrow tea is a strong antipyretic.

- *Headache and muscle soreness:* Treat headaches and muscle soreness with OTC acetaminophen, ibuprofen, or naproxen.

Differential Diagnostic Table
for Common & Urgent Expedition Medical Problems

Major S/Sx & History	Possible Problems	Page
Non-traumatic, Substernal Chest Pain	Heart Attack & Angina ⚑	178
	Congestive Heart Failure (CHF) ⚑	179
	Heartburn	205
	Aortic Aneurysm/Dissection ⚑	180
	Pulmonary Embolism (PE) ⚑	182
	Spontaneous Pneumothorax ⚑	185
Abrupt & Severe Headache	Subarachnoid Hemorrhage (CVA) ⚑	181
Awake & Confused to V P U	Intracerebral Hemorrhage (CVA) ⚑	182
Speech Impediment	Ischemic Stroke (CVA) ⚑	182
Partial Paralysis	Transient Ischemic Attack (TIA) ⚑	182
Acute Respiratory Distress	Asthma ⚑	186
	Anaphylaxis ⚑	151
	Congestive Heart Failure (CHF) ⚑	179
	Pulmonary Embolism (PE) ⚑	182
	Spontaneous Pneumothorax ⚑	185
	Infectious Disease Index	225
General Malaise	Lower Airway Infection ⚑	183
Productive Cough	*Infectious Disease Index*	225
Sore Throat	Throat Infection ⚑	182
Bloody Nose	Nosebleed	201
	Broken Nose ⚑	201
Inattention	Seizure Disorder ⚑	192
Automatic Repetitive Behavior		
Seizures		
Awake & Confused to V P U	Hypoglycemia ⚑	189
History of Diabetes	Hyperglycemia ⚑	189
Burning Pain with Urination	Sexually Transmitted Disease (STD) ⚑	212
	Vaginitis ⚑	215
	Urinary Tract Infection (UTI) ⚑	212
	Prostatitis ⚑	217
Abnormal Vaginal Bleeding	Ectopic Pregnancy ⚑	214
	Miscarriage ⚑	214
Vaginal Itching or Irritation	Vaginitis ⚑	215
Testicular Pain & Tenderness	Testis Torsion ⚑	216
	Epididymitis ⚑	217

⚑ Always a Level 1 or Level 2 Evacuation
⚐ May be a Level 2 or Level 3 Evacuation depending on the severity of the patient's S/Sx
⚑ Typically a Level 3 Evacuation

174 Medical Illnesses

Major S/Sx & History	Possible Problems	Page
Ear Pain	Insect in External Ear Canal External Ear Infection Middle & Inner Ear Infections ▪ Ruptured Eardrum ▪	193 193 193 193
Eye Irritation or Pain	Foreign Body Open Globe Injury ▪ Subconjunctival Hemorrhage Corneal Abrasion Corneal Ulcer ▪ Chemicals (sunscreen, insect repellent) Photokeratitis Conjunctivitis ▪ Stye *Infectious Disease Index*	197 197 197 197 197 197 114, 197 197 197 225
Teeth or Gum Pain & Tenderness	Fractured/Broken Tooth ▪ Avulsed Tooth Lost Filling or Crown ▪ Tooth Infection ▪ Gum Infection ▪	202 202 202 202 202
Skin Rash	Fungal Infection (Tinea & Candida) ▪ *Infectious Disease Index* Allergic Reaction ▫ Toxic Reaction ▫	204 225 149 140
Abdominal Pain & Tenderness ± Nausea & Vomiting ± Diarrhea ± Fever	*Abdominal Pain & Tenderness Table* *Infectious Disease Index* Gastroenteritis (Intestinal Infection) ▫ Abdominal Aortic Aneurysm/Dissection ▪ Appendicitis ▪ Constipation Diverticulitis ▪ Ectopic Pregnancy ▪ Gall Stones ▫ Inguinal Hernia ▫ Intestinal Gas Kidney Stones ▫ Ovarian Cyst ▫ Pancreatitis ▫ Pelvic Inflammatory Disease (PID) ▪ Peptic Ulcer ▫	176 225 206 180 209 211 209 214 208 210 210 211 216 208 213 207
Red Blood & Pain with Stool	Constipation Hemorrhoids	211 211

▪ Always a Level 1 or Level 2 Evacuation
▫ May be a Level 2 or Level 3 Evacuation depending on the severity of the patient's S/Sx
▪ Typically a Level 3 Evacuation

Field Assessment of Abdominal Pain & Tenderness

Onset	Quality	Character	Region	Radiate	Severity	Additional History, S/Sx, & Notes	Possible Problem	Page
Slow	Crampy	Diffuse	RLQ LLQ		1-10	Hx: gas-producing food, altitude; S/Sx: cramps, relief after flatulence	Intestinal Gas	210
Slow	Bloated	Diffuse	LLQ		1-5	Hx: no bowel movement, dehydration, no/low fiber diet; S/Sx: cramps, distended abdomen	Constipation	211
Rapid	Crampy	Diffuse	Entire Abdomen		5-10	Hx: ± poor hygiene, ± contaminated food or water; S/Sx: nausea, vomiting, diarrhea & fever	Gastroenteritis	206
Sudden	Burning Sharp	Local early Diffuse late	Epigastric	Back	8-10	Hx: antacid, aspirin or NSAID use; S/Sx: nausea & vomiting, ± blood in vomitus or stool	Peptic Ulcer	207
Variable	Colicky	Local	Epigastric RUQ	Scapula Back	8-10	Hx: ± gallstones, recent fatty meal; S/Sx: ± nausea, vomiting & fever	Gallstones	208
Slow Steady	Dull Ache	Diffuse early Local late	RUQ LUQ	Back	5-10	Hx: alcohol abuse; S/Sx: nausea, vomiting, loss of appetite, ± diarrhea; fever, increased pulse, guarding if severe	Pancreatitis	208
Sudden	Sharp	Local	RLQ LLQ		1-10	Hx: ± hernia, lifting heavy object; S/Sx: bulge in scrotal sac or inguinal crease	Inguinal Hernia	210
Slow Mod	Ache	Local	RLQ LLQ		5-10	Hx: sexually active; S/Sx: ± fever, weakness, abnormal vaginal bleeding, green/yellow vaginal discharge	Pelvic Inflammatory Disease	213
Rapid	Variable	Diffuse early Local late	RLQ LLQ		5-10	Hx: ± ovarian cyst; S/Sx: nausea, vomiting, ± guarding	Ovarian Cyst	216
Sudden	Sharp Stabbing	Local	Flank Back	RLQ LLQ Groin	8-10	Hx: ± kidney stones; S/Sx: ± blood in urine	Kidney Stones	211
Slow	Ache	Local	LLQ		1-5	Hx: straining at defecation; typically male > 40 y/o; S/Sx: fever, diarrhea, bloody stools	Diverticulitis	209
Slow	Ache	Diffuse early Local late	RLQ		1-5	Hx: no appendectomy; S/Sx: ± fever, guarding, rebound pain, + heel drop test	Appendicitis	209
Variable	Variable	Diffuse early Local late	RLQ LLQ Pelvis	Shoulder	1-5	Hx: missed period, ± morning nausea, sexually active; S/Sx: cramping & spotting prior to rupture; Notes: Rule-out with negative pregnancy test	Ectopic Pregnancy	214

RUQ = Right Upper Quadrant   LUQ = Left Upper Quadrant   RLQ = Right Lower Quadrant   LLQ = Left Lower Quadrant

NOTE: There is considerable overlap in the above categories, and the conditions described can present in an atypical manner not covered in this chart. When in doubt, begin an urgent (2/1) evacuation for physician evaluation. See evacuation levels on pages 55 and 172-173.

Field Assessment of Abdominal Pain & Tenderness continued...

Onset	Quality	Character	Region	Radiate	Severity	Additional History, S/Sx, & Notes	Possible Problem	Page
Abrupt	Sharp	Local	RLQ LLQ	Back	10	Hx: None S/Sx: ± tenderness over site prior to rupture, pain appears with rupture and is often followed by death. Notes: Typically 50-80 y/o males or due to extreme exertion/stress	Abdominal Aortic Aneurysm	180
Abrupt	Tearing Ripping	Local	RLQ LLQ	Back	10	Hx: None S/Sx: No early S/Sx. S/Sx are variable depending on the location; death from volume shock is possible Notes: Rule out with negative pregnancy test	Abdominal Aortic Dissection	180

RUQ = Right Upper Quadrant   LUQ = Left Upper Quadrant   RLQ = Right Lower Quadrant   LLQ = Left Lower Quadrant

NOTE: There is considerable overlap in the above categories, and the conditions described can present in an atypical manner not covered in this chart. When in doubt, begin an urgent (2/1) evacuation for physician evaluation. See evacuation levels on pages 55 and 172-173.

Circulatory System Problems

Atherosclerosis

Pathophysiology

Over time healthy arteries may become obstructed by plaque, as fats—cholesterol and triglycerides—are deposited within their walls. The depositions lead to inflammation and scarring, and the normal elastic nature of the arterial walls is eventually lost. As the plaque thickens, the blood flow at the site of the constriction is reduced, slowing the delivery of blood and nutrients to the downstream tissue, and blood pressure increases. The process is so gradual that the body accepts the existence of arterial plaque as a normal development. If the plaque ruptures, the body senses an "abnormal" disturbance in the arterial wall and initiates the clotting process at the site of the disturbance. Once the clot is fixed in place, it cuts off perfusion to the tissue serviced by the artery. If the tissue is not adequately supplied by collateral circulation, it will die. Clots may also break-off, travel, and lodge in a smaller artery anywhere in the body (arterial embolism). Note that embolotic clots may also originate in the venous vessels for other reasons than atherosclerosis; see the discussion on Pulmonary Embolism, page 182. An embolus, regardless of its origin, that becomes trapped in the vasculature of the lung or brain, can rapidly cause death. Risk factors for atherosclerosis include obesity, a high-fat diet, high blood pressure, smoking, no or low exercise, chronic stress, and a family history of atherosclerosis.

Prevention

- Eliminate the associated risk factors by eating a healthy diet, by engaging in a daily aerobic exercise program, by not smoking, by treating high blood pressure, and by limiting stress.
- Trace minerals that help strengthen the circulatory system include copper, chromium, calcium, magnesium, and selenium.
- Additional supplements include Vitamins E and C, lecithin, and coenzyme Q. Avoid excess vitamin D.
- Herbs that support circulation include raw garlic, ginger, and licorice.
- Medications are available to decrease serum cholesterol and to control high blood pressure.

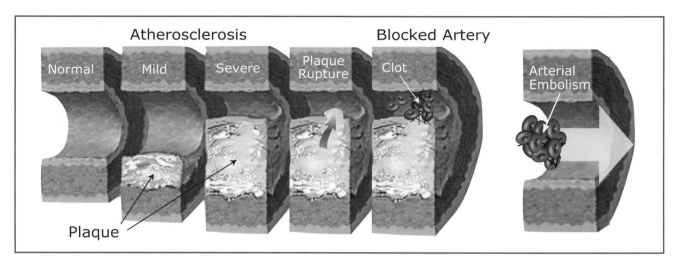

Atherosclerosis | Blocked Artery

Normal | Mild | Severe | Plaque Rupture | Clot | Arterial Embolism

Plaque

Heart Attack

Pathophysiology

Developing atherosclerosis, plaque rupture, and subsequent clotting of a coronary artery is the most common cause of a heart attack. Signs and symptoms commonly appear immediately and are due to a lack of oxygen in the affected tissue. Cardiac arrest evolves along a continuum and is not predictable. Arrest is ultimately due to a change in the electrical impulses and conduction pattern (cardiac arrhythmia) in the specialized cardiac nerves that stimulate normal cardiac contractions. An injury to these nerves blocks the conduction pathway. The block prevents or delays the electrical impulses from reaching their destination and causes cardiac arrest. The potential for arrest from a heart attack is directly related to the type, location, and size of the compromised tissue. If the blocked artery services the specialized conduction cells that coordinate the pumping action of the heart, arrest occurs within seconds or minutes. If the blocked artery services the heart's contractile fibers rather than its specialized conduction cells, the pumping action of the heart may be compromised. A reduction in the heart's ability to pump blood efficiently may cause a back pressure in the pulmonary vessels and force fluid into the alveoli; this causes respiratory distress (congestive heart failure), fatigue, swelling in the hands and feet, indigestion and loss of appetite. Complete pump failure and arrest may develop if a significant amount of heart muscle has been injured and the heart cannot continue to meet the body's demands for nutrients (cardiogenic shock). The longer arrest is delayed, the more likely the patient will survive without immediate hospital treatment. Patients who survive heart attacks are usually tired and "feel sick" with slightly elevated pulse and respiration rates. Recovery often takes months or years. Subsequent heart attacks are possible.

Atherosclerosis reduces the amount of oxygen available to the heart by effectively shrinking the size of the arteries with plaque deposits. Exercise and stress can increase the heart's need for oxygen beyond the delivery capacity of the restricted arteries. The resulting hypoxia causes heart pain or angina. Once the exercise or stress is removed, the oxygen requirements of the patient's heart will return to normal levels and the chest pain will subside, usually within 20 minutes.

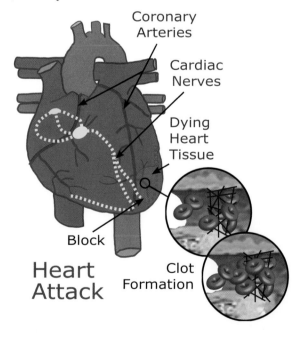

Coronary Arteries

Cardiac Nerves

Dying Heart Tissue

Block

Heart Attack

Clot Formation

Prevention

- Eliminate the risk factors for atherosclerosis.
- Herbs that help control blood cholesterol levels, triglyceride levels, and blood pressure include hawthorn, globe artichoke, black cohosh, evening primrose, and lily of the valley.
- In consultation with a physician, persons with atherosclerosis should consider taking two tablets of chewable baby aspirin per day to prevent coronary clotting.
- In consultation with a physician, persons with atherosclerosis should consider medications for controlling serum cholesterol levels and high blood pressure.
- Rx cardiac medications—vasodilators like nitroglycerin—are available to relieve angina, but do nothing to treat the underlying plaque.

Assessment

- The classic signs and symptoms of a heart attack are non-traumatic chest pain or pressure accompanied by shortness of breath and diaphoresis (pale sweating skin). ***Initially it is difficult to tell the difference between angina and a heart attack.***

Assessment of Angina

- The patient complains of non-traumatic chest pain when exercising, under stress, or if unstable, at rest.
- The chest pain will usually resolve within 20 minutes after stopping the exercise or removing the stressor.
- The chest pain is relieved within 3-5 minutes after administering nitroglycerin.

Assessment of Heart Attacks

- The patient complains of non-traumatic chest pain. The pain may mimic indigestion and is typically described as pressure or squeezing. The pain may radiate to the patient's neck or arms (classically the left arm, but can be either arm, or both).
- Rule out musculoskeletal mechanisms.
- Shortness of breath is common, as are sweating and pale skin.
- Fatigue and weakness are present.
- Many patients deny the possibility of a heart attack.

Assessment of Cardiac Arrest

- Cardiac arrest evolves along a continuum and is not predictable. From the onset of chest pain, arrest may occur within seconds to minutes if the heart's conduction cells are affected or within hours if a "large" area of cardiac muscle is damaged and pump performance is decreased (cardiogenic shock). Arrest is unlikely if a very small area of cardiac muscle is affected and pump performance remains relatively unaffected.

Assessment of Cardiogenic Shock

- Cardiogenic shock occurs when pump performance is decreased after tissue damage from a heart attack. If severe enough, it will lead to cardiac arrest.
- Rising pulse and respiration rates, decreasing mental status, and a falling blood pressure are the hallmarks S/Sx of cardiogenic shock.

Assessment of Congestive Heart Failure

- CHF occurs when the left ventricle is damaged from a heart attack and can no longer effectively pump blood to the body. The blood backs up in the pulmonary vein, increasing pressure in the pulmonary capillaries and forcing plasma into the alveoli.
- Increased respiratory distress and developing edema (fluid) in the lungs, hands, and feet indicate congestive heart failure.
- Fatigue, weakness, and fainting, accompanied by weight gain, are common S/Sx of CHF, as are loss of appetite, indigestion, nausea and vomiting.

Field Treatment

Treatment of Angina & Heart Attacks

- Because it is difficult to distinguish between angina and a heart attack in the initial stages, field treatment is identical.
- If respiratory distress is present, allow the patient to sit or support them in a sitting position. Provide rest, reassurance, and oxygen.
- Begin a Level 1 Evacuation with ALS for all patients with a suspected heart attack.
- Administer 160-325 mg of chewable baby aspirin with the onset of chest pain. The aspirin acts as an anticoagulant and may help minimize cardiac damage, especially in patients with partial blockages.
- Administer nitroglycerin in awake patients who have a current prescription. Adult dose is one tablet (.4 mg) dissolved under the patient's tongue OR .4 mg delivered as a metered spray. The dose may be repeated every 5 minutes for three doses. Nitroglycerin will cause a tingling or burning

sensation in the patient's mouth if it is active. Headaches are common following the administration of nitroglycerin and rarely last longer than 20 minutes. Chest pain should resolve within a 3-5 minutes if due to angina.

Treatment of Cardiac Arrest

• Begin CCR (chest compressions only) if the patient's arrest is due to heart attack and rapid defibrillation—less than five minutes—and ALS intervention are possible. Compress hard and fast.

• Begin CPR (chest compressions and rescue breathing) if defibrillation and ALS intervention may be delayed for more than five minutes. Compress hard and fast. Ventilate until the patient's chest begins to rise; do not overinflate. The ratio of compressions to ventilations is thirty compressions to two breaths. Use high-flow supplemental oxygen if available. Be prepared for vomiting.

• If a defibrillator is available and VF or pulseless VT have been confirmed, defibrillate regardless of core temperature (an AED will advise shock).

• If resuscitation is successful, begin a Level 1 Evacuation to the nearest hospital.

• Consider stopping resuscitation efforts after 30 minutes of pulselessness.

Treatment of Cardiogenic Shock

• Support critical systems and begin a Level 1 Evacuation with ALS to a major hospital.

Treatment of Congestive Heart Failure

• Allow the patient to sit or support them in a sitting position. Provide rest, reassurance, and high-flow oxygen.

• If the patient has a history of CHF and their own diuretic medication, allow them to continue taking it on schedule.

• If the patient has a prescription for nitroglycerin, they should take it.

• Begin a Level 1 Evacuation with ALS to a major hospital.

Aortic Aneurysm & Dissection

Pathophysiology

Aneurysms tend to occur at weak spots in an arterial wall as the patient's blood pressure forces the weak area to bulge and balloon outward. While aneurysms can develop in any artery, the majority occur in the abdominal and thoracic aortas where the pressure is greatest. Blood flow slows as it passes through an aneurysm and clot formation at the site is common. Once formed, a clot may break off, travel downstream, and become lodged in a small artery, cutting off the local blood supply. Large aneurysms may rupture causing internal bleeding and potentially volume shock. A large rupture is usually fatal, while a small leak may provide enough warning for evacuation and treatment.

In an aortic dissection, the inner lining of the aortic wall slowly deteriorates and then finally, and abruptly, rips. As blood erupts through the tear, it separates the inner and outer layers forming a new channel within the arterial wall. From there, a number of things can happen. If the tear is close to branching arteries, the dissected portion of the wall can block blood from entering. Both damage and S/Sx will reflect the location of the blockage: stroke, heart attack, sudden abdominal pain, low-back pain, and nerve damage are possible. If blood leaks into the stuff sacks surrounding the heart, it will prevent the heart from filling and pumping effectively. If the blood leaks into the chest or abdominal cavity, it will cause local pain and potentially, volume shock.

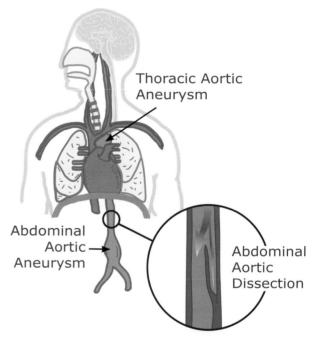

Thoracic Aortic Aneurysm

Abdominal Aortic Aneurysm

Abdominal Aortic Dissection

Prevention

• Eliminate the risk factors for atherosclerosis.

• Strongly consider taking medications for controlling serum cholesterol levels and high blood pressure.

Assessment

- Most aneurysms and dissections have no early S/Sx.
- Upon rupture or dissection, patients generally report sudden, severe pain.

Assessment of Thoracic Aortic Aneurysms

- Patients with thoracic aneurysms may report chest pain or pain between their shoulder blades. Some develop coughing and wheezing.
- If a thoracic aneurysm is high enough to affect the subclavian arteries, the patient's blood pressure tends to have more than a 10-point spread between arms. If you don't have a BP cuff, simply feel the pulse in each radial artery; if you notice a difference in strength, treat as a potential dissection.
- Upon rupture, pain tends to begin high in the back and radiate down the back into the abdomen as the rupture progresses. Patients may also report chest pain that radiates to the arms as per a heart attack. Rapid death from volume shock is common.

Assessment of Abdominal Aortic Aneurysms

- An abdominal aortic aneurysm may occur at any age, but is most common in men aged 50-80 years.
- Some patients with abdominal aneurysms report a pulsing sensation within their abdomen and/or a deep, penetrating pain in their back. Rapidly enlarging aneurysms that are about to rupture commonly hurt or feel tender when pressed during an abdominal examination.
- Upon rupture, there is usually excruciating pain in the lower abdomen and back and tenderness over the site of the aneurysm. Rapid death from volume shock is common.

Assessment of Aortic Dissections

- Aortic dissections occur with no early S/Sx.
- Pain may be variable, but tends to be abrupt, excruciating, often described as tearing or ripping. The pain follows the dissection as it advances along the aorta. Additional S/Sx vary and depend upon whether the dissected portion blocks a branching artery and/or if blood leaks into the chest or abdomen. The patient may present with the S/Sx of a stroke, heart attack, sudden abdominal pain, low-back pain, nerve damage, and volume shock are possible.

Field Treatment

- Begin a Level 1 Evacuation if either an aortic aneurysm or dissection is suspected.

Stroke

Pathophysiology

Most strokes are caused by either embolotic clots breaking off from the carotid arteries and drifting downstream into the cerebral vasculature, or by the rupture of a cerebral artery (cerebral aneurism). With an ischemic stroke (clot), the tissue serviced by the blocked artery loses perfusion and dies within a few minutes. Hemorrhagic strokes (bleeding) may lead to increased ICP. The signs and symptoms reflect the amount of brain damage. In extremely mild cases, the patient has no noticeable loss of function and the stroke may go undetected. Serious cerebral blocks or aneurysms may be large enough to be instantly fatal. The loss of sensation and motor function in the patient is proportional to the severity and location of the stroke. Because the cerebrum is divided into two hemispheres by the corpus callosum (right and left brain), and each hemisphere is serviced by a separate arterial supply, tissue damage caused by a stroke is usually confined to a single side. Motor and sensory functions for the head and face are serviced by cranial nerves, while the remainder 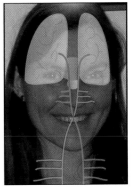 of the body is serviced by spinal nerves. Because the spinal nerves cross in the brain stem, loss of sensation and motor function in the head and face reflect damage to the same side of the brain, while a loss of function below the head reflects damage to the opposite side of the brain.

Prevention

- Eliminate the risk factors for atherosclerosis.
- Consider taking medications for controlling serum cholesterol levels and high blood pressure.

Assessment

Assessment of Subarachnoid Hemorrhages

- The patient will complain of abrupt and severe headache, with or without stiff neck, nausea, and vomiting. Death may occur rapidly or may be delayed 2-5 days. Subarachnoid bleeds may occur in young, healthy people.

Assessment of Intracerebral Hemorrhagic or Ischemic Strokes

- Awake patients may show a decrease in motor and sensory skills on one side of face and the opposite side of the body, slurred speech, partial paralysis, lethargy, with or without a headache and amnesia. Ask the patient to smile and repeat a simple rhyme; test arm and grip strength for equality.
- Most awake patients are lethargic and tired immediately following a stroke.
- Some patients may present with a depressed level of consciousness. These patients generally have a poorer prognosis.
- S/Sx may disappear within 24 hours. Medically, this is known as a Transient Ischemic Attack (TIA) and in a remote setting is treated as a stroke.

Field Treatment

- Administer oxygen.
- Sleep is a necessary part of the recovery process. A stroke patient should be permitted to sleep, be closely monitored while sleeping, and be awakened every few hours during the 24-hour period following the event.
- ***Begin a Level 1 Evacuation for all stroke patients to a major hospital; small strokes may be followed by more serious ones.*** IV thrombolytic medications are indicated ASAP and typically must be given within three hours if the stroke is caused by a blocked blood vessel and there are no contraindications. Mechanical clot removal may be of benefit up to 12 hours after the initial insult. Surgery may be indicated if the stroke is due to a ruptured vessel. A CAT scan is required to distinguish between the various treatment options.

Pulmonary Embolism
Pathophysiology

A pulmonary embolism (PE) is a complication arising from blood clots that primarily form in the deep veins of the lower legs, but occasionally form in the pelvis, upper extremities, kidneys, or the right ventricle. Parts of the clots break off and travel with the venous blood through the right side of the heart and into the lungs, where they become lodged in the pulmonary vasculature. The immediate effects of the blockage are decreased blood oxygen levels and increased respiratory and pulse rates. If the condition is not treated, the affected tissue will die. Pulmonary arterial pressure also increases because of the blockages; if severe enough, the pressure and blood back up into the right ventricle causing right ventricular failure and death. Presenting S/Sx depend on the size of the clots, their number and their location. While the majority of cases of pulmonary embolisms are associated with bedridden and postsurgical patients, a pulmonary embolism should be considered in all patients who present with unexplained respiratory distress or chest pain.

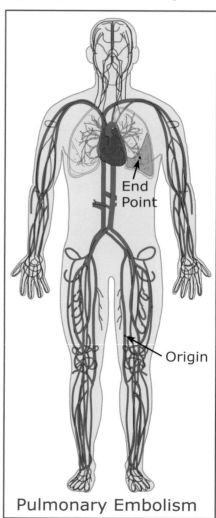

End Point

Origin

Pulmonary Embolism

Risk factors:

- Immobilization—in a litter, cast, or as a result of bed rest—slows venous circulation and increases the chance of clot formation.
- Trauma predisposes patients to clot formation by activating clotting factors and causing immobility. Femur and tibia fractures have the highest risk,

followed by pelvic, spinal, and other fractures. Severe burns also increase risk in a similar manner.

- Estrogen-containing birth control pills increase the potential for clots in healthy women. The risk is proportional to the estrogen content and is further increased in postmenopausal women on hormonal replacement therapy.

- Blacks are at 50% greater risk than whites for PE while whites are at 50% greater risk than other races.

Assessment

S/Sx are highly variable and are often mistakenly attributed to other causes; atypical S/Sx are common and make diagnosis difficult, even for physicians. S/Sx may include:

- Shortness of breath. Rales are possible.
- Increased pulse and respirations.
- Coughing with or without blood.
- Pleuritic chest pain (chest pain upon deep inhalation); chest pain may be indistinguishable from a heart attack.

Field Treatment

- Begin an Level 1 Evacuation if a pulmonary embolism is suspected.

Respiratory System Problems

Respiratory Tract Infections

(Sinus, Throat, & Lower Airway Infections)

Pathophysiology

Most respiratory tract infections are transmitted through close contact with an infected patient, usually through shared water bottles, coughing, sneezing, or poor sanitation. These infections commonly infect most members of small expeditions where close contact is unavoidable. Respiratory infections are also associated with near-drowning episodes and rib fractures. Most respiratory tract infections are either bacterial or viral in origin. Viral infections destroy the integrity of the infected tissue and are often followed by secondary bacterial infections. While bacterial infections often produce yellow- or green-colored phlegm, in viral infections the mucus is usually clear; however, phlegm color is not a reliable diagnostic tool. A culture may provide definitive diagnosis.

Sinus Infection Pathophysiology

The sinuses are normally sterile. Inflammation is secondary to obstruction and subsequent infection by a virus in the nasopharynx; a secondary bacterial infection often follows. Sinus infections are often transmitted by sneezing and are characterized by a runny nose (increased mucus production), sneezing, congestion, headache, and in rare cases, fever. Severe sinus infections may travel up the eustachian tubes and become established in the middle or inner ear.

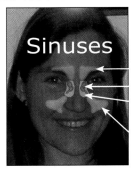

Pathophysiology of Throat Infections

In throat infections, the infecting organism becomes established in the soft tissue of the throat, causing inflammation, a sore throat, and dry cough. More serious infections may become systemic. Most sore throats are caused by a viral infection and resolve on their own without consequence. A few however, result from a group A streptococcus bacterial infection, known simply as "Strep." Some people are asymptomatic carriers. Untreated Strep can cause a variety of life-threatening illnesses: kidney inflammation, toxic shock, skin and soft tissue infections, and rheumatic fever. Rheumatic fever can, although rarely does, lead to inflamed and painful joints and damage heart valves. Strep is highly contagious and primarily transmitted via skin contact or respiratory droplets, depending on the strain; food and water-borne outbreaks have occurred. Strep can be difficult to diagnose without a lab. Throat infections may spread to include the middle ear and sinuses.

Pathophysiology of Lower Airway Infections

Inflammation of the trachea and bronchi is due to a viral or bacterial infection. In most lower respiratory tract infections (bronchitis) the microorganism makes its way into the lower airway causing increased mucus secretion, a productive cough, and mild respiratory distress. This is usually accompanied by muscle soreness, a low-grade fever, and general fatigue. If the infection becomes well established, it may spread into the alveoli (pneumonia) and respiratory signs and symptoms will increase. Rales, or wet lung sounds, are often heard and increased fever, chills, and chest pain may develop; death is possible, but rare.

Prevention

- Avoid close contact with infected persons and maintain good expedition hygiene.
- Nutrition and rest strengthen the immune system and are useful in preventing respiratory tract infections.

Assessment

General Assessment

- The patient has a recent history of close contact with another infected patient, usually through coughing, sneezing or sharing water bottles.
- Although bacterial infections tend to produce yellow- or green-colored phlegm, in viral infections the mucus is usually clear, however, phlegm color is not a reliable diagnostic tool. A culture may provide definitive diagnosis.

Assessment of Sinus Infections

- Patient may have a recent history of severe throat infection.
- Patients usually present with a persistent cold, nasal congestion, colored discharge, facial pain and tenderness, headache, and eye pain, if ethmoid sinus is involved. Pain is often exacerbated by leaning forward or by any head movement.
- An anticipated problem is a middle or inner ear infection if the infecting organism travels up the eustachian tubes.

Assessment of Throat Infections

- A sore throat may be caused by post nasal drip and NOT by a throat infection. Post nasal drip is usually caused by allergies; although birth control medication or pregnancy may also be causes because they contribute to elevated levels of estrogen hormones.
- Signs and symptoms include local inflammation, a sore throat, dry cough, or possibly no cough, and no congestion. Fever and swollen lymph glands occur with more severe infections.
- In addition to the above S/Sx, strep typically presents with red and swollen tonsils, with or without white patches or streaks of pus, and petechiae (tiny red spots) at the back and on the roof of the

mouth. Heart and kidney complications related to bacterial strep throat, although very rare are possible if improperly assessed and treated. Depress the patient's tongue with a clean spoon handle and use an otoscope, penlight, or head lamp to view the back of their throat.

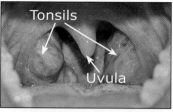
Normal

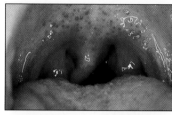
Inflammation & Petechiae

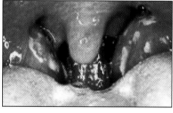
Pus patches on tonsils

- An anticipated problem is a middle or inner ear infection if the infecting organism travels up the eustachian tubes.

Assessment of Lower Airway Infections

- The patient may have a recent history of near drowning, fractured ribs, or contact with an infected person.
- A productive cough, fever, malaise, nasal congestion, shortness of breath, chest pain, wheezing, and sore muscles are common; severe cases may develop rales.
- An anticipated problem is pneumonia.

Field Treatment

General Treatment

- Provide rest and assistance with thermoregulation.
- Replace fluids and electrolytes. Encourage patients to increase their normal fluid intake (force fluids). Monitor the patient's urine to assess their hydration status.
- Fevers above 102° F are best controlled with acetaminophen using the OTC dose. Herbs that help control fever include yarrow and bark from white and black willows (aspirin). Because of the

potential for developing Reye's syndrome, aspirin is contraindicated in children under age 17.

- Do not use an antihistamine in the treatment of symptoms associated with cold, flu, or sinus infection. Antihistamines inhibit mucus production, and the associated runny nose, and restrict drainage permitting the infecting microorganism to multiply.

- Herbs that stimulate the immune system include echinacea/golden seal combination, ginseng/astragalus combination, and hyssop; all have antibiotic and antiviral properties.

- Herbal teas specific to relieving the symptoms of colds and flu include: catnip, bone set, osha, sage, thyme, and angelica.

- Because of the potentially serious complications of leaving respiratory tract infections untreated in a backcountry setting, a broad spectrum antibiotic may be indicated if evacuation is not possible. Indications for antibiotic use include local infections that do not respond to supportive treatment, infections that appear to get worse, and all systemic infections. The extended-range erythromycins (clarithromycin, azithromycin) are expensive, but target most respiratory tract infections. Clarithromycin is given by mouth at 250-500 mg 2 times a day for 10-14 days. Azithromycin is given by mouth at 500 mg 4 times a day on day 1 then 250 mg 4 times a day for four more days.

- Begin a Level 3 Evacuation if rest is not possible, S/Sx worsen, or strep is suspected.

Treatment of Sinus Infections

- Sinus infections usually resolve with symptomatic treatment in healthy people within 7-10 days; antibiotics may be required for acute bacterial infections.

- Steam inhalation therapy may ease congestion and pressure headaches.

- A systemic OTC decongestant is useful to relieve general congestion and to promote drainage. Eyebright tea may also be used to relieve nasal congestion.

- A local OTC decongestant (nasal spray) is helpful before bed to promote rest. Have the patient inhale the spray deeply into their sinuses and hold for ten seconds.

- Consider sinus flush using a Neti pot and warm salt water 2-4 times per day until S/Sx resolve.

Regular flushing has proven to be as effective as antibiotic treatment.

- TMP/SMX or amoxicillin are the drugs of choice, but azithromycin and clarithromycin are also effective.

Treatment of Throat Infections

- An OTC cough suppressant or cough drops may be useful to suppress irritation caused by a dry nonproductive cough. Mullein and black cherry bark are effective herbal cough suppressants. Give as syrup, tea, or lozenge.

- Gargling with warm salt water or thyme tea may help reduce inflammation.

- Begin a Level 3 Evacuation if strep is suspected; the patient cannot remain in field. Isolate the patient from the rest of the group; DO NOT let them handle or cook group food, or clean dishes after eating. Penicillin VK is the drug of choice; however, azithromycin and clarithromycin are also effective.

Treatment of Lower Airway Infections

- Most lower respiratory tract infections are self-limiting in healthy people within 7-10 days; antibiotics are not indicated.

- An OTC expectorant may be useful during the day. Herbal expectorants include skunk cabbage, pleurisy root, and lungwort.

- An OTC non-narcotic cough suppressant may be administered before bed to permit rest. Black cherry bark or mullein taken as a tea are two effective herbal cough treatments.

- Steam inhalation therapy may ease daily episodes of respiratory distress. Sage or eucalyptus oil may be added for their antimicrobial properties.

Spontaneous Pneumothorax

Pathophysiology

A spontaneous pneumothorax occurs when a weak spot in the stuff sack covering the lung (parietal pleura) forms a small blister and eventually ruptures. The rupture occurs without warning—usually at the top of the lung—and permits air to leak into the pleural space, collapsing the lung. Healthy patients with no underlying lung disease or damage tolerate the loss of lung capacity fairly well; some may be asymptomatic. Those with an underlying lung problem tend to present with respiratory distress at rest. Alternately, air can escape into the surrounding tissue and present as small crackling bubbles within the tissue of the chest, neck, and throat (subcutaneous emphysema). Severity of the S/Sx varies depending on the size of the rupture; some are asymptomatic. Reoccurrence is common and patients may have a history of a similar episode, typically in the same lung. Smoking greatly increases the risk for both conditions. Males are at greater risk than females.

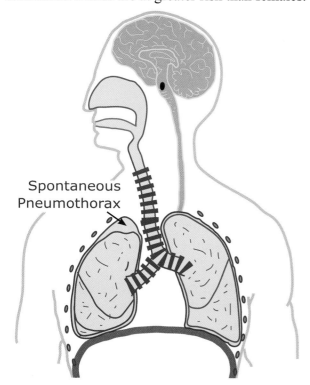

Spontaneous Pneumothorax

Assessment

Assessment of Spontaneous Pneumothorax

• A spontaneous pneumothorax is more common in tall, thin, young males.

• The patient experiences abrupt chest pain upon rupture on the same side as the rupture.

• The pain may radiate down the arm if the pneumothorax puts pressure on the brachial plexus. The pain is sharp and different from the squeezing chest pain of MI. Pain generally diminishes after rupture and completely resolves within 24 hours.

• Respiratory distress may be present upon exercise or at rest with patients who have an underlying lung disease (asthma, pneumonia, respiratory infection, emphysema, etc.). Most patients complain of shortness of breath. Many will assume a standing tripod position during exertion and be unable to speak normally without taking a breath.

Assessment of Pneumomediastinum

• Subcutaneous emphysema

• The patient may present with jaw or neck pain, difficulty swallowing, sore throat, and/or coughing. Some patients will experience mild respiratory distress.

Field Treatment

General Treatment

• If available, administer oxygen; it increases blood oxygen levels and enhances the reabsorption of free air.

Treatment of Spontaneous Pneumothorax

• Begin a Level 2 Evacuation for patients with mild S/Sx. Mild cases (less than 15% of lung capacity) often resolve on their own over the next three months. More serious cases require needle aspiration or a chest tube.

• Begin a Level 1 Evacuation for patients with moderate or severe respiratory distress or patients with mild respiratory distress and an underlying lung condition such as asthma or a respiratory infection.

Treatment of Pneumomediastinum

• Begin a Level 3 Evacuation with mild S/Sx. Pneumomediastinum is generally benign and will resolve without complications with rest; however, more serious complications, for example, tension pneumothorax, are possible and the patient should be evacuated for further evaluation.

• Begin a Level 2 Evacuation for patients with more serious S/Sx.

Asthma

Pathophysiology

Asthma is a chronic disease of the respiratory tree that, with exposure to a causal agent, produces an immediate bronchial spasm, increased mucus production, and subsequent bronchial constriction. Secondary swelling due to the inflammatory response is possible during the first 24 hours following the attack. In persons suffering from chronic and severe asthma, the smooth muscular walls of the bronchi thicken, making subsequent attacks increasingly more dangerous. The primary agents for inducing an asthmatic episode are cold, exercise, allergens, and stress. Patients present with the signs and symptoms of respiratory distress immediately following exposure. Severe asthma attacks may be fatal, if not treat-

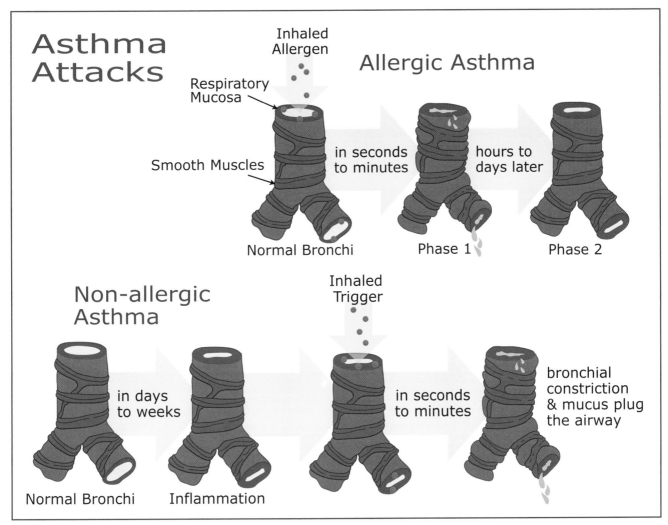

Asthma Attacks

Inhaled Allergen

Respiratory Mucosa

Smooth Muscles

Normal Bronchi

Allergic Asthma

in seconds to minutes

hours to days later

Phase 1

Phase 2

Non-allergic Asthma

Inhaled Trigger

Normal Bronchi

Inflammation

in days to weeks

in seconds to minutes

bronchial constriction & mucus plug the airway

ed. The disease falls into two basic categories: allergic and non-allergic asthma. Many asthma patients have components of both types. In allergic asthma, IgE attaches to mast cells within the respiratory mucosa. Within seconds of exposure to an inhaled allergen, the mast cells degranulate and release histamine into the local tissue, causing a local allergic reaction that leads to increased permeability, inflammation, mucus production, and bronchial constriction. The initial phase of the attack tends to respond well to inhaled bronchodilators. The second phase occurs hours to days later as inflammatory cells accumulate in the respiratory mucosa; the second phase may be prevented using inhaled or oral corticosteroids. Either phase may result in respiratory arrest and death.

In most non-allergic asthma attacks, inflammation starts and builds days to weeks prior to the attack. Common inflammatory triggers are stress, chemicals (including the sulfating agents commonly used to preserve food), respiratory infections, and general respiratory tract irritants. Exercise-in-

duced asthma usually occurs within 5-20 minutes after exercise with inhalation of cold and/or dry air increasing the severity of the response. A severe attack may result in respiratory arrest and death.

Regardless of the precipitating event or trigger, ALL types of asthma share the following pathophysiologic and treatment components:

- Inflammation and swelling of the respiratory mucosa.
- Bronchial constriction.
- Extreme mucus production.
- A severe attack may result in respiratory arrest.
- Therapy focuses on prevention and emergency treatment.

Prevention

- Prior to the trip, persons responsible for the ongoing care of asthmatic trip members should consult with the patient's personal physician and procure written standing orders for and training in the emergency assessment and treatment of their disease.

- Avoid exposing people who have a prior history of asthma to their triggers.
- Short-acting bronchodilators (albuterol, levalbuterol, and pirbuterol) do not have any effect on inflammation and are used to prevent exercise-induced asthma when administered 15 to 30 minutes before physical activity. The normal dose is 2 puffs every 4-6 hours as needed, delivered by a MDI; a spacer is often prescribed.
- Low-to-medium-dose inhaled corticosteroids are often used with long-acting bronchodilators for persons with moderate-to-severe asthma. Dose varies with medication, delivery system (MDI or DPI), and patient. Patients using a MDI should also use a spacer to enhance the delivery of the medication. All patients should rinse their mouth after each use to help prevent a local fungal infection (thrush) and systemic absorption of the drug.
- Long-acting bronchodilators (salmeterol and formoterol) DO NOT have any effect on inflammation and are ONLY used in conjunction with inhaled corticosteroids delivered with an MDI using a spacer or DPI. These act to lower the dose of corticosteroids needed for effective prevention.
- Mast cell stabilizers (cromolyn sodium and nedocromil) are primarily used by persons having allergy-induced asthma who cannot avoid the allergen, or those with exercise-induced asthma, who cannot avoid exercise. They are delivered with an MDI.

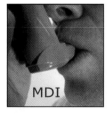 MDI 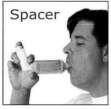 Spacer 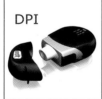 DPI

Assessment

- Most asthma patients have a prior history and are familiar with the disease and treatment procedures.
- Most patients will present with mild respiratory distress accompanied by wheezing that may or may not progress depending on the severity of the attack.
- In severe cases, a patient typically assumes an erect, eyes forward, sitting position and is focused on their breathing. Acute episodes may quickly develop into severe respiratory distress accompanied by a decrease in AVPU levels and cyanosis; respiratory arrest is possible.

- Severe asthma attacks may be fatal if left untreated.

Field Treatment

Emergency Field treatment

- Separate the patient from the trigger: stop exercise, warm and humidify the patient's air, remove the stressor, remove the allergen or irritant, etc.
- Reassure the patient, to both help slow their breathing rate and to permit more complete lung expansion. Supplemental oxygen is helpful.
- Short-acting bronchodilators are delivered using an MDI and spacer at 4-8 puffs every 20 minutes for up to four hours, then every 1-4 hours as needed. Wait 1 minute between puffs.
- Give an epinephrine injection to patients who do not respond to short-acting bronchial dilators; adult dose is 0.3 cc 1/1000 IM for a maximum of three doses.
- Oral corticosteroids (prednisone) may be used to speed recovery from severe asthma attacks and to help prevent reoccurrence.

Evacuation

- No evacuation is required for patients who respond to the normal dose of their bronchodilators.
- Begin a Level 3 Evacuation for patients who have more than 2 attacks per week, require frequent/emergency doses of their bronchodilator to successfully treat an attack, OR whose respiratory distress limits their participation in the trip.
- Begin a Level 2 Evacuation with ALS for patients who obtain only partial relief from frequent/emergency doses of their bronchodilator to successfully treat an attack OR experience respiratory distress at rest that interferes with normal conversation.
- Begin a Level 1 Evacuation with ALS for patients who obtain no relief from frequent/emergency doses of their bronchodilator and require epinephrine to successfully treat an attack, experience respiratory distress at rest and cannot speak, and/or are faint/unresponsive OR have any risk factor for death due to asthma.

Risk Factors for Death from Asthma

Asthma History

- Includes previous severe attacks that required intubation or ICU admission.
- Includes two or more hospitalizations for asthma in the past year.

- Includes three or more emergency room visits for asthma in the past year.
- Includes hospitalization or emergency room visit for asthma in the past month.
- Includes use of more than 2 canisters of short-acting bronchodilator per month.
- Includes difficulty perceiving asthma symptoms or severity of attacks.

Additional Risk Factors
- Lack of a written asthma action plan.
- Sensitivity to Alternaria, a plant fungus and major airway allergen or irritant.
- Moderate-to-severe attack at altitude.

Endocrine System Problems
Diabetic Emergencies
Pathophysiology

Diabetes is a multisystem disease with both biochemical and anatomical consequences. Diabetes is a disease of the pancreas and results from insufficient insulin production. The pancreas is a mixed gland with two functions: it releases digestive enzymes into the first part of the small intestine and it produces and releases the hormones glucagon and insulin into the blood to control blood sugar (glucose) levels. Glucagon facilitates the release of sugar stored in the liver into general circulation and raises blood sugar levels. Insulin facilitates the entry of sugar into cells, protein synthesis, and fat storage; insulin lowers blood sugar levels. Sugar is used by cells to synthesize the proteins and chemicals required for homeostasis. Normal blood sugar levels fall between 70-125 mg/dl; levels should be below 100 mg/dl in the morning prior to breakfast and rise after eating. Diabetes is typically diagnosed when blood sugar levels exceed 180 mg/dl or with two fasting glucose level test results of over 125 mg/dl. Blood sugar levels are measured from a pin-prick of blood using a glucometer.

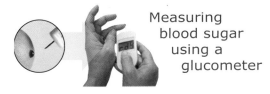
Measuring blood sugar using a glucometer

There are two forms of diabetes: Type 1 (insulin-dependent diabetes) and Type 2 (non-insulin-dependent diabetes).

Pathophysiology of Type 1 Diabetes

The primary cause of Type 1 diabetes is an autoimmune disease that attacks and kills the insulin-producing beta cells in the pancreas. In most cases, this eventually results in complete insulin dependence. In some cases (± 20%), the alpha cells that produce glucagon are also destroyed. When insulin is no longer available, blood sugar levels rise above normal levels; levels of 300-500 mg/dl are common in hyperglycemic diabetics. Protein synthesis and fat storage are severely inhibited or cease altogether. In an effort to maintain balanced concentration levels between the intra- and extra-cellular fluids, water moves from the cells into the extracellular space, dehydrating the cells and decreasing their function. Urine output significantly increases and excess sugar spills into the urine, making it sweet. When cells cannot uptake sugar, the body metabolizes fats. Fat metabolites (ketones) are strong organic acids capable of altering blood pH and often lead to coma and death.

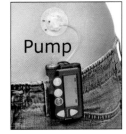
Pump

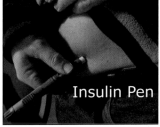
Insulin Pen

Type 1 diabetics control their blood sugar with regular insulin injections or an insulin pump. They must carefully monitor their blood sugar on a regular basis in order to balance their insulin dosing with their diet and energy requirements. Potentially life-threatening complications associated with the control of Type 1 diabetes include hypoglycemia, hyperglycemia, and diabetic ketoacidosis (DKA)

Pathophysiology of Type 2 Diabetes

Type 2 diabetes accounts for approximately 90% of all diabetes mellitus and tends to occur in mature adults; heredity, obesity, and low exercise are predisposing factors. Insulin production declines and insulin receptors fail to respond normally (insulin resistance), causing the characteristic rise in blood sugar. Treatment tends to focus on diet, weight loss, and exercise. Oral medications may include drugs that stimulate the pancreas to produce more insulin, lower insulin resistance, or decrease the amount of sugar released from the liver. The standard treatment regime is not always effective and some patients eventually require insulin injections to maintain control of their blood sugar. Potentially life threatening complications associated with the control of Type 2 diabetes, include hypoglycemia, hyperglycemia, diabetic ketoacidosis (DKA is rare in Type 2 diabetics), and hyperosmolar hyperglycemic state (HHS). The S/Sx of HSS are similar to DKA; however, no ketones are produced.

Complications

Hypoglycemia (low blood sugar)

Hypoglycemia or low blood sugar—less than 50 mg—may affect both Type 1 and Type 2 diabetics. It typically results from a combination of not eating and too much exercise or, rarely, too much insulin. Insulin causes cells to uptake glucose. Brain cells rely on glucose for normal functioning. If insulin levels are too high and corresponding blood glucose levels too low, brain cells will not get the glucose they need and will die. Onset occurs within minutes and if not quickly corrected, it can be fatal. Hypoglycemia is commonly encountered in a wilderness setting with insulin-dependent diabetic participants when the environmental conditions are harsh or the activity is new.

Hyperglycemia (high blood sugar)

Well-controlled diabetics may participate in wilderness activities, however, they MUST take extreme care to balance their blood sugar with their medications, food intake, and energy output. If their blood sugar level rises above 180 mg/dl, they should take steps to lower it ASAP. Left untreated, high blood sugar levels in a Type 1 diabetic lead to dehydration, an increase in ketones, and a potentially fatal drop in blood pH known as diabetic ketoacidosis (DKA). Hyperglycemia left untreated in a Type 2 diabetic will lead to severe dehydration and death (HHS) if water intake is not sufficient to balance the loss. Severe hyperglycemia is rare in a wilderness setting because most Type 1 diabetics who engage in wilderness activities know their personal patterns and have a good handle on their disease. When hyperglycemia does occur, it is usually due to loss of insulin or sudden illness and its onset is slow enough to detect and correct. Illness, especially infection, alters glucose requirements and increases susceptibility.

Prevention of Diabetic Emergencies

- *Control and treatment of diabetes is highly individualistic. Prior to the trip, persons responsible for the ongoing care of diabetic trip members should consult with the patient's personal physician and procure written standing orders for, and training in, the control and emergency assessment and treatment of their disease. Every diabetic patient should have a written "Sick Day Plan" prior to going into the field.*

- Balance food intake (complex carbohydrates and proteins) with energy output; if a diabetic's alpha cells have been destroyed, they will not produce glucagon and will not be able to access stored glucose. Most diabetics, who are new to outdoor pursuits/sports, severely underestimate the amount of energy required for the activity and commonly do not eat enough to avoid hypoglycemia. Avoid simple sugars, alcohol, and fats.

- Diabetics participating in outdoor activities should check their blood sugar numerous times (8+) during the day and adjust their diet and activity level accordingly.

- Both participants and trip leaders should carry glucose tabs and glucose paste for treatment of hypoglycemia; GU® energy gel works well.

- Maintain the patient's water balance; monitor urine output and color. Avoid dehydration.

- The patient should closely monitor and balance their blood insulin levels with their energy and sugar requirements. Some diabetics are more sensitive than others and require multiple adjustments of their insulin dose to maintain a balance. Any activity that requires additional energy will require more sugar and perhaps more insulin. Unless you have been thoroughly trained, you should not attempt to balance a participant or patient's blood insulin levels.

- Extremes in environmental temperatures affect insulin requirements. Plan wilderness outings and expeditions with diabetics to minimize exposure to temperature extremes.

- Bring additional diabetes-care supplies and ensure

Normal Blood Sugar	Low Blood Sugar	High Blood Sugar

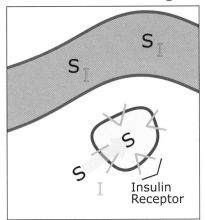

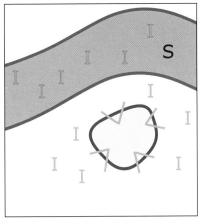

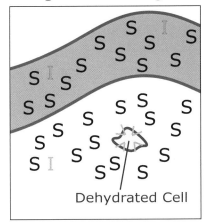

Insulin Receptor

Dehydrated Cell

Blood sugar 70-125 mg/dl

Blood sugar < 50 mg/dl

Blood sugar >180 mg/dl

Prevention

Type 1 diabetics should check their blood sugar levels 8+ times per day in order to balance caloric intake, exercise, and insulin levels.

Hypoglycemia

Too much insulin or not enough calories will cause a rapid and potentially fatal drop in blood glucose levels.

Hyperglycemia

Above 180 mg/dl, dehydration begins leaving the diabetic predisposed to heat illnesses, hypothermia, and AMS. If prolonged this will lead to DKA (Type 1) or HHS (Type 2).

---

that they are carried in different locations (packs, boats, etc.) to prevent accidental loss.

- Type 1 diabetics participating in outdoor activities should carry a glucagon kit for emergency treatment of hypoglycemia and urine test strips (Ketostix®, Chemstrip K®) for checking ketone levels in urine when sick or hyperglycemic.

Assessment

General Assessment

- All diabetics who travel in a wilderness environment will have a previous history, be in a treatment program, and may be taking insulin to control the disease. Some will be wearing a Medical Alert Tag or tattoo on their chest, wrist, or ankle. Have a complete patient history, including medications, dosages, and schedule, for any diabetic participants on wilderness trips.

 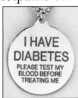 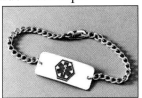

- *Most diabetic emergencies are due to hypoglycemia. Hyperglycemia is rare in a wilderness environment. When in doubt, treat for hypoglycemia.*

Assessment of Hypoglycemia

- In most cases, the patient has been taking their insulin, but has not eaten enough to maintain their blood sugar levels. In rare cases, the patient may have taken too much insulin with the same results. Blood sugar is less than 50 mg/dl for a hypoglycemic patient.

- Onset of acute hypoglycemia may occur within minutes once the patient has run out of sugar.

- Watch for a change in normal mental status to awake and lethargic, irritable, or confused. Patients often complain of headache, hunger, weakness, and dizziness. Respirations are normal or shallow; seizures are common.

- Assume any voice-responsive, pain-responsive, or unresponsive diabetic patient is suffering from hypoglycemia.

- Death is possible as brain cells starve and die from a lack of sugar. Although brain cells can use fat as an alternate energy source, the process is often too slow (hours) to prevent permanent brain damage or death.

Assessment of Hyperglycemia

- The patient has not taken their usual dose(s) of insulin or has an infection or illness.

- Blood sugar is greater than 180 mg/dl and frequently as high as 300-500 mg/dl.
- Check urine for ketones every 4-6 hours if blood sugar is greater than 240 mg/dl, using a ketone urine test strip (Ketostix®, Chemstrip K®).
- The onset of hyperglycemia S/Sx is delayed 24 to 72 hours or more as the controlled diabetic reverts back into an uncontrolled state. Patient is initially awake, restless, and usually thirsty with abdominal pain, nausea, and vomiting. The patient's urine output increases as blood sugar increases; dehydration is likely. Their skin is warm, flushed, and dry.
- Fruity breath and/or rapid, deep respirations indicate the patient's changing blood pH and diabetic ketoacidosis (DKA). Check the patient's urine for ketones. If not immediately corrected, the patient may die.

Field Treatment

Treatment of Hypoglycemia

- STOP and restrict exercise until blood sugar levels are normal for 24 hours.
- Feed awake diabetic patients. Begin with simple sugars (sugar tabs or paste, honey, candy, juice) and follow with complex carbohydrates and a protein-based meal (peanut butter works well).
- IV glucose is the definitive treatment for V, P, or U patients.
- If IV glucose is unavailable and the patient is V, P, or U, administer 0.5-1 unit of glucagon IM. If the patient does not respond in 10-20 minutes, repeat the dose for a maximum of 3 injections. If successful, glucagon administration will elevate the patient's blood sugar for several days. Maintain fluid balance; monitor urine output and color.
- DO NOT GIVE INSULIN. Once the patient has fully recovered, they should check their blood sugar and adjust their diet and insulin dose accordingly.
- Protect the patient from all environmental insults.
- Diabetics, who have a brief hypoglycemic episode that was easily corrected, are usually safe to stay in the field, but need to take additional care with insulin dosing and food intake to prevent a recurrence. Begin a Level 3 Evacuation if a second hypoglycemic episode occurs.
- Begin a Level 1 Evacuation with O₂ and ALS for all diabetic patients who remain V, P, or U.

Treatment of Hyperglycemia

- If the patient is awake, administer water and electrolytes (ORS) by mouth at 1 L per hour to flush ketones and to help raise blood pH during evacuation.
- DO NOT EXERCISE if ketones are high and blood sugar is greater than 240 mg/dl.
- Protect the patient's airway, suction as necessary.
- Begin a Level 1 Evacuation with O₂ and ALS.

Nervous System Problems
Seizures
Pathophysiology

Seizures are a disturbance of the brain's normal electrical activity; while they can have many causes, they may be subdivided into non-recurring and recurring seizures. Non-recurring seizures are typically part of a clinical pattern associated with a brain injury or illness, such as increased ICP, toxins, hypoglycemia in the insulin-dependent diabetic, lack of oxygen, heat stroke, HACE, and electrolyte sickness. Recurring seizures are collectively called seizure disorders or epilepsy. These fall into three main categories depending on their location in the brain: partial (or focal), generalized, and continuous.

While most partial or generalized seizures begin spontaneously, some require triggers, including flashing lights, specific sounds, etc. Control is usually achieved using anticonvulsant medications; the type and dose of the medications vary with each patient. Common medications used in the control of epilepsy are diphenylhydantoin (Dilantin®), phenobarbital, and diazepam (Valium®). The primary cause of seizures in patients undergoing treatment for seizure disorders is failure to take their anti-seizure medications. Seizure activity tends to follow patterns specific to individual patients. Seizures that fall outside their "normal" pattern should be evaluated. Exposure to new environments, participation in new activities, and alcohol withdrawal may trigger a seizure, even in patients current with their medications. Most seizures are self-limiting and are followed by an indeterminate recovery period dependent upon their cause. Initial field treatment is supportive, while definitive care must address the cause. People with seizure disorders are predisposed to depression and anxiety disorders, migraine and other headaches, and attention-deficit/hyperactivity disorder (ADHD).

Absence seizures are a type of generalized seizure that primarily occur in early childhood through adolescence. They begin with no warning, last 15-20 seconds and may lead to tonic-clonic seizures (described below) later in life. During an absence seizure, patients typically become very quiet and stare into space; the seizure may be accompanied by small subtle movements of the eyes, lips, and/or fingers. Immediately after the seizure, patients are often tired. While they have no memory of the seizure itself, they may be aware that a seizure has taken place.

Pathophysiology of Partial Seizures

Partial seizures remain focused in the area of the brain where they originate. S/Sx vary depending on the function of the cells affected. The patient usually remains conscious throughout the event and can later describe it. Many patients report weakness, numbness, unusual smells or tastes, visual changes, and vertigo. Motor symptoms, if they occur, tend to spread slowly from one part of the body to another. More complex partial seizures cause altered consciousness, although NOT unresponsiveness, and automatic repetitive behavior (walking in circles; sitting, then standing, again and again; smacking the lips repeatedly, etc.).

Pathophysiology of Generalized & Continuous Tonic-clonic Seizures

Generalized tonic-clonic seizures affect the entire brain and are often preceded by an aura, a subtle feeling that warns of an imminent attack. They typically begin with a loud cry and strong muscular contraction (tonic). The patient is unresponsive, not breathing and often becomes cyanotic, bites their tongue, and may lose bladder and/or bowel control. During the seizure, the patient's muscles alternate between periods of contraction (tonic) and relaxation (clonic), with each part of the cycle lasting about 30 seconds. Most generalized seizures are short-lived, ending within 2-5 minutes; however, continuous seizures lasting more than 20 minutes are possible (status epilepticus) and may cause permanent brain damage or death. During the postictal period, after the seizure passes, patients are confused, may have trouble talking, and commonly complain of head and body aches before falling into a sound sleep.

Prevention
- Patients under treatment for epilepsy should closely follow their medication schedule.

Assessment
- A clonic/tonic seizure is characterized by severe and repetitive muscular contractions, unresponsiveness, and a loss of bladder and bowel control.
- Causes may vary. Persons under treatment for epilepsy or diabetes will have a medical history and may wear a medic alert tag.

Field Treatment
During the seizure
- Protect the patient from injury but DO NOT restrain them or place anything in their mouth.
- Continuous seizures require immediate intervention. If available, administer rectal Diazepam at 0.5 mg/kg, not to exceed 10 mg total. If rectal Diazepam is unavailable begin a Level 1 Evacuation with ALS. Respiratory arrest and death are possible.

After the seizure
- Provide BLS as necessary.
- Place the patient on their side in the recovery position during the postictal period.
- Separately assess and treat any associated traumatic injuries.
- Begin a Level 3 Evacuation if the seizure is outside of the patient's normal pattern.

Ears, Eyes, Nose, Teeth, & Gum Problems
Ear Infections & Problems
Hearing

Sound waves are collected by the external ear and directed toward the eardrum via the ear canal. There, they bombard the eardrum and cause it to vibrate. The vibrations are transmitted into mechanical energy and then amplified by the auditory bones of the middle ear. When the stirrup, one of three auditory bones in the middle ear, hits the thin membrane separating the middle ear from the fluid-filled chamber of the inner ear, the energy is converted into pressure waves. The waves cause small hairs in the cochlea to move and send electrical impulses to the brain via the otic nerve. Small hairs in the semicircular canals respond to changes in head position and are responsible for balance.

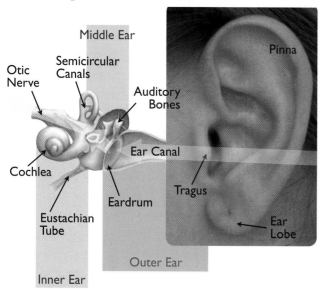

Pathophysiology

Internally, each ear is a single tube divided by a thin membrane. The external ear canal is open to the general environment and ends with the eardrum. The middle ear begins at the eardrum and contains the specialized hearing apparatus of the body, while the inner ear contains the balance center. Both are connected to the throat and sinuses via the eustachian tubes. Invading bacteria or viruses are confined to the external ear canal unless the eardrum has ruptured. Infecting organisms may also travel from the sinuses or throat, through the eustachian tubes, and into the middle ear. External ear infections are usually caused by water trapped in the external ear canal. Middle ear infections are usually secondary to sinus infections, throat infections, or a ruptured eardrum. Dizziness and fever are characteristic of both middle and inner ear infections. In very rare instances, infections may spread to the brain and cause death.

Pathophysiology of Insects in the External Ear

Insects occasionally crawl or fly into the external ear canal. Depending on their size, they can be mildly irritating to painful.

Pathophysiology of External Ear Infections

The primary cause of external ear infections is bacterial infection. These are typically caused by getting water trapped in the ear, such as from swimming or from being in a humid environment. Fungal infections are also possible. Inflammation due to an infection causes the ear canal and drum to redden, swell and discharge pus.

Pathophysiology of Middle & Inner Ear Infections

In children, viruses or bacteria tend to migrate up the eustachian tube from a throat or sinus infection. In adults, bacteria enter from a ruptured eardrum with the introduction of water while swimming or bathing.

Pathophysiology of Ruptured Eardrums

Common causes include puncture by a foreign object, abrupt ascent while SCUBA diving, rapidly expanding air (thunder) or pressure, or a severe middle ear infection.

Prevention

Prevention of External Ear Infections

• Avoid swimming in contaminated water.

• Avoid "cleaning" ears using a cotton swab; they irritate the lining of the external canal, making it susceptible to infections.

• Thoroughly remove all water from the external ear canal using a few drops of alcohol in each ear or flush with a 1:1 diluted vinegar solution.

Prevention of Middle & Inner Ear Infections

• Monitor and treat all sinus infections.

• Do not flush or use ear drops when a ruptured eardrum is suspected.

Prevention of Ruptured Eardrum

• Avoid abrupt pressure changes.

• Avoid rapid twisting and turning of the head when in thick brush; consider wearing a hat or hood to protect the ear canal.

Assessment

Otoscope Use

With a little practice, external ear infections and ruptured eardrums are easily seen with an otoscope; unless the eardrum is clearly bulging, an insufflator (air) bulb is usually required—and generally unavailable in a wilderness setting—to accurately diagnose a middle ear infection. The inner third of the ear canal (near the eardrum) is composed of bone and is covered with a thin layer of skin; the skin is highly innervated, sensitive, and easily damaged. The speculum of the otoscope should never touch the inner ear canal wall. Follow the guidelines below.

- Stabilize the hand holding the otoscope against the patient's head.
- Place the speculum tip in the entrance of the canal. While looking through the otoscope, slowly advance the speculum into the ear canal until you see the eardrum. The speculum of the otoscope should never touch/scrape the inner ear canal wall.
- Use your other hand to pull on the pinna and straighten the ear canal. In adults, pull the pinna *up*; with children, pull the ear lobe *down*. DO NOT use the speculum to press around the bend; the skin on the inner ear canal is easily abraded and pressure is extremely painful.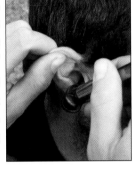
- When squeezed gently, an insufflator bulb blows a puff of air against the patient's eardrum. A normal adult eardrum is flexible and will abruptly move 1-2 mm when "hit" with the air; movement is significantly decreased or absent with a middle ear infection.
- When no infection is present, the eustachian tube is open and the eardrum will move slightly if the patient closes their mouth, holds their nose, and blows. There will be no movement, if the tube is swollen closed from a bacterial infection.

Assessment of External Ear Infections

- External ear infections are common in children and often follow swimming.
- Pus drains from the canal and dries on the outer ear.
- Both the ear canal and drum are inflamed and red.

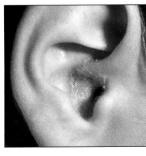
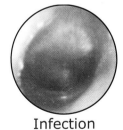

Infection

- The canal itches and hearing may be affected by the accumulation of swelling, drainage, and wax.
- The patient experiences a mild-to-severe earache.

Pain increases when the ear canal is manipulated by pushing the tragus or pulling the ear lobe.

- In rare cases, severe infections may cause fever and swollen lymph glands.
- In extremely rare cases usually reserved for diabetics and immune-suppressed patients, an external ear infection can progress to infect the temporal bone. Toxins produced by the bacteria may cause facial nerve paralysis and progress to involve the brain. S/Sx include disproportionate and severe ear pain, temporal headaches, and an on-going discharge of pus, in spite of treatment. Difficulty swallowing, hoarseness, and facial paralysis are possible. The soft tissue behind the jaw is typically extremely tender.

Assessment of Middle or Inner Ear Infections

- The patient may have a recent history of a severe sinus infection or ruptured eardrum.
- The patient experiences a moderate-to-sever earache accompanied by a full feeling in the ear. Pain does NOT change when the ear canal is manipulated by pushing the tragus or pulling the ear lobe.
- When "hit" with air from an insufflator bulb, normal movement of the patient's eardrum is significantly decreased or absent with a middle ear infection.
- During a bacterial infection, the eustachian tube swells, traps the bacteria in the middle ear, and prevents drainage. Pressure builds in the middle ear as bacteria multiply. Ask the patient to close their mouth, hold their nose, and blow outward. The eardrum will move slightly if the eustachian tube is open; there will be no movement if the tube is blocked. As pressure behind the eardrum builds, it begins to bulge. Rupture is possible if left untreated. Pain decreases with pressure after a rupture.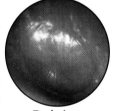

Bulging

- Fever, chills, swollen lymph glands, nausea, and vomiting are common with severe bacterial infections. If the infection reaches the inner ear, balance may be affected and a brain infection (meningitis or encephalitis), although rare, is possible.

Assessment of Ruptured Eardrums

- A ruptured eardrum causes immediate, moderate-to-severe pain that may be accompanied by a hearing loss. Common MOI include foreign objects, an abrupt ascent while SCUBA diving, or an abrupt pressure change.

- There is a sudden relief of pain if the rupture is caused by a middle or inner ear infection.

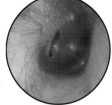
Perforated

- Dizziness and nausea, with or without vomiting, may occur.

Field Treatment

Ear Wax Removal

A normal eardrum is thin and pearly white and some of the auditory bones can be seen beneath it. The view may be obstructed by wax build up and the wax may need to be removed for an accurate assessment and treatment of external ear infections.

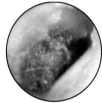 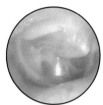

Ear Wax   Normal

- Apply a few drops of warm mineral oil into the external ear canal.
- Wait 5-15 minutes for the oil to soften the wax.
- Using an irrigation syringe, gently flush the ear canal with warm water; the wax will come out with the water. DO NOT insert the tip of the irrigation syringe into the ear canal; aim the stream of water so that it "bounces" off the ear canal. DO NOT flush if the eardrum is ruptured or if the MOI indicates a possible rupture.
- Apply a few drops of alcohol to break the surface tension of the water and to encourage the canal to dry.
- Repeat, as necessary, until the ear canal is clean.

Treatment of Insects in the External Ear

- Most insects will leave on their own within 10-15 minutes. If they do not or the patient cannot wait due to irritation or pain, gently flush the ear with warm water. Alternately, kill the insect with a few drops of mineral or vegetable oil and then flush.

Treatment of External Ear Infections

- Remove ear wax.
- Mild infections, those where the patient has no fever or swollen lymph glands, may be treated with diluted vinegar or GSE. Alternately, an infusion of warm oil and strained garlic works well.

- When the patient has a severe infection with fever and swollen lymph glands, administer antibiotic drops containing hydrocortisone. In addition, consider a systemic antibiotic: penicillin VK or the extended-range erythromycins (clarithromycin, azithromycin). Penicillin VK and clarithromycin are given by mouth at 250-500 mg two times a day for 10-14 days. Azithromycin is given by mouth at 500 mg four times a day on day 1, then 250 mg four times a day for four more days. Begin a Level 3 Evacuation if antibiotics are unavailable.
- If a temporal bone infection is suspected, start a course of ciprofloxacin and begin a Level 3 or 2 evacuation depending on the severity of the patient's S/Sx. The adult dose for ciprofloxacin is 500 mg per day by mouth three times a day.

Treatment of Middle or Inner Ear Infections

- Viral infections often resolve on their own, however, a secondary bacterial infection may follow.
- A systemic OTC decongestant is useful to relieve general congestion and promote drainage.
- The patient should rest. Provide assistance with thermoregulation.
- Replace fluids and electrolytes. Encourage patients to increase their normal fluid intake (force fluids). Monitor the patient's urine to assess their hydration status.
- Fevers above 102° F are best controlled with acetaminophen using the OTC dose.
- Many middle or inner infections will resolve with supportive treatment (described above) in 2-3 days. Initiate antibiotic therapy, if conditions worsen or do not improve. If antibiotics are not available, consider a Level 3 Evacuation.
- If the infection appears to be bacterial, with worsening S/Sx despite supportive treatment, consider administering one of the following antibiotics: clarithromycin, azithromycin or TMP/SMX. Clarithromycin is given by mouth at 250-500 mg two times a day for 10-14 days. Azithromycin is given by mouth at 500 mg on day 1, then 250 mg per day for four more days. The adult dose for TMP/SMX is one double strength (960 mg) two times a day for 10 days. Begin a Level 2 Evacuation if antibiotics are unavailable and the patient is unable to self-evacuate.
- Avoid swimming, washing hair, and showers if a ruptured eardrum is present or suspected.

196 Medical Illnesses

Treatment of Ruptured Eardrums

- Consider a Level 3 Evacuation.
- Cover the affected ear to prevent contamination; do not flush. Avoid swimming, washing hair, and showering, until the eardrum is completely healed, as determined by visual inspection.
- Administer OTC ibuprofen, naproxen sodium, or acetaminophen for pain. Avoid aspirin in children and teens under 17 because of the potential for Reye's syndrome.
- Monitor for a middle or inner ear infection as the MOI warrants. Most ruptured eardrums heal on their own in 3-4 weeks without complications.

Eye Problems

Pathophysiology

The globe of the eye is muscular and filled with a gel-like fluid that transmits light and maintains the internal pressure necessary for the eye to function properly. Light enters the eye through the pupil, is focused by the lens, absorbed by the rods and cones of the retina, and then the information is transmitted to the brain via the optic nerve. The conjunctiva is a mucous membrane that covers the cornea and the inside of the eyelids. Tears are produced in glands located above and to the outside of each eye. They flow across the eye to a drain in the inside corner of each eye. The drain empties into the nasal cavity.

The musculature surrounding the eyes and the eyeball itself are reasonably tough. Penetrating injuries are extremely rare, and must be attended to by a specialist. Injury from blunt trauma is also rare in a wilderness setting and if it occurs, it tends to be mi-nor. The most common injuries associated with the eyes are general irritation, sunburn (ultraviolet photokeratitis), or irritation from small foreign bodies, corneal abrasions, and infection. All of these problems involve the conjunctiva and, if more severe, the cornea. S/Sx often include itching, redness, a burning sensation or pain, tearing, headache, and light sensitivity. Normal movement of the injured eye is usually uncomfortable, but possible. Eyes are highly vascular and minor injuries usually heal within 24-72 hours.

Prevention

Prevention of Ultraviolet Photokeratitis

- Protective eyewear is mandatory in mountain, river, ocean, and desert environments where sunlight and glare are unavoidable. All types of protective eye wear, including prescription glasses, contact lenses, and intraocular lens implants, should absorb the entire UVR spectrum (280-400 nm).
- Consider wearing goggles, wraparound glasses, or glasses with side protection. Carry an extra pair of sunglasses in case of loss or damage. For emergency short-term protection, improvise a pair of "slit lens glasses" from duct tape and nylon cord.
- Polarization or photosensitive darkening are additional sunglass features that are useful under specific circumstances, but do not by themselves provide UVR protection. They are helpful in snow, ocean, and desert environments where sunlight and glare are unavoidable.
- A wide-brimmed hat blocks about 50% of UVR and significantly reduces the amount of light entering above or around glasses.

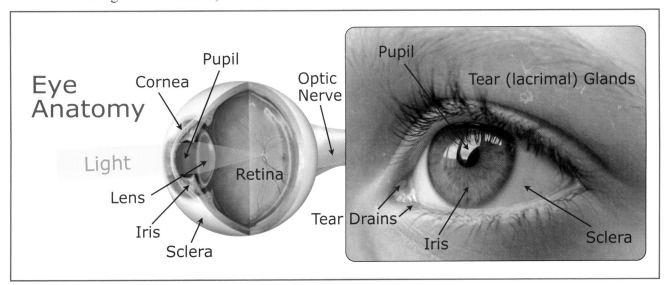

Prevention of Foreign Bodies

- Common foreign bodies found in the eye include wind-blown sand, dirt, or small insects.
- Protective goggles are helpful for protection in brushy areas and while working with machinery.
- Seek shelter from windstorms and from helicopter rotor wash, when sand or dirt is present.
- Contact lens wearers should consider wearing glasses instead of contact lenses.
- Consider wearing a head net when bugs are bad.

Prevention of Conjunctivitis

- If contact lenses are worn, wearers should take care to maintain a clean environment when working with their lenses.

Assessment

Fluorescein Use

Fluorescein is a dye used to highlight damage to the conjunctiva or cornea. It is available as a solution or in dry strips. To use a strip, wet it using a sterile saline solution and touch it to the eye near the tear gland. Have the patient blink a few times; their tears will carry the dye across the eye. The solution is applied in a similar manner. Shine a cobalt blue light across the eye from the side; damage is visible as a green fluorescence.

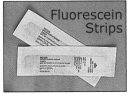
Fluorescein Strips

Assessment of Chemical Irritation of the Eye

- Smoke and chemicals, typically sunscreen and insect repellent, often irritate the conjunctiva, but rarely the cornea.
- Signs and symptoms are usually nonspecific, with redness, tearing, and general irritation.

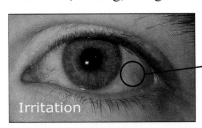
Irritation

Assessment of Ultraviolet Photokeratitis

- UV photokeratitis usually requires direct exposure to the sun for more than an hour. Travel at high altitude, or on snow, water, or white sand, increases the potential for injury.
- S/Sx are usually delayed for 6-12 hours after exposure and often accompany a sunburned face.
- The patient complains of bilateral eye pain, grit or dirt in their eyes, headache and light sensitivity.
- Due to extreme pain, assessment may require a SINGLE dose of a topical ophthalmic anesthetic. Use only once; multiple doses significantly impair healing.
- The affected eyes appear red; surrounding tissue may be swollen.
- A horizontal band is commonly seen with fluorescein stain in patients who squint in an attempt to shield their eye from bright sunlight (see below).

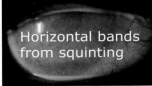
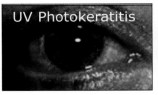
UV Photokeratitis   Horizontal bands from squinting

Assessment of Foreign Bodies

- The onset of S/Sx from a foreign body is abrupt, with immediate irritation or pain, tearing, and redness.
- The patient may have difficulty opening their eye and submitting to an eye exam without a topical ophthalmic anesthetic.
- If a foreign body is not immediately obvious upon inspection, check under eyelids; invert using cotton-tipped applicator.

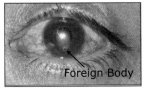
Foreign Body

- If the MOI is trauma, inspect and rule-out an open globe injury.

Assessment of Styes

A stye is a bacterial infection in one of the oil glands at the edge of the eyelids. External styes form on the outside of the lids and can be seen as small red bumps; internal styes appear on the lining underneath the eyelids. They contain water and pus; the bacteria will spread, if the stye is forcefully ruptured.

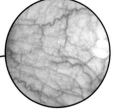
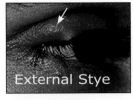
External Stye   Internal Stye

- A stye appears as a swollen, painful, tender, red bump at the top or bottom of an eyelid.
- A stye may cause crusting of the eyelid margins, similar to conjunctivitis.

- A stye may also cause general eye irritation, similar to that from a foreign body, tearing, and discomfort while blinking.

Assessment of Conjunctivitis

- Conjunctivitis is caused by a bacterial or viral infection, and may result from a systemic infection of chlamydia, gonorrhea, or candida.
- Risk factors for conjunctivitis include corneal abrasion and wearing extended-wear contact lenses.
- The onset of the infection may be acute or sub-acute, with minimal pain, foreign-body-type irritation and pus, with or without itching.
- The infection may also redden the inner surface of the eyelid and cause surface changes.
- Blurred vision from conjunctivitis is typically caused by pus; visual acuity is not affected. Pus often "glues" eyelids together during sleep.

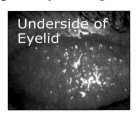 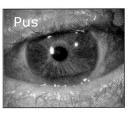

- Conjunctivitis is *highly* contagious. Thoroughly wash hands after patient assessment and treatment.

Assessment of Corneal Abrasion

- Abrasions may occur on the conjunctiva through contact with branches, foreign bodies, etc.
- Foreign body sensation or gritty feeling (in spite of thorough flushing), pain of varying severity, light sensitivity, and excessive tearing are common symptoms of corneal abrasion. A topical ophthalmic anesthetic may facilitate examination.

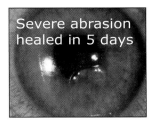 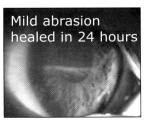

- Only large scratches will be visible on examination; most corneal abrasions cannot be seen without fluorescein staining. The patient will continue to report a foreign body or general irritation.

Assessment of Corneal Ulcers

- A corneal ulcer is an ophthalmic emergency with the potential to develop permanent eye damage or blindness within 24 hours.
- Most corneal ulcers are have a traumatic history. Even a small break in the surface of the cornea may lead to serious infection.
- Risk factors for developing a corneal ulcer include wearing extended-wear contact lenses, smoking, cold and wind exposure, and a vitamin A deficiency; corneal ulcers are more common in males.
- A topical ophthalmic anesthetic may facilitate examination.
- Foreign body sensation or gritty feeling, pain, light sensitivity, visible pus under cornea and impaired vision are common S/Sx of a corneal ulcer.

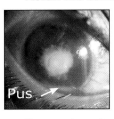 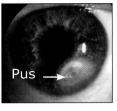 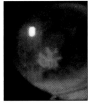

- Cornea is red; ulcer is opaque and cream-colored or hazy. Fluorescein staining is often unnecessary.

Assessment of Open Globe Injuries

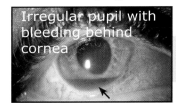 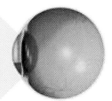

- With a traumatic MOI to the eye, it is crucial to distinguish between essentially harmless sub-conjunctival bleeding and an open globe injury, which is an ophthalmic emergency.
- DO NOT palpate or put pressure on the eye during physical exam.
- An open globe injury presents with pain, bleeding behind the cornea, irregular pupil, and blurred vision.

Assessment of Sub-conjunctival Hemorrhages

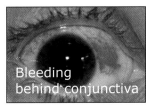 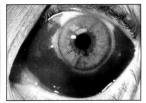

- A sub-conjunctival hemorrhage presents with bleeding between conjunctiva and sclera. No eye pain and normal vision. Facial or orbital pain is possible, depending on the MOI.

Field Treatment

General Treatment

- If the patient presents or develops any vision impairment, begin a Level 2 Evacuation to an ophthalmologist.

Treatment of Chemical Irritation of the Eye

- Thoroughly wash the patient's face.
- Immediately flush the eye and underneath the eyelids. *Flush away from the nose and the other eye;* use sterile saline. Clean water works as well, but leaves the eye feeling "dry." After flushing, moisten the eye with artificial tears.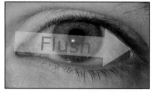
- If pain persists after flushing, use a topical ophthalmic antibiotic ointment to prevent superinfection and to lubricate the conjunctiva. Apply the ointment to the inside of lower eyelid and have the patient blink their eye a few times to spread the ointment. Ophthalmic antibiotic solutions are easier to apply, but do not provide lubrication.
- Use NSAID ophthalmic solutions for treating pain. DO NOT use anesthetics to control pain beyond the initial assessment.
- If possible, avoid patching the eye; eye patches slow healing and eliminate depth perception. Base your decision on the patient's comfort and the terrain requirements.
- Monitor for a corneal abrasion.

Treatment of Ultraviolet Photokeratitis

- Remove from sunlight until the S/Sx subside, usually within 24 to 48 hours.
- Severe cases may require bandaging. Treat with bacitracin ophthalmic ointment four times a day until S/Sx are relieved. Monitor for corneal ulcer.
- Treat headaches with NSAIDs (aspirin, ibuprofen, naproxen sodium) or acetaminophen.
- While cold compresses may offer some relief from the pain, consider using topical ophthalmic NSAIDs (Rx: ketorolac 0.5% ophthalmic solution) to control mild to moderate pain. Stronger pain medications (Rx: oxycodone with acetaminophen) may be required in severe cases.

Treatment of Small Foreign Bodies

- If there is no globe damage then, lightly flush the eye and underneath eyelid toward nose (in the di-

rection of tearing); use sterile saline. Clean water works as well, but leaves the eye feeling "dry." After flushing, moisten the eye with artificial tears. A moistened cotton-tipped applicator can also be used.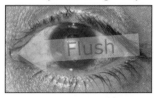

- Use a topical ophthalmic antibiotic ointment to prevent superinfection and to lubricate the conjunctiva. Apply to inside of lower eyelid and have patient blink their eye a few times to spread the ointment. Ophthalmic antibiotic solutions are easier to apply, but do not provide lubrication.
- Use NSAID ophthalmic solutions for treating pain. DO NOT use anesthetics to control pain beyond the initial assessment.
- DO NOT patch the affected eye. Eye patches slow healing and eliminate depth perception.
- Monitor for a corneal abrasion and/or conjunctivitis.

Treatment of Styes

- Most styes are harmless and heal on their own without special treatment in 5-10 days.
- Avoid wearing contact lenses until the stye is completely healed.
- Apply warm compresses for ten minutes, four times a day.
- DO NOT squeeze or puncture a stye; this will spread the infection.
- Antibiotic creams may help recurrent or persistent styes. Some large styes may need to be lanced to drain the infection.
- Begin a Level 3 Evacuation if irritation persists beyond a week or vision becomes blurry.

Treatment of Corneal Abrasions

- Most corneal abrasions heal rapidly (within 1-5 days). Consider a Level 3 Evacuation.
- Use a topical ophthalmic antibiotic ointment to prevent superinfection and to lubricate conjunctiva. Apply to inside of lower eyelid and have patient blink their eye a few times to spread the ointment. Ophthalmic antibiotic solutions are easier to apply, but do not provide lubrication.
- Use NSAID ophthalmic solutions for treating pain. DO NOT use anesthetics to control pain beyond the initial assessment.
- DO NOT patch the affected eye; eye patches slow

healing and eliminate depth perception.
- Monitor for a corneal ulcer and/or conjunctivitis.

Treatment of Conjunctivitis
- Discontinue contact lens use until the infection heals; replace the lenses and use new solution.
- Herbs that can be used as an eye wash to treat infection include: chamomile, agrimony, and eyebright.
- Mild infections may be treated with repeated flushing using saline or fresh tea from chamomile, agrimony, cats claw, or eyebright. Begin a Level 3 Evacuation if unsuccessful and if ophthalmic antibiotics are unavailable.
- Bacterial infections may be treated with antibiotic ointment or drops every two hours while the patient is awake. Ophthalmic antibiotic solutions are easier to apply than ointments; however, ointments provide some pain relief. Consider using Rx medications, ophthalmic gentamicin or neomycin-polymyxin B-gramicidin ophthalmic. Do not use antibiotics containing steroids.
- If infection is secondary to systemic STD, treat the STD and the conjunctivitis concurrently; remember to treat the patient's sexual partner for the STD.

Treatment of Open Globe Injuries
- For open globe injuries, do not disturb any impaled objects and do not flush the eye. Cover the affected eye with a durable shield, preferably metal, and begin a Level 2 Evacuation; surgery is required.

Treatment of Sub-conjunctival Hemorrhages
- Sub-conjunctival hemorrhages heal without treatment in 1-3 weeks. Avoid treating the patient with NSAIDS, as these may increase bleeding. The coloration in the eye may spread and may also change to green or yellow over time as the bruise heals.

Nasal Problems
Pathophysiology
The nasal cavity is complex and consists of numerous boney structures, cartilage and connective tissue. Nasal cartilage has no blood supply and receives all of its nutrients and oxygen from its connective tissue. The septum is part bone, part cartilage, and divides the nose vertically into two separate cavities and is lined with a mucous membrane. In addition to detecting odors, the nose is designed to filter and humidify incoming air. Its lining is filled with blood vessels and is somewhat fragile. Anterior nosebleeds are

common in dry and/or cold air, those who chronically sneeze or pick their nose, or following trauma to the nose or face. Assess for concussion and increased ICP. Posterior nosebleeds are unusual, more serious, and cannot be treated in the field without advanced training and materials.

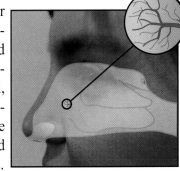

Prevention
- Coat the nasal lining with petroleum jelly, saline gel (Ayr nasal gel®) or aloe vera gel before exposure to unusually cold and/or dry air.

Assessment
Assessment of Nosebleeds
- The severity of bleeding varies greatly between individuals and MOI. Bilateral bleeding is highly unusual.
- Nausea occurs if blood is swallowed.

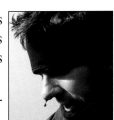

Assessment of Broken Noses
- The septum is capable of absorbing significant amounts of kinetic energy before breaking. Damage, when it occurs, can be to the cartilage and/or bone.
- Nosebleeds are common with a broken nose; severity of bleeding varies greatly between individuals. Bilateral bleeding is possible.
- Nausea occurs if blood is swallowed.
- Pain, tenderness, swelling, crepitus, deformity, bruising of the nose or under the eyes, lacerations, and difficulty breathing through the nose are all possible; mouth breathing is common. NOTE: The nose can visually appear straight but the septum can be internally deviated; if this is the case, it is very difficult to detect unless you have a nasal speculum and some experience. Realignment is much easier if done early.

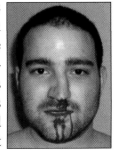

Treatment
Treatment of Nosebleeds
- Have the patient sit upright to reduce blood pres-

sure lean forward to keep from swallowing blood, pinch the lower nostrils closed between thumb and forefinger, and hold for at least 10-15 minutes. Pinching higher on the boney part of the nose doesn't work, because it doesn't apply pressure to the septum. Ice does NOT help. The application of a vasoconstricting nasal spray or drops (Afrin®, Neosynepherine®) will speed clotting.

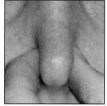

• After bleeding stops, gently blow out clots and AVOID heavy lifting/straining, smoking, nose picking, alcohol, sneezing (cough instead), dust/irritants, and spicy foods for 3-5 days.

• Treat with acetaminophen for pain; avoid NSAIDs as they may increase bleeding.

• Consider nasal packing if bleeding does not stop.

Treatment of Broken Noses

• Treat nosebleed as described above.

• Acetaminophen for pain; avoid NSAIDs as they may increase bleeding.

• Consider a Level 3 Evacuation. Reduction/repair is usually done within 72 hours, 5-10 days after injury when swelling has gone down, or repaired surgically after the initial damage has healed.

• Begin a Level 3 Evacuation if pain or swelling remains after three days, if the patient develops a fever, if nasal breathing remains restricted after swelling goes down, or if the patient's nose is crooked.

Nasal Packing

• Consider nasal packing if bleeding does not stop.

• Packing materials include commercial nasal tampons (Sheppard AbsorbENT Nasal Tampons®, Nasal-CEASE®), gauze packing/strips, and small vaginal tampons.

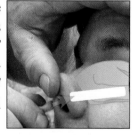

• Prepare the packing materials by lubricating Sheppard AbsorbENT Nasal Tampons®, gauze, or vaginal tampons with petroleum jelly and spraying with topical vasoconstrictor (Afrin®, Neosynepherine®) prior to insertion. DO NOT use petroleum jelly or nasal spray on NasalCEASE®. Twist gauze and NasalCEASE® material prior to insertion.

• Have patient gently clear their nose by blowing.

• If possible, examine the nasal passage using an otoscope before packing.

• The nasal cavity goes straight back, not up. Press up with your thumb on the tip of the patient's nose to access and insert the packing material straight back until fully inserted. Leave strings or part of the packing material accessible to facilitate removal.

• Bleeding should stop within a few seconds with packing; clotting will take longer. If bleeding persists, apply outside pressure over septum and consider packing the other nostril to increase pressure.

• Remove the packing material after 30 minutes. Repack if bleeding reoccurs.

• Begin a Level 3 Evacuation if repacking is necessary. Leave the packing in until arrival at the hospital. Nasal packing may remain in place for 24-72 hours. Because the packing blocks sinus drainage, administer prophylactic antibiotics to prevent sinusitis and staphylococcal toxic shock syndrome. DO NOT over pack. The nasal cartilage has no blood supply and receives all of its nutrients and oxygen from its connective tissue. Over packing or pressure on both sides of the cartilage can kill it within 24 hours.

Teeth & Gum Problems
Pathophysiology

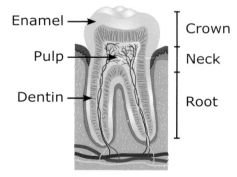

Teeth rest in boney sockets in the jaw and are connected to a root via ligaments. Canals in the root house the nerves and blood vessels necessary to keep the pulp alive. The pulp supplies nutrients to the tooth tissue and contains the nerves responsible for sensation. The pulp is surrounded by dentin, a mineral substance similar to bone. Dentin does not contain living cells and is secreted by specialized cells located in the pulp. The crown of the tooth is covered in enamel, which is responsible for protecting the surface of the tooth exposed to the outside. Enamel is the hardest substance in the body. The gums surround each tooth like a collar, providing additional support to the ligament and helping to hold the tooth in its socket. Problems associated with teeth and gums can be mildly irritating to unbearable. Fillings or caps can loosen and fall out. Teeth may be broken or knocked out. Broken teeth or gums can become infected. Once established, a local infection may become severe, systemic, and difficult, if not impossible to effectively treat in the field.

Prevention

- Have all dental work done well in advance to leaving on a expedition. Floss and brush on a regular basis.

Assessment

Assessment of Broken Teeth, Lost Fillings or Crowns, & Knocked Out Teeth

- A broken tooth is sensitive and painful. If the pulp is exposed, there is a risk of infection.
- A tooth may become loose or knocked out. If out, the socket is exposed, painful, and at risk for infection.
- A filling or crown may loosen or fall out.

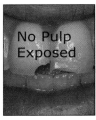
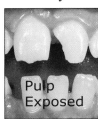
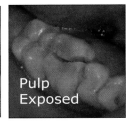

Assessment of Tooth or Gum Infections

- Severe tooth pain on percussion indicates a tooth infection. Lightly tap a normal tooth on the top of its crown first, then progress toward the suspected tooth.

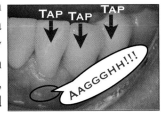

- The surrounding soft tissue is red, tender and swollen; swelling may progress to include the entire jaw. The patient may have swollen lymph glands and a fever. An abscess may be noticeable in the gums.

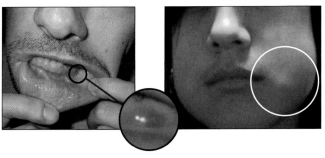

Field Treatment

Treatment of Broken Teeth & Lost Fillings or Crowns

- The pain may be controlled with oil of clove (eugenol) and OTC medications (aspirin, ibuprofen, naproxen sodium, or acetaminophen), or in severe cases with codeine-based drugs. Soak a small piece of cotton or finely chopped gauze with eugenol and pack into the hole.
- There are two basic types of temporary filling materials, while Cavit® and DenTemp®. DenTemp® contains eugenol; Cavit® does not. Cavit® sticks better than DenTemp® and is easier to remove. Either can remain in place for days or weeks. Caution the patient not to chew hard or sticky foods.
- To repair a broken tooth or lost filling, first flush the broken area thoroughly with salt water, a dilute vinegar solution, or an iodine solution. Dry. If using Cavit®, place eugenol-soaked cotton/gauze into the hole first. Wear gloves. Roll a small amount of putty into a ball and press it firmly into place. If the putty is on top of a tooth, have the patient bite down gently to mold the putty to their natural bite. When dry, sand or file any rough edges off the temporary filling. Coat the filling and tooth with cavity varnish.
- To repair a crown, use DenTemp® or Cavit® to cement the crown in place. Wear gloves. Roll a small amount of Cavit® or DenTemp® into a ball and press firmly onto the crown, then press the crown into position. Have the patient bite firmly to set the crown. For additional security, use putty to splint both sides of the crown to adjacent teeth.
- Begin a Level 3 Evacuation to a dentist for all patients who have exposed pulp; they will require a root canal. Monitor for infection.

Treatment of Loose or Knocked Out Teeth

- Replace teeth that have been knocked out if they are clean and have been out for less than 15 minutes.
- To replace a tooth, first rinse both the socket and the tooth with normal saline, then place firmly in the socket. Handle the tooth by the crown and do not scrub the connective tissue from the tooth.

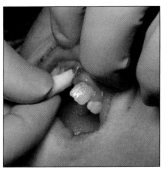

- Do not replace teeth of patients who have not had a tetanus booster within the past five years.
- Secure loose or avulsed teeth to the adjacent teeth using Cavit® or by "lashing" in place with dental floss or fishing line. Monitor for infection. The tooth should remain splinted for 7-10 days.
- Administer NSAIDs for pain.
- To insure proper alignment and receive antibiotic prophylaxis, begin a Level 3 Evacuation; if possible, patients should be seen by a dentist within 48 hours.
- If evacuation is not possible, begin antibiotic prophylaxis. Administer oral penicillin VK or erythromycin. Both are dosed at 250-500 mg 4 times a day for 10 days.
- If an infection develops, remove the tooth and treat for an infection.

Treatment of Tooth or Gum Infections

- Apply hot, moist compresses to the infected area inside the patient's mouth. Do not apply heat to the outside of a patient's face when their tooth or gum is infected; abscesses move towards heat.
- Carefully lance any obvious pustule heads with a sterile scalpel blade or knife, by making a quick horizontal cut to the bone. If available, infiltrate with a local anesthetic before making the incision; ice applied directly to the site for a few minutes also works.
- Thoroughly clean the infected area with saltwater, a dilute vinegar solution, or an iodine solution. Follow with saline rinses every 2 hours.
- Administer a systemic antibiotic. Consider penicillin VK or erythromycin. The adult dose for both drugs is 500 mg 4 times a day for 10 days.
- Use codeine-based analgesics to treat severe pain.
- Begin a Level 3 Evacuation if antibiotics are unavailable; upgrade to Level 2, if fever is present.

Integumentary System Problems
Fungal Infections
Pathophysiology

Numerous types of fungi live on and in our bodies without causing harm; they are held in check by competing bacteria and our immune system. Disease-causing fungi can be divided into two groups: filamentous fungi and yeasts. Filamentous fungi are made up of branching threads, known as hyphae; yeasts are single-celled organisms. The most common fungal infections are superficial and caused by either Tinea, a filamentous fungi, or Candida albicans, a yeast. Heat, humidity, immunocompromised states, long-term antibiotic use, diabetes, and steroid therapy predispose people to both types of fungal infections. Fungal infections are more common in the summer and are exacerbated by wearing synthetic clothing and by sweating.

Tinea Infections

Tinea infections are caused by a group of fungi (ringworm) that live on keratinous structures and invade dead layers of the host's skin, hair, and nails; the transmission routes are direct contact with an infected person or animal or with contaminated soil. Clinically, tinea infections are classified according to the body region involved/infected: tinea capitis (scalp), tinea corporis and versicolor (trunk and extremities), tinea manuum and tinea pedis (palms, soles, and interdigital webs), tinea cruris (groin), tinea barbae (beard area and neck), tinea faciale (face), and tinea unguium (nails).

Candida Albicans (Yeast) Infections

Candida albicans skin infections may closely mimic tinea crurisare, but are usually more moist, more inflammatory, and associated with satellite macules, pustules, and scales. Unlike Tinea, Candida may also infect the mucous membranes of the mouth, vagina, penis, and eye. These infections are red, itchy, moist and often associated with a yeasty odor and a white cheese-like discharge. Most mucosal infections result from long-term antibiotic use.

Prevention
- Avoid communal baths.
- Keep areas that may potentially become affected, such as between the toes, around the genitals, and between skin folds, clean and dry.
- People participating in contact sports are predisposed to tinea infections.

Assessment
- Both Tinea and Candida skin infections present with localized itching and red rash. Candida may exhibit satellite lesions and pustules.
- Vaginal Candida infections typically present with white, cheesy discharge and yeasty smell.

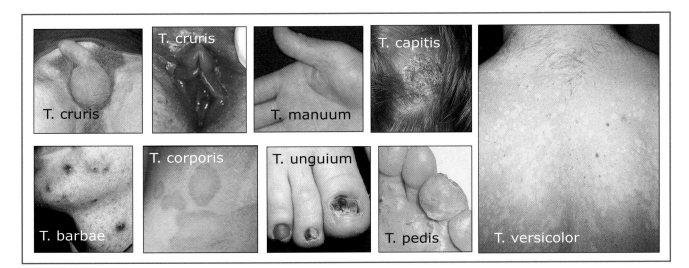

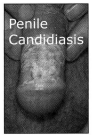

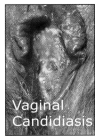

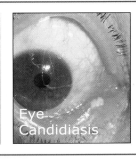

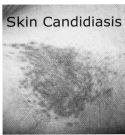

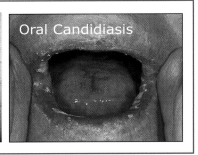

- In the mouth, Candida shows up as thick, white lacy patches on the tongue, lips, gums, or inside of the patient's cheeks. The lesions are painful and swallowing may be difficult.
- Candida infections on the scrotum often present as red bumps.

Treatment

- Treatment varies and is based on the anatomic location of the infection. Most localized fungal infections may be treated with numerous topical antifungal agents, such as clotrimazole, econazole, ciclopirox, miconazole, ketoconazole, or nystatin, prepared as creams, suppositories, lozenges, etc. Systemic or persistent infections are treated with oral antifungal therapy using either fluconazole or itraconazole. These more potent agents may affect the liver, and require periodic liver function tests.
- For skin rashes from either both Tinea or Candida, apply topical lac-hydrin and clotrimazole twice a day for 3-4 weeks; wash and dry thoroughly before each application.
- For oral Candida infections, dissolve a clotrimazole lozenge twice a day for 7-14 days.
- Begin a Level 3 Evacuation if S/Sx are mild and antifungals are unavailable or the patient does not respond. Begin a Level 2 Evacuation if patient is immunosuppressed or a systemic Candida infection is suspected.

Gastrointestinal System Problems
Heartburn & Acid Reflux

Pathophysiology

Stomach acids leak into the esophagus due to a failure of the lower esophageal sphincter.

Assessment

- Occasional pain after a big meal is common; more than once a week indicates Acid Reflux Disease.
- Sub-sternal burning pain often mimics a heart attack. CAUTION: Without a previous history, it may be difficult to assess and rule out angina and heart attack.
- Mild respiratory distress associated with heartburn and acid reflux may mimic asthma.
- A chronic cough and nausea may be present.
- The presence/history of hiatal hernia increases risk.

Treatment

- Drugs: antacids, baking soda and water, acid reducers (H-2 blockers), seaweed alginates (forms protective coating). Proton pump inhibitors (PPI) stop stomach cells from producing acid.
- Sleep on the left side with the head of the sleeping platform raised at least 6-8 inches. Avoid slouching.
- Do not eat 3-4 hours prior to lying down or sleeping.
- Avoid coffee, alcoholic beverages, and high doses of vitamin C before lying down, as these stimulate gastric secretion. Avoid chocolate, peppermint, and chamomile tea taken before sleeping because they relax the stomach. Also avoid fatty foods, which slow emptying of the stomach, milk products, and difficult to digest cruciferous vegetables. And finally, avoid acidic foods, such as citrus, tomato products, and carbonated drinks.
- Consider a Level 3 Evacuation if treatment is unsuccessful.

Gastroenteritis

Pathophysiology

Gastroenteritis is a nonspecific term for intestinal illnesses that produce diarrhea. In the majority of cases, the diarrhea is accompanied by nausea, vomiting, and abdominal pain. Causes include viral (50-70%), bacterial (15-20%), and parasitic (10-15%) infections with severities ranging from mild to life-threatening. A number of the more severe infections are discussed in detail in Section IX, Infectious Diseases. Gastroenteritis occurs when a microorganism directly invades the cells of the intestinal lining, causing inflammation (Salmonella, Yersinia) or death (Shigella, Campylobacter, enteroinvasive E coli). Gastroenteritis produces toxins that destroy or irritate the intestinal lining (Shigella dysenteriae, Vibrio parahaemolyticus, Clostridium difficile, enterohemorrhagic E coli). Gastroenteritis also occurs when invading organisms adhere to the intestinal walls, colonize, and displace the normal flora (V cholera, enterotoxigenic E coli). Diarrhea ensues when the microorganisms overwhelm normal body defenses.

Prevention

Almost all diarrheal illnesses are a result of poor personal or expedition hygiene, poor food preparation, or contaminated food or water. Rigorous attention to basic travel and expedition hygiene, water purification, and food handling guidelines cannot be overstated and bears repeating:

- Wash hands before cooking or eating. Maintain hand-washing stations in the kitchen and at the field toilet.
- DO NOT touch your eyes, nose, mouth or any food after touching any contaminated surfaces, until after washing hands.
- Avoid sharing water bottles.
- Keep cutting boards, cooking pots, dishes, utensils and food preparation areas clean by washing them with soap and water and by allowing them to dry thoroughly.
- Thoroughly cook meats and seafood. Cooking to a temperature of 180°F (82°C) will kill disease-causing organisms. Use a meat thermometer when cooking roasts or whole turkeys in a Dutch oven to be sure food is cooked to a safe temperature.
- Keep raw food away from cooked food. Avoid cross-contamination by using separate plates and utensils for the cooked and the raw food.
- Thoroughly wash raw vegetables such as, carrots, lettuce, tomatoes, etc. and soak in a diluted vinegar or GSE solution for 30 minutes to kill bacteria.
- Wash melons and similar fruits and vegetables to avoid transferring any dirt or contamination from the rind or skin to the inside of the fruit during cutting or peeling.
- Drink purified water and use purified water for washing hands and cleaning food-preparation areas.
- Don't let cooked food sit at room temperature; to slow bacterial growth, promptly pack in shallow containers and cool at or below 4°C/40°F. If refrigeration is unavailable, cook only the amount of food you or your group can consume. Do not eat spoiled food, or any food that has an unpleasant smell or taste. When in doubt, throw it out.

Assessment

- Abdominal pain, which is NOT accompanied by diarrhea is NOT gastroenteritis and may be a serious problem requiring a Level 2 or 1 evacuation. Refer to the assessment table on pages 176-177.
- Norovirus is the leading cause of viral gastroenteritis in the United States. It has a 12-48 hour incubation period. Onset is abrupt, with violent episodes of vomiting, moderate diarrhea, headache, fever

(~50%), chills, and general muscle soreness. S/Sx resolve spontaneously within 12-60 hours.

- Rotavirus may cause severe dehydration and is the leading cause of viral gastroenteritis in children worldwide.

- Shigella, Salmonella, C jejuni, Yersinia enterocolitica, E coli, V cholera and Aeromonas are the leading bacterial agents that cause gastroenteritis.

- Giardia, Amebiasis, Cryptosporidium, and Cyclospora are the leading parasitic agents.

- It is extremely important to complete a thorough abdominal exam to rule out serious abdominal problems from other causes that may require surgical intervention.

- A thorough patient history is extremely helpful in determining the specific agent.

- In adults, a fever, with or without chills, typically suggests that an invasive organism is the cause of the diarrhea.

- Pain in the lower quadrants or lower back indicates an infection in the large intestine, while pain in the umbilical region suggests an infection in the small intestine.

- Vomiting, without diarrhea, indicates a noninfectious cause rather than gastroenteritis.

- Large volume stools are usually associated with an infection of the small intestine, whereas an infection of the large intestine causes many small stools.

- The presence of blood in the stool indicates ulceration of the large intestine.

- Copious "rice water" diarrhea is a hallmark of cholera.

- Bulky, white feces that float indicate a high fat content that is typically due to a small bowel pathology and malabsorption.

Treatment

- Treatment for gastroenteritis includes aggressive fluid replacement with electrolytes via an oral rehydration solution at roughly 8 ounces every 15 minutes (1 L/hour) until the patient is rehydrated and their urine is clear. Once they are hydrated, give roughly 1.5 L of oral fluid per L of stool excreted. Consider a Level 3 Evacuation and upgrade, if you are unable to keep the patient hydrated.

- Begin feeding the patient complex carbohydrates and lean meats to speed mucosal repair ASAP after vom-

iting has been controlled and the patient rehydrated.

- Antiemetics may be used to treat nausea and vomiting in adults, but are not recommended for children.

- Grapefruit Seed Extract, at 6-8 drops/L for a maximum of 32 drops per day, has successfully treated mild-to-moderate bacterial and parasitic infections.

- A single dose of trimethoprim-sulfamethoxazole (TMP/SMX) at 1 DS tablet OR 500 mg of ciprofloxacin can shorten the course of bacterial infections (traveler's diarrhea). Give the same dose twice a day for 3-5 days, if S/Sx persist beyond the first day.

Peptic Ulcer
Pathophysiology

A peptic ulcer is a breakdown of the lining of the stomach or of the first portion of the small intestine, commonly caused by long-term use of NSAIDs or an H-pylori bacterial infection.

Assessment

- Epigastric pain and tenderness 2-3 hours after eating.

- Nausea, with or without vomiting, is a common symptom.

- Vomited blood: resembles coffee grounds (bleeding and perforated ulcers).

- The patient's stool will look black and tar-like if a bleeding or perforated ulcer is present.

- Patients often have a history of long-term NSAID use.

Treatment

- Begin a Level 3 Evacuation if the S/Sx are not relieved by symptomatic treatment.

- If due to NSAIDs, *stop* NSAID use.

- Administer an antacid or rantidine (Zantac®); both are H-2 blockers. Alternately, administer proton pump inhibitors (Prilosec®, Prevacid®, Nexiumetc®).

- If due to H-pylori infection, administer proton pump inhibitors (PPI) plus antibiotics (commonly amoxicillin and clarithromycin) for 7-14 days.

Anticipated Problems
- The ulcer may bleed or perforate.

- Begin a Level 2 Evacuation for abdominal pain and tenderness accompanied by stomach or intestinal bleeding (e.g.: coffee-ground vomitus or black tar-like stools).

• Begin a Level 1 Evacuation if a perforated ulcer is suspected; death is possible. Monitor for S/Sx of internal bleeding.

Gallstones

Pathophysiology

Gallstones are crystallized cholesterol deposits or calcium crystals and bilirubin, that block the bile ducts and/or pancreatic duct of the gallbladder or pancreas. The stones can be as small as sand grains or as large as golf balls.

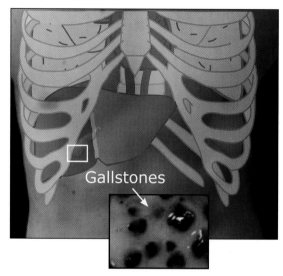
Gallstones

Gallstones can temporarily block the bile duct during a contraction or permanently block it. A permanent block permits bacteria to flourish, causing inflammation and perforation. Females are at greater risk than males. The difference in risk between the sexes is due to the increased levels of estrogens and progesterone in women. Estrogens increase cholesterol formation, which supersaturate the bile, leading to precipitation of cholesterol stones. Progesterone inhibits gallbladder motility and promotes stone formation. Pregnancy increases the amount of circulating estrogens and progesterone and exacerbates the problem. Obesity, a high-fat diet, and high triglycerides further increase the risk.

Assessment

• A gallbladder attack is characterized by gradually increasing abdominal pain, that usually begins after eating a high-fat meal. The pain tends to localize in the Right Upper Quadrant within 10 minutes.

• The pain may be constant or intermittent. It is NOT relieved by vomiting, taking antacids, after defecation, or with positional changes.

• Nausea and vomiting are common.

• Fever and increased pulse are possible.

• Patients often exhibit tenderness during inhalation as steady pressure is applied to the Right Upper Quadrant along the costal arch (Murphy's sign). Inhalation expands the lungs and pushes the gall bladder down below the ribs, where it can be palpated; an inflamed gallbladder is tender.

• Temporary blockages typically last 30-90 minutes; pain resolves quickly after stone dislodges.

• Localized rebound tenderness and guarding indicate perforation.

Treatment

• Begin a Level 3 Evacuation if S/Sx are mild, quickly resolve, and do NOT indicate an infection.

• Begin a Level 1 Evacuation if fever or other S/Sx of an infection are present. Treatment usually requires surgery.

Pancreatitis

Pathophysiology

Pancreatitis is an inflammation of the pancreas caused by a gallstone blocking the pancreatic duct at the common entrance to the small intestine or by long-term alcohol abuse. Pancreatitis due to alcohol abuse is more common in males over age 40, while pancreatitis due to gallstones is more common in females over age 50.

Assessment

• S/Sx often begin after a heavy meal or drinking binge.

• Nausea, vomiting, and lack of appetite are common; diarrhea is possible.

• Fever and increased pulse accompanied by abdominal pain, tenderness, and guarding.

• The onset of pain is gradual and steady, eventually reaching a dull ache. Pain may radiate through to the back and typically lasts more than a day

• Some patients develop respiratory distress or jaundice.

Treatment

• STOP all alcohol consumption.

• Have the patient consume a liquid diet or fast until their appetite returns, then restrict fats and protein.

• Maintain fluid and electrolyte balances.

• Begin a Level 3 or Level 2 Evacuation depending on severity.

Diverticulitis

Pathophysiology

Diverticula are small pouches in the intestinal wall that develop as a result of muscular/intestinal weaknesses. The pouches may become infected and rupture or bleed internally. Risk factors include being male over age 40 and a diet high in fat/low in fiber.

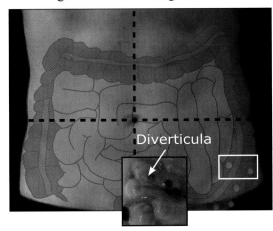

Diverticula

Assessment

- The patient often has a history of previous dull, colicky, and diffuse abdominal pain accompanied by flatulence, bloating, diarrhea, and/or constipation.
- Abdominal pain is usually specific to the Left Lower Quadrant; the pain is steady, severe and deep.
- Nausea, vomiting, and low-grade fever are common.
- The abdomen may be distended and feel drum-like.
- A red- or wine-colored stool indicates internal bleeding. Bright red blood issuing from the rectum in patients over age 60 is often caused by bleeding associated with diverticula and can be quite severe.
- Localized pain that becomes diffuse indicates rupture. The pain may or may not be accompanied by back or lower-extremity pain,
- Localized rebound tenderness and guarding indicate perforation.

Treatment

- Begin a Level 2 Evacuation if diverticulitis is suspected.
- Begin a Level 1 Evacuation if large amounts of bright red blood issue from the rectum or if perforation or rupture is suspected.
- Surgery may be required; the patient should not have any food for 6 hours prior to their arrival at a hospital.

Appendicitis

Pathophysiology

An appendicitis occurs when the appendix is blocked by a mucus plug or the patient's stool. The blockage encourages bacterial growth that leads to inflammation and often rupture. If the appendix ruptures, it precipitates an infection of the abdominal lining that may ultimately lead to death. S/Sx may disappear with spontaneous healing; however, the risk of rupture increases with surgical delay. Perforation and rupture are more likely to occur for patients under 18 years of age or over age 50.

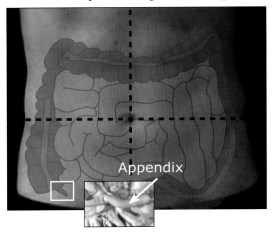

Appendix

Assessment

- The early S/Sx of appendicitis can be vague and similar to those of many other abdominal problems. Consider appendicitis if the MOI is unclear. When in doubt, take them out.
- Abdominal pain and tenderness are diffuse early when the inflammation is confined to the appendix. The pain localizes to the Right Lower Quadrant as the abdominal lining becomes irritated. The pain becomes diffuse again after rupture.
- The S/Sx of appendicitis include fever with or without nausea and/or vomiting; vomiting tends to develop after the onset of pain. Diarrhea or constipation is possible.
- The heel-drop test is the most sensitive of the field tests for appendicitis. Have the patient stand on their toes and drop jarringly onto their heels. If the patient reports sharp abdominal pain when their heels hit the ground, the test is positive. The pain occurs when an infected appendix bounces off the floor of the abdominal cavity.
- The right psoas muscle runs over the pelvis near

the appendix. Apply resistance to the right knee as the patient tries to lift their right thigh while lying down. If the appendix is inflamed, this will hurt.

- The right obturator muscle also runs near the appendix. Ask the patient to lie down with their right leg bent at the knee. Move the bent knee left and right. This requires flexing the obturator muscle and will cause abdominal pain if the appendix is inflamed.
- Sharp pain with a voluntary cough indicates inflammation of the abdominal lining.
- Rebound tenderness and guarding are common prior to rupture. Pain felt in the Right Lower Quadrant upon the release of pressure on the Left Lower Quadrant indicates an inflamed appendix (Rovsing's sign).
- Rule out ectopic pregnancy with an early pregnancy test (EPT).

Treatment

- Begin a Level 2 Evacuation if appendicitis is suspected.
- Begin a Level 1 Evacuation if perforation or rupture is suspected.
- Surgery is usually required; the patient should not have any food for 6 hours prior to their arrival at a hospital.

Intestinal Gas
Pathophysiology

Large amounts of gas produced in the intestinal tract are poorly transported by peristalsis and result in bloating and pain. Causes include lactose intolerance, sulfur-dried foods, improperly rehydrated foods, cruciferous vegetables, and legumes. The pain is exacerbated by lower pressure at high altitude.

Prevention

- Avoid consumption of gas-producing foods.
- Ensure complete rehydration of all dried foods prior to consumption.
- Use milk enzymes (Lactaid®) with dairy products.
- Use alpha-D-galactosidase, a mold enzyme (Beano®), when consuming gas-producing foods.

Assessment

- The patient presents with bloating, stomach distention, abdominal cramps, and/or gas (flatulence).
- Colicky abdominal pain is relieved by flatulence.

Treatment

- Simethicone liquid, tablets, or capsules (Phazyme®, Flatulex®, Mylicon®, Gas-X®, Mylanta Gas®, etc.).
- Use activated charcoal tablets.
- Kneel with the butt in the air (gas does indeed rise).
- No evacuation is necessary.

Inguinal Hernia
Pathophysiology

An inguinal hernia is caused when a part of the small intestine breaks through the abdominal wall into the scrotal or femoral area due to increased pressure, typically from straining or lifting, and/or an abdominal weakness.

Assessment

- The pain from an inguinal hernia is variable; it may radiate to hip, back, or leg, and increases significantly with activity, obstruction or strangulation.
- The hernia presents as a soft lump in the scrotal or femoral area.
- The size of the hernia often increases when the patient coughs or strains and decreases when the patient is relaxed or lies on their back.
- If obstructed, the patient may develop colicky abdominal pain, distension and vomiting.
- If strangulated, the lump will become red and increasingly tender; femoral hernias are more common in women and are more prone to strangulation.

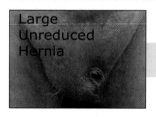
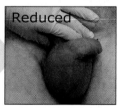

Treatment

- Position the patient on their back with their knees bent and supported with the leg on the herniated side rotated outward.
- Apply a cold pack to the site to reduce swelling and blood flow.
- Place two fingers at the edge of the break in order to prevent the hernia from riding over it during reduction.
- Apply firm steady pressure to the side of the hernia closest to the break to guide it back in; avoid putting pressure on the apex of the lump.

- Once reduced, support the groin and begin a Level 3 Evacuation.
- Begin a Level 2 Evacuation if reduction is unsuccessful or if an obstruction/strangulation is suspected.

Constipation
Pathophysiology
Constipation occurs when fecal matter hardens over time until defecation is difficult or impossible. Common causes are lack of a perceived opportunity, dehydration, low-fiber diet, stress, disruption of normal routine, and stopping smoking.

Prevention
- Avoid dehydration and ensure that the expedition diet includes high quantities of fiber.
- Trip leaders must ensure that all group members are informed and understand the importance of proper diet, hydration, and the necessity to relieve their bowels on a regular basis. They should also create daily opportunities for regular elimination. Strategies include taking regular breaks from daily travel and announcing "Now is a good time to go to the bathroom" or setting up the river toilet making an announcement that "The toilet is ready."

Assessment
- Constipation causes abdominal pain, bloating and lack of appetite.
- The patient has hard stools or incomplete evacuation more than 25% of the time or less than three bowel movements in a week.

Treatment
- Constipation can be avoided through education, adequate hydration, and a high-fiber diet.
- Administer a bulking agent, stool softener, lubricating agent, osmotic agent, an intestinal stimulant, or a warm-water enema.
- Begin a Level 3 Evacuation for manual removal of fecal impact.

Hemorrhoids
Pathophysiology
Hemorrhoids are caused by swelling, inflammation, and subsequent bleeding of the veins in the rectum and anus. Constipation is the major contributing factor. Most hemorrhoids are internal.

Assessment
- Presentation may be acute, chronic, or relapsing.
- Bright red blood covering the stool or toilet paper. Dark blood or blood mixed with the stool indicates bleeding higher in the intestinal tract.
- Painful swelling occurs in more severe cases. Pain peaks in 2-3 days.

Treatment
- Treat the patient as for constipation. Most hemorrhoidal S/Sx will disappear within a few days.
- Cold compresses and/or topical analgesic (Nupercainal®) will provide temporary relief.
- Consider a Level 3 Evacuation if S/Sx worsen during the fourth day.

Genitourinary System Problems
Kidney Stones
Pathophysiology
Kidney stones form within the kidneys, as mineral salts precipitate from supersaturated urine. The stones pass from the kidneys to the ureters where they become lodged until pressure or surgery removes them. The male to female ratio is 3:1.

Assessment
- The patient presents with uninterrupted flank pain with a gradual or abrupt onset. The pain typically increases during the first few hours, remains constant for hours, and then slowly fades.
- Patients with severe pain are writhing and unable to lie still. The pain may radiate to back or groin and stops when the stone reaches the bladder; most stones pass painlessly through the urethra.
- Nausea, with or without vomiting, is common.
- Fever is rare and indicates an infection.
- In patients over 60 with no prior history, the S/Sx may indicate an abdominal aortic aneurysm.

Treatment
- Roughly 85% of kidney stones pass spontaneously within 18 hours; the rest require hospitalization.
- The cessation of pain after 24 hours does NOT mean that the stone has passed; verification requires

advanced technology. Permanent kidney damage begins within 5-14 days if the stone is not removed.

- Begin a Level 3 Evacuation if the stone does not pass within 18 hours.
- Begin a Level 1 Evacuation if the patient is over 60 years of age, with no prior history of kidney stones or if the S/Sx are accompanied by a fever.

Urinary Tract Infection
Pathophysiology

Urinary tract infections (UTIs) are bacterial infections that may migrate to the patient's kidneys if untreated. UTIs are common in women because their urethras are short and close to their vagina and anus. Bacteria, usually e-coli, migrate from the vagina; incidence increases with sexual activity. UTIs are rare in men younger than age 50 because their urethras are longer and at a greater distance from their anus than women; however, the incidence increases with age and history of an enlarged prostate.

Prevention

- Maintain hydration and urinate on a frequent basis to flush bacteria. Don't "hold it in."
- Women should wash a minimum of twice a day, keep their genital area cool and dry, and wear clean cotton underwear or skirts without underwear whenever possible.
- Good hygiene is important. Women should consider using "pee rags" to pat dry after urination; avoid "drip drying." Wipe from front to back after a bowel movement to prevent contamination of the vagina.
- Direct trauma to the urethra from a bicycle seat, a climbing harness, or vigorous sexual activity contributes to the development of UTIs. A significant number of UTIs occur from bacteria exchanged during oral sex. In addition to washing, women prone to UTIs should urinate before and after sex to help flush unfriendly bacteria.

Assessment

- UTIs present with internal burning pain with urination accompanied by increased urgency, frequency, and decreased output.
- Urine may be cloudy or bloody with a strong odor. *There is no vaginal discharge.* The sensation of a full bladder and/or lower abdominal discomfort are common.

- A positive (pink) urine nitrite dipstick test indicates a UTI; however, false negatives are possible.

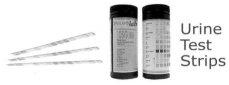

Urine Test Strips

- Fever, chills and general malaise, combined with flank or low-back pain, indicate a kidney infection.

Treatment

- Force fluids to flush bacteria.
- Cranberry juice or vitamin C (both with colloidal silver) may successfully treat very mild infections; severe infections require antibiotics.
- Herbs useful in treating UTIs include gravel root, couch grass, boldo, and parsley. These herbs act as a diuretic and have antimicrobial properties. Prickly pear juice may be used to alleviate the pain, but has no antimicrobial action.
- UTIs should be treated aggressively with antibiotics to prevent spreading to the kidneys and blood. Consider administering trimethoprim with sulfamethoxazole (TMP/SMX) or ciprofloxacin. The adult dose for TMP/SMX is one double-strength tablet (960 mg) twice a day for 7-10 days. Do not give TMP/SMX to patients allergic to sulfa drugs. The adult dose for ciprofloxacin is 250 mg twice a day for 7-10 days.
- Women taking antibiotics should take oral acidophilus or eat yogurt with live cultures to help avoid vaginal yeast infections.
- Begin a Level 3 Evacuation if antibiotics are unavailable. Over-the-counter phenazopyridine (AZO®, Uristat®) relieves UTI S/Sx but is not a cure; use for a maximum of two days during evacuation.
- Begin a Level 2 Evacuation if a kidney infection is suspected.

Sexually Transmitted Diseases
Pathophysiology

Gonorrhea, chlamydia and genital mycoplasma infections are the three most common sexually transmitted bacterial diseases. Most carriers are asymptomatic, therefore, S/Sx indicate a serious infection. If left untreated in women, they often lead to pelvic inflammatory disease (PID) and ectopic pregnancies. The local inflammation and scarring of the uterus common in PID may lead to tumors followed by scarring of and adhesions between the fallopian tubes and ovaries, causing infertility. PID may progress to include the liver and inflammation of the abdominal lining. The bacteria that cause gonorrhea may infect any mucous membrane; severe cases of gonorrhea-caused conjunctivitis may lead to blindness. If a systemic gonorrhea infection occurs (rare), death is possible. Gonorrhea and chlamydia account for most cases of epididymitis in men younger than age 35. The herpes simplex virus causes outbreaks of open sores. Finally, herpes is extremely contagious during an outbreak and predisposes people to other sexually transmitted diseases.

Prevention

- Use condoms.
- If an STD is suspected, get tested, and, if necessary, treated, prior to the start of any expedition.
- Know your partner's sexual history or abstain.

Assessment

Assessment of Gonorrhea, Chlamydia, & Genital Mycoplasma Infections

- S/Sx are similar for all three diseases. A culture is required for definitive assessment.
- All three diseases cause burning pain with urination.
- Secondary gonococcal bacterial conjunctivitis may follow accidental inoculation by fingers in either sex and is usually unilateral. Mild pharyngitis is common.
- Chlamydia infection is also frequently found in patients having gonorrhea.
- In males, a yellow or green penile discharge, with or without scrotal swelling, is associated with gonorrhea, while a clear or milky, white discharge is associated with chlamydia and mycoplasma infections. If the bacteria infect the prostate lining, they will cause the classic S/Sx of a UTI, including flank and back pain. The three diseases will all present with a positive (pink) urine nitrite dipstick test.
- In females, all three diseases will present with a greenish-yellow vaginal discharge and a strong fishy odor. Lower abdominal and cervical motion tenderness are common.

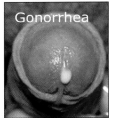
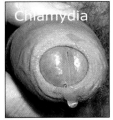
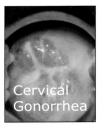

Gonorrhea   Chlamydia   Cervical Gonorrhea

Assessment of Genital Herpes

- In males having genital herpes, sores appear on the penis and occasionally on the scrotum, thighs, and buttocks. In dry areas, the lesions progress to pustules and then encrust. The urethra becomes infected in 30-40% of affected men and is characterized by extremely painful urination and clear mucoid discharge.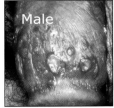

Male

- In females having genital herpes, sores appear on the external genitalia. In moist areas, the sores rupture, leaving tender ulcers. The vaginal mucosa is inflamed with a watery discharge. The cervix is involved in 70-90% of cases and is characterized by ulcerated mucous membranes. A cervical infection may be the only symptom in some women. Extremely painful urination may lead to urinary retention.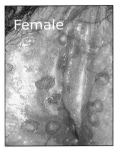

Female

- Recurrent genital herpes begins with tenderness, pain, and burning at the site of eruption that may last from 2 hours to 2 days.

Assessment of Pelvic Inflammatory Disease

- Acute PID is highly unlikely if the patient has no history of recent intercourse or IUD use.
- The onset of PID tends to be towards the end of menses and during the first 10 days following the menstrual period.
- Lower abdominal pain and tenderness may radiate to the lower back.
- Other symptoms include an unusual vaginal discharge, tenderness following cervical motion, irregular menstrual bleeding, and painful intercourse.
- Fever, nausea, vomiting, and severe pain are possible and indicate a serious infection.

Treatment

General

• Treat sexual partners concurrently if possible.
• Women taking antibiotics should take oral acidophilus or eat yogurt with live cultures to help avoid vaginal yeast infections.

Treatment of Gonorrhea, Chlamydia & Genital Mycoplasma Infections

• Administer a single 400 mg dose of cefixime by mouth AND 100 mg of doxycycline twice a day by mouth for 7 days. Begin a Level 3 Evacuation if antibiotics are unavailable.

Treatment of Genital Herpes

• Initiate wound care; treatment for secondary bacterial skin infections may be required.
• Genital herpes is treated with oral antiviral medications (acyclovir, valacyclovir, and famciclovir). The dosage depends upon the severity of the infection.

Treatment of Pelvic Inflammatory Disease

• Mild PID may be treated with 1 gram of azithromycin weekly for 2 weeks OR 100 mg doxycycline twice a day by mouth for 14 days. Severe infections are treated by a combination of IV and oral antibiotics. Begin a Level 3 Evacuation if antibiotics are unavailable and upgrade if S/Sx become severe.

Miscarriage

Pathophysiology

Pregnant women may undergo a spontaneous abortion that is usually NOT physically significant, unless accompanied by severe bleeding or followed by an infection. Miscarriage typically occurs in a wilderness environment when a woman is unaware that she is pregnant. More than 75% of miscarriages occur within the first trimester and are unlikely thereafter unless secondary to trauma. Fetuses with chromosomal defects tend to miscarry within 13 weeks.

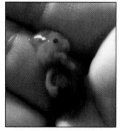

Assessment

• The patient has a history of pregnancy, delayed menses, and/or sexual intercourse within the past three months.
• Spotting, abdominal pain, and cramping are followed by heavy vaginal bleeding prior to and during the abortion of the fetus and placenta.
• Fever, chills, nausea, and vomiting after a miscarriage indicate an infection caused by a decomposing portion of fetal tissue attached to the uterine wall.
• Feelings of grief and loss are common.

Treatment

• The herb agrimony, given as a tea, increases clotting and may be useful in the treatment of heavy menstrual bleeding or bleeding due to miscarriage.
• The patient needs rest. Administer acetaminophen for pain. Exercise caution using aspirin, ibuprofen, and naproxen sodium; they may worsen bleeding.
• Consider a Level 3 Evacuation and monitor for S/Sx of systemic infection for 3-4 days.
• Begin a Level 1 Evacuation for infection or if bleeding is in excess of 5 soaked maxi-pads per day.

Ectopic Pregnancy

Pathophysiology

In an ectopic pregnancy, a fertilized egg implants outside the uterus, usually in a fallopian tube, which can lead to internal bleeding and infertility. Ectopic pregnancies are the leading cause of pregnancy-related death in the first trimester. Risk factors include prior PID/Chlamydia infection, ectopic pregnancy, and/or tubal surgery, use of fertility drugs or an IUD, and smoking; women over age 35 are at higher risk than younger women. Ectopic pregnancies tend to occur in a wilderness environment when a woman is unaware she is pregnant.

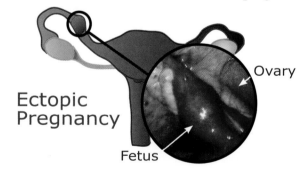

Ectopic Pregnancy

Ovary

Fetus

Assessment

• The patient has a history of delayed menses and sexual intercourse within the past two months and a Positive Early Pregnancy Test (EPT).
• The patient experiences abdominal pain, cramping, with or without spotting, and painful intercourse.
• Heavy vaginal bleeding usually indicates a tubal

miscarriage; there is no inflammation of the fallopian tube.

- Pain is caused by prostaglandins released at the site and by free blood leaking into and irritating the abdominal cavity. Shoulder pain indicates severe internal bleeding; monitor for S/Sx of volume shock.

Treatment

- 50% of ectopic pregnancies resolve without treatment by spontaneous abortion.
- If early in the pregnancy and the fallopian tube is still intact, the drug, methotrexate, will safely induce a miscarriage. Surgery is required if the tube is near rupture or has ruptured.
- Begin a Level 3 Evacuation for mild S/Sx.
- Begin a Level 1 Evacuation for moderate to severe S/Sx or suspected internal bleeding.

Vaginitis

Pathophysiology

Vaginitis is caused by a yeast, bacteria or protozoans. Fluctuations in the acid/base balance within the vagina due to diet and the women's menstrual cycle, may predispose some women to one type of infection or another. Within a woman's vagina, bacteria and yeast coexist in a balanced state. If the bacteria are destroyed, the balance is disturbed, and the yeast will grow unchecked, causing a vaginal yeast infection. All antibiotics are capable of upsetting the vaginal balance and women taking antibiotics are at risk for yeast infections. Bacterial infections are usually due to an increasingly alkaline vaginal environment and may be sexually transmitted. Untreated vaginal infections may lead to a UTI or PID. Protozoan infections are rare and usually sexually transmitted.

Prevention

- Take supplemental bacteria (yogurt, acidophilus capsules, etc.) concurrently with antibiotics.
- Rigorously maintain personal hygiene.

Assessment

General Assessment

- The patient experiences burning pain with urination, with or without an inflamed, itchy, and sore vagina and vulva; intercourse may be painful.
- Definitive assessment requires a vaginal smear.

Assessment of Vaginal Yeast Infections

- Yeast infections are caused by candida albicans and present with a thick, white, cheesy discharge with or without a slight yeasty odor. Recent history often reveals antibiotic therapy. Women who have previously been treated for yeast infections easily recognize the signs and symptoms.

Assessment of Vaginal Bacterial Infections

- Bacterial infections present with a thin, white or gray discharge having a foul, fishy odor that is stronger after intercourse. Bacterial infections may be accompanied by low pelvic pain.

Assessment of Vaginal Protozoal Infections

- Protozoal infection are caused by trichomonas and present similar to bacterial vaginitis but with an abundant foamy discharge; the odor is stronger after menstruation. The infection may spread to include abdominal pain and fever.

Treatment

Treatment of Vaginal Yeast Infections

- OTC medications are highly effective for yeast infections, including clotrimazole (Gyne-Lotrimin®) or miconazole nitrate (Monistat®) vaginal suppositories, tablets, or cream. Shorter courses with a higher dose increase compliance and cost; follow package directions.
- Begin a Level 3 Evacuation if drugs are unavailable.

Treatment of Vaginal Bacterial Infections

- For bacterial vaginitis (Gardnerella) treat the patient with Rx intravaginal metronidazole (MetroGel-Vaginal®) given as a 5 gram vaginal insert twice daily for 7 days OR intravaginal clindamycin 5 gram vaginal cream insert at bedtime for 7 days.
- Alternately 300 mg clindamycin can be given by mouth four times a day for 7 days OR metronidazole at 250 mg by mouth three times a day for 7 days or 500 mg by mouth twice a day for 7 days.
- Begin a Level 3 Evacuation if drugs are unavailable.

Treatment of Vaginal Protozoal Infections

- For protozoal infections (Trichomoniasis) treat the patient with Rx oral metronidazole and treat their sexual partner concurrently. Therapy has been successful using a single 2 gram dose of metronidazole. If unsuccessful, give 500 mg twice a day by mouth for 7 days. Alternately, use a single 2 gram dose of tinidazole taken by mouth with food. For resistant infections, use 2 grams twice a day for 14 days.

- Begin a Level 3 Evacuation if drugs are unavailable.

Ovarian Cyst

Pathophysiology

Most ovarian cysts function as a normal part of a women's menstrual cycle. Rarely, cysts may become too large, tumorous or cancerous; some twist and cut off circulation to the ovary and others rupture blood vessels, causing internal bleeding.

Assessment

- Lower abdominal pain is accompanied by abdominal fullness, pressure or bloating. The pain may radiate to lower back. The severity varies. Onset tends to be at the beginning, during or after the menstrual period. *Abrupt, sharp, severe pain indicates rupture and if benign, will improve within 45 minutes.*
- The patient will report irregular periods or spotting, nausea, with or without vomiting, and fatigue.
- The patient will have increased frequency of urination or difficulty with bowel movements due to intra-abdominal pressure from the cyst.

Treatment

- 95% of ovarian cysts are benign and require no treatment other than rest and NSAIDs for pain. NSAIDs are more effective when given early.
- Maintain hydration to avoid constipation.
- Avoid caffeine, alcohol, sugar and foods that cause gas.
- Limiting activity may reduce the risk of torsion or rupture.
- Consider Level 3 Evacuation if discomfort persists.
- Begin a Level 1 Evacuation if patient exhibits severe abdominal pain and tenderness with guarding.

Testicular Torsion

Pathophysiology

The spermatic cord that provides blood to the testis is twisted usually due to sudden exposure to cold, as in getting out of a sleeping bag, trauma, or exercise. The affected testis will die if not untwisted. Success approaches 100% if treated within 6 hours, 70% within 12 hours, 20% within 24 hours, and near 0% after 24 hours. Adolescents aged 12-18 through early adulthood (± 30) are at highest risk.

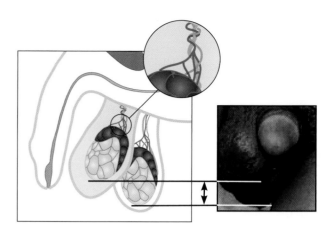

Assessment

- Testicular torsion is characterized by a sudden onset of severe scrotal pain; 50% of patients have a history of prior episodes that have spontaneously resolved. Pain may radiate from the flank to the groin.
- The patient will exhibit scrotal swelling and redness. Cord is typically thickened and extremely tender. The affected testis is usually elevated.
- Nausea and vomiting are common.
- Increasing pain and swelling after 24 hours, when the testis is already dead, indicates an infection or tumor.

Treatment

- Manually rotate the affected testis outward, as if opening a book. If the testis hangs lower but the pain persists, continue to rotate up to 2 full turns. If pain does not resolve, reverse direction and rotate inward.
- If detorsion is successful, provide scrotal support, limit activity and evacuate at Level 3 for surgical tacking.
- If detorsion is unsuccessful, begin a Level 2 Evacuation for removal of the affected the testis and surgical tacking of opposite testis.

Epididymitis

Pathophysiology

Epididymitis is an inflammation of the epididymis that is usually caused by a bacterial infection. In males under age 14 or over age 35, it is typically caused by an E-coli infection; in males aged 14-35, it is typically caused by chlamydia or gonorrhea. Epididymitis is the most common cause of scrotal pain and tenderness. Epididymitis may be difficult to distinguish from testicular torsion.

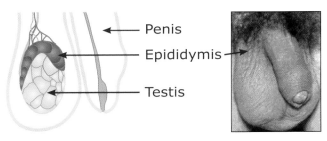

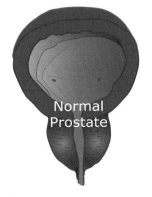

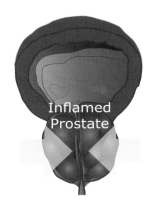

Assessment

- The onset of pain is slow, often over 24 hours. This helps to distinguish epididymitis from testicular torsion.
- Testes are not elevated and remain equal in size.
- The scrotum is painful, tender, and red, with or without swelling. The pain is behind and above the testis, with no pain felt in the testis itself. The pain may be aggravated during a bowel movement.
- The testis is increasingly sensitive to pressure and traction; scrotal elevation and support may decrease pain.
- Abdominal and/or flank pain may be present.
- S/Sx of a UTI are usually present and may be accompanied by an abnormal penile discharge.
- A positive (pink) urine nitrite dipstick test indicates bacterial infection.
- Fever and chills are common; nausea and vomiting are unusual.

Treatment

- The patient should rest and remain well hydrated.
- NSAIDS and ice packs should be used to control pain and inflammation.
- Doxycycline is the oral antibiotic of choice, given at 100 mg by mouth twice a day for 10-14 days.
- Begin a Level 3 Evacuation if antibiotics are unavailable.

Prostatitis

Pathophysiology

Prostatitis is inflammation of the prostate gland that may be caused by either bacterial infections and non-bacterial causes; it can be acute or chronic. The size of the prostate increases with the amount of inflammation, squeezing the urethra; bladder dysfunction and the accompanying thickening of its walls also contribute significantly to the S/Sx.

Assessment

- The patient presents with the S/Sx of a UTI with or without a positive urine nitrite test. A positive (pink) urine nitrite test indicates an active bacterial infection.
- Trouble starting and/or maintaining a urine stream, with dribbling.
- The patient experiences vague genital and pelvic pressure and/or discomfort.
- Low-back pain, fever, generalized muscle soreness, and painful ejaculation, with or without blood in the semen, indicate a serious bacterial infection.

Treatment

- Rest. Hydrate.
- Begin a Level 3 Evacuation if S/Sx interfere with the trip.
- Begin a Level 2 Evacuation if S/Sx are serious and/or a bacterial infection is suspected. Antibiotics are required for treatment of bacterial infections. Levofloxacin is the drug of choice because it has good concentration in the prostate; adult dose is 500 mg by mouth 4 times a day for 14-28 days. An alternate medication is trimethoprim/sulfamethoxazole DS dosed at 1 DS tab (160 mg TMP) by mouth twice a day for 10-28 days.

SECTION IX

Infectious Diseases

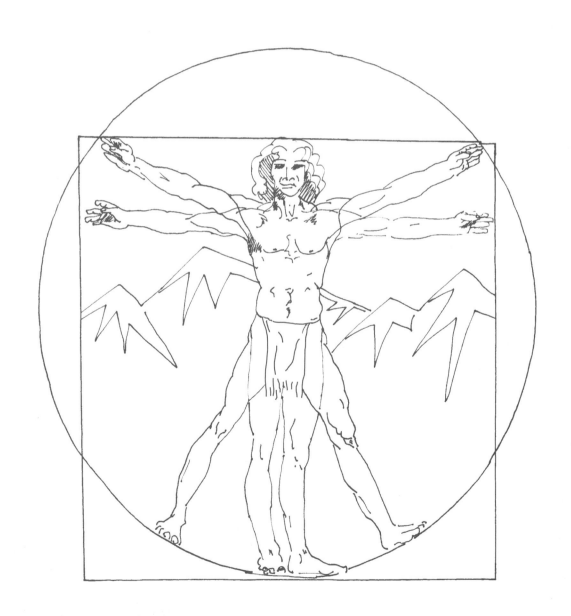

Infectious Diseases

The following information on infectious diseases is offered to help you understand the importance and methodology of prevention. Pathophysiology of each disease is offered because definitive diagnosis often depends upon a complete understanding of a patient's potential contact history, which hinges upon your understanding of the disease. *Unless stated otherwise, there are no effective field treatments for the infectious diseases discussed in this text. Patients exhibiting the signs and symptoms of any infectious disease should be evacuated to the nearest medical facility.* Specific treatments for adults are included for two reasons: first, to help you to understand the significance of the disease, and second, to assist with its treatment when hospital or clinical care is limited or not available. Treatments for children and pregnant women differ from the normal adult treatments and are not included in this text. Current treatment guidelines are available from:

- Centers for Disease Control (CDC) at www.cdc.gov
- International Association of Medical Assistance to Travelers (IAMAT) at www.iamat.org
- World Health Organization (WHO) at www.who.int

The following general information, together with Section X, Basic Pharmacology, should be read and understood before referring to the Infectious Disease Index and a specific disease.

Infectious Organisms

Infectious diseases are caused by viruses, bacteria, parasites, and fungi. Each infectious organism is briefly discussed in the following pages.

Viruses

Viruses are NOT alive; their size, shape, and behavior are similar to molecules. Viral DNA or RNA organisms are surrounded by a protein shell. The shell has "hooks" on the outside to attach to cell membranes. Once docked, virus particles inject their DNA or RNA into the cell's cytoplasm; the viral shell remains outside the cell. The virus's DNA or RNA then hijacks the cell's reproductive mechanisms to reproduce itself. Eventually the cell becomes a "viral packet," bursts, and releases new viral particles into the tissue. While vaccines are available for some viral diseases, few effective antiviral drugs have been developed; treatment is primarily supportive.

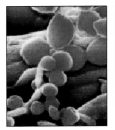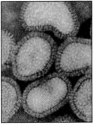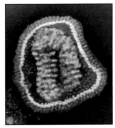

Examples:

• Hepatitis A, B, C	• SARS
• Herpes Simplex	• Rabies
• West Nile Encephalitis	• Dengue Fever
• Yellow Fever	• Influenza

Bacteria

Bacteria are 10-1,000 times larger than viruses and 100 times smaller than most human cells. They destroy human cells by producing toxins, feeding directly on the cell's cytoplasm, or feeding on nutrients in the extracellular fluid. Antibiotics are available for treating many bacterial diseases and are usually successful if the disease is diagnosed and treated early.

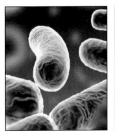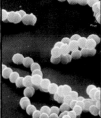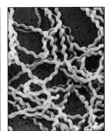

Examples:

• Leptospirosis	• Tetanus
• Cholera	• Diphtheria
• Bacterial Dysentery	• Pertussis
• Typhoid Fever	• Lyme Disease

Parasites

Single-celled parasites are 10 times larger than bacteria and can only be seen using a microscope. Most multi-celled parasites may be seen clearly with the naked eye.

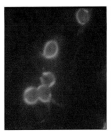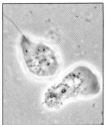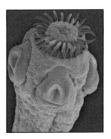

Examples:

- Malaria
- Giardia
- Amoebic Dysentery
- Cryptosporidium
- Chagas Disease
- Blood Flukes

Parasites damage organs and organ systems by producing toxins, feeding directly on body tissue, or robbing tissue of nutrients. Antimicrobial drugs are available for treating many parasitic diseases and are often highly successful if the disease is diagnosed and treated early.

Fungi

Fungi include single-celled yeasts slightly bigger than bacteria and multi-celled mushrooms and molds. They release enzymes and toxins to disable, kill and dissolve their food sources so that they can absorb the nutrients through their cell walls. Fungi continuously grow from their tips into fresh zones of nutrients and can easily penetrate human skin. Anti-fungal drugs are available for treating many fungal diseases and treatment is usually successful.

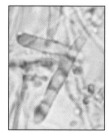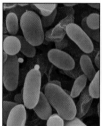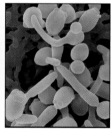

Examples:

- Candida
- Tinea

Transmission Routes & Prevention

Infectious diseases are transmitted via direct contact with infected body fluids, contact with animal or insect vectors, and contact with, or ingestion of, contaminated food or water. Prevention lies primarily in avoidance; research and study potential diseases, endemic areas, transmission routes, signs, symptoms, and treatment prior to leaving for a trip. Common transmission routes and avoidance tactics are briefly discussed in the following pages.

Vaccines are available for many infectious diseases; some are required for foreign travel or travel into endemic areas; visit the CDC, IAMAT and WHO websites for current information. Since many immunizations require multiple doses over a potentially lengthy period of time and planning is necessary, complete your research as early as possible. When vaccines are not available, preventive drug therapy is occasionally effective.

Body Fluids & Patient Care

Many infectious diseases (refer to the table below for those covered in this text) are transmitted through direct contact with an infected person's blood, mucus, genital secretions, saliva, feces, urine, sputum, and respiratory droplets. Prevention is possible by avoiding contact with these "wet and slippery" body fluids.

Fluid-Borne Diseases	Type	Page
Meningococcal Meningitis	bacteria	226
Diphtheria	bacteria	227
Hepatitis B	virus	228
Bacterial Dysentery	bacteria	242

Personal Protection

- Gloves, masks, glasses, and clothing may act as a physical barrier and offer protection.
- Chloroprene or nitrile gloves may be effectively carried in a wilderness setting by storing a pair inside a film canister or similar plastic container. Avoid latex gloves; they are less durable and many people have latex allergies.
- Wear a surgical face mask and glasses—or put a mask on the patient—when treating coughing or sneezing patients. Breathe clean air; if possible, treat coughing or sneezing patients outside.
- Wash your body and clothing with soap and water immediately after exposure. Regularly wash clothing and bedding that is in contact with infectious patients.
- Dispose of contaminated materials in a sealed and clearly marked container (usually a zip-lock bag).

Personal & Group Hygiene

While seemingly mundane, basic expedition hygiene procedures are critical to the success of any outdoor endeavor lasting longer than 24 hours.

- Wash hands before cooking or eating and after using the toilet. Maintain hand-washing stations in the kitchen and field toilet.
- DO NOT touch your eyes, nose, mouth or any food after touching any contaminated surfaces until after washing hands.

- Avoid sharing water bottles.
- Avoid reaching directly into snack bags; instead, pour snacks into clean hands.
- Brush and floss teeth daily to prevent gum diseases and dental decay.
- To prevent wart infections and athlete's foot, avoid walking barefoot in public areas such as showers or communal changing rooms. Avoid sharing shoes and socks.

Animal Vectors

In addition to sometimes devastating wounds, animal bites may transfer disease. Avoidance is protection; become familiar with specific animal habitat and behaviors. Once a patient is bitten, the wound should be thoroughly flushed with water and povidone-iodine. Thorough wound cleansing significantly reduces the risk of transmission.

Animal-Borne Diseases	Type	Page
Rabies	virus	228
Tetanus	bacteria	229

Insect Vectors

Many insect bites have the potential to transmit disease; common carriers are fleas, mosquitoes, ticks, chiggers, lice, sand flies and assassin bugs. The general preventive measures described below apply to all insects:

- Use no-see-um netting in tents and bug nets to protect against all biting insects; consider soaking the netting in permethrin.
- Use an insect repellent containing DEET or picaridin on exposed skin to repel mosquitoes, ticks, fleas, and other arthropods. EPA-registered repellents include products containing DEET (N,N-diethylmetatoluamide) and picaridin (KBR 3023). DEET concentrations of 30% to 50% are effective for several hours. Picaridin, available at 7% and 15% concentrations, needs more frequent application. DEET formulations as high as 50% are recommended for both adults and children over 2 months of age.
- When using sunscreen and an insect repellent together, apply sunscreen first and then repellent. Repellent should be washed off at the end of the day before going to bed.
- Apply permethrin-containing insecticide, such as Permanone®, to clothing, shoes, tents, mosquito nets, and other gear for greater protection. While permethrin kills most insects on contact, it has low mammalian toxicity, is poorly absorbed through the skin, and is rapidly inactivated by the body; skin reactions are uncommon. It is regularly used to kill head lice and the mites responsible for scabies.

Since prevention is primarily avoidance, it's important to understand the natural history of insect vectors. The following pages describe in detail most of the biting insects responsible for transmitting infectious diseases in humans. Each description is accompanied by a table that lists the disease, type, and page number for each vector.

Mosquitoes

Mosquito-Borne Diseases	Type	Page
Malaria	parasite	232
Yellow Fever	virus	233
Japanese Encephalitis	virus	233
West Nile Encephalitis	virus	235
Dengue Fever	virus	234

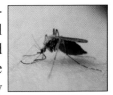
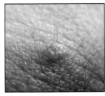

Mosquitoes are found worldwide in tropical and subtropical areas; some species have adapted to cooler environments; most are found below 6,000 feet. They typically feed on nectar and plant juices. In some species, blood serves as a protein source for egg production in females; males do not bite. Most feed between dawn and dusk and are attracted by carbon dioxide and 1-octenol, a chemical contained in human breath and sweat. Mosquito saliva contains proteins that may cause an allergic reaction. During the heat of the day, most mosquitoes rest in a cool place, such as grass, shrubbery, or other foliage, and then are active again in the evening; they may still bite if disturbed. Avoid mosquito bites by wearing head nets and appropriate clothing, by using insect repellents, and by being inside a tent as much as possible between dusk and dawn when mosquitoes are most active. Protect infants less than 2 months of age by using a carrier draped with mosquito netting with an elastic edge for a tight fit.

Ticks

Tick-Borne Diseases	Type	Page
Lyme Disease	bacteria	236
Rocky Mountain Spotted Fever	parasite	235
Colorado Tick Fever	virus	237
Q-fever	bacteria	237
Tularemia	bacteria	237
STARI	unknown	238
Heartland Virus	virus	239
Relapsing Fever	bacteria	238
Ehrlichiosis	bacteria	238

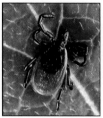 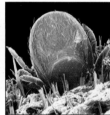 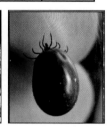

Ticks can be found in most grasslands and forests worldwide. Outbreaks of tick-related illnesses follow seasonal patterns as ticks evolve from larvae to adults. Ticks require blood to survive and have multiple hosts throughout their lifespan. As such, they act as vectors for numerous infectious diseases hosting different forms of bacteria, viruses, and parasites that they deliver via saliva when they feed. In addition to transmitting numerous diseases, proteins in their saliva may cause allergic reactions. Tick size ranges from those that are easily seen to almost undetectable. Hard ticks, so called because they have a hard back plate, attach and feed for hours to days. Disease transmission usually occurs near the end of a meal, as the tick becomes full of blood. Soft ticks do not have a back plate and typically feed for less than an hour; disease transmission may occur in seconds. While most tick bites are painless, some soft-tick bites produce intense pain. It is important to find and immediately remove any ticks. Do a thorough check for ticks periodically during the day, before sleeping, and upon waking. Remove and shake clothing before going inside a tent or shelter. Wear light-colored long pants, long-sleeved shirts, and socks so that ticks can be more easily seen; pull socks over pant cuffs. Use DEET on skin and permethrin on clothing.

Tick Removal

Ticks have barbed mouthpieces that firmly anchor them to a host while feeding. Using a small pair of tweezers or forceps, grasp the tick as close to its head as possible and gently pull straight out; avoid twisting. Ideally the head will come free with the body leaving a small crater behind. Destroy the tick and thoroughly wash your hands, instruments, and the bite site with soap and water and apply 10% povidone iodine to the site; contact with tick tissue and fluids can transmit disease. Circle the site with a felt-tipped marker and monitor it over the next few days for a rash or infection.

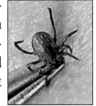

Chiggers

Chigger-Borne Diseases	Type	Page
Scrub Typhus	bacteria	239

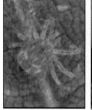 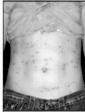 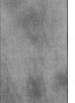 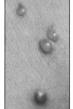

Chiggers belong to a family of mites and are related to ticks. They live in grasslands, scrub, and low, damp areas with thick vegetation. The larvae feed on the skin cells, but not the blood, of animals, including humans. The mites inject digestive enzymes into the skin that cause severe irritation, swelling, and small red lesions or blisters after the larvae detach. Wash with soap and warm water to remove.

Fleas

Flea-Borne Diseases	Type	Page
Murine Typhus	bacteria	239
Plague	bacteria	231

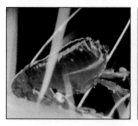 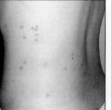 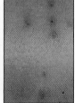

Fleas are dark-reddish-brown in color with hard, flat, fish-like bodies well adapted to moving easily through hair. The short spines on their bodies and legs resist removal. Fleas are wingless, but capable of jumping great distances. They live in the bedding and clothes of infected persons. Flea bites are irritating and can become swollen or inflamed; only the adults feed on blood. Scratching can lead to secondary infection. Outbreaks of bubonic plague or typhus tend to occur when people are in close proximity to wild rodents (rock squirrels, ground squirrels, prairie dogs, chipmunks, and rats). Select your campsites with care.

Lice

Lice-Borne Diseases	Type	Page
Epidemic Typhus	bacteria	239

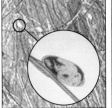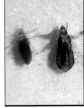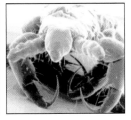

Humans host three different species of lice: head lice, pubic lice, and body lice. Head and pubic lice attach their eggs to the base of the hair shaft and feed on skin debris. Body lice live and lay eggs on clothing—often in the seams—and move to the skin to feed. Only the body louse spreads disease. Lice move by crawling and cannot hop or fly. They are easily spread by close contact and by sharing bedding or clothing. Animals do not play a role in the transmission of human lice.

Assassin Bugs

Assassin Bug-Borne Disease	Type	Page
Chagas Disease	parasite	239

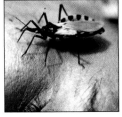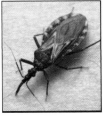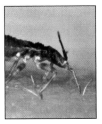

Assassin bugs can be found in tropical and subtropical areas worldwide. Most insects in this family prey solely on other insects and are considered beneficial; however, the blood-sucking species may carry the parasite, Trypanosoma cruzi, and transmit Chagas Disease. Insects in the blood-sucking species are also known as kissing bugs (because they tend to bite the lips or eyes of their victims) or conenose bugs and feed exclusively on the blood of vertebrate animals. Natural reservoirs of the Trypanosoma parasite are maintained in nature among small vertebrate animals, notably armadillo, opossums, rodents, bats, cats, and dogs. Assassin bugs commonly feed on several different hosts during their life cycle, become infected with the parasite, and later transmit it to an unsuspecting host. While feeding, the insect may defecate on the victim's skin. If the victim touches the feces, parasites may be transferred to the bite site or the victim's eyes and mucous membranes. Scratching increases the chance of transmission. Assassin bug bites are gentle and painless and occur at night while the victim is asleep. They cannot bite through clothing. They tend to infest primitive living quarters.

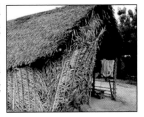

Sand Flies

Sand Fly-Borne Diseases	Type	Page
Cutaneous Leishmaniasis	parasite	240
Mucocutaneous Leishmaniasis	parasite	241
Visceral Leishmaniasis	parasite	241

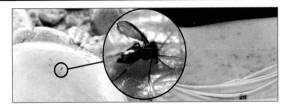

Sand flies are small—roughly one third of the size of mosquitoes—and difficult to detect; "no-see-um" netting is required for tents and head nets in order to prevent sand fly access. Similar to mosquitoes, the female sand fly requires blood proteins to produce eggs. Unlike mosquitoes, female sand flies use their mouth parts to create a pool of blood and then suck it up. They are active from dusk until dawn and bite mainly at night; they will bite during the day if they are disturbed. Sand fly bites are usually painless and leave a small, round, reddish bump that starts itching hours or days later. Leishmaniasis is caused by a protozoan that lives in the sand fly gut and is transmitted to people during feeding.

Contaminated Water

Water-Borne Diseases	Type	Page
Cholera	bacteria	241
Bacterial Dysentery	bacteria	242
Hepatitis A	virus	243
Typhoid Fever	bacteria	243
Giardia	parasite	244

Waterborne transmission of disease is both common and easily avoidable by using one of the following water-treatment methods or a combination. Clarification removes suspended particulate matter and many microorganisms. Clarify cloudy water prior to purification. Purification ideally renders the water free from all infectious microorganisms. Always have a back-up purification system.

Clarification Options

• *Sedimentation:* Let water stand for a minimum of one hour. Decant from the surface; pour decanted water through a coffee filter.

• *Coagulation/ Flocculation*: Add 1/8-1/4 teaspoon of aluminium sulfate (Alum, pickling powder) to each gallon of water, stir for 5 minutes, and allow floc to settle. Decant from the surface; pour decanted water through a coffee filter and purify.

• *Filters:* Filters clarify water and improve the taste by absorbing chemicals. A filter size of .2 microns effectively removes parasites, protozoans and bacteria. ***Viruses are not removed by filtration and filtration alone is not considered a purification method. Even filters that use an iodine resin should not be considered completely reliable because of the short contact time.*** That said, it's worthy of mention that within the United States, waterborne transmission of viruses is rare and filtering alone is generally considered safe. Ceramic filters can be cleaned; most charcoal filters are disposable.

Purification Options

• *Boiling:* Bringing water to 185° F for several minutes kills all intestinal pathogens; therefore, bringing water to a boil at any altitude renders it safe to drink.

• *Ultraviolet Light Pens:* UVC radiation (240-290 nm) prevents microorganisms from reproduc- ing by interfering with their ability to read and copy their own DNA. UVC purifies 16 ounces of water (one pint) in about 45 seconds and 32 ounces (one quart) in about 90 seconds. Clarify before the water before using the pen. Follow the manufacturer's instructions; bring extra batteries.

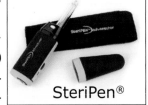

SteriPen®

• *Halogens:* iodine or chlorine is *NOT* effective against Cryptosporidium cysts. Dirty water may be clarified and then treated as described in the table below or treated directly by doubling the dose. Add a small amount of powdered ascorbic acid (vitamin C) to the water after it has been treated to eliminate the poor taste.

Halogens: Concentration vs.Contact Time

Method	4 ppm	8 ppm
Iodine tablets	1/2 tab	1 tab
2% Tincture of iodine	5 drops	10 drops
10% Povidone-iodine	8 drops	16 drops
Halazone tablets	2 tab	4 tab
Bleach (5% sodium hypochlorite)	2 drops	4 drops

Concentration	Contact Time		
	41° F 5° C	59° F 15° C	86° F 30° C
4 ppm per liter	3 hrs	1 hr	45 min
8 ppm per liter	1 hr	30 min	15 min

• *Grapefruit Seed Extract:* Follow the manufacturer's instructions. GSE is not approved by the FDA.

Contaminated Food

Food-Borne Diseases	Type	Page
Cholera	bacteria	241
Bacterial Dysentery	bacteria	242
Hepatitis A	virus	243
Typhoid Fever	bacteria	243

The Centers for Disease Control (CDC) recommends that any raw food found in areas of poor sanitation should be assumed to be contaminated. Salads, uncooked vegetables and fruits, unpasteurized milk and milk products, and raw meat and shellfish are considered high risk. Raw food that has been thoroughly washed and rinsed in potable water, peeled vegetables and fruits, and food that is still hot, are considered reasonably safe. Tropical fish should not be considered safe even when cooked because of the presence of toxins in their flesh. Ice made from contaminated water will also transmit disease. Cordon off expedition kitchens to promote safe management, food preparation, and cleanup. Adhere to the following guidelines:

- Keep cutting boards, cooking pots, dishes, utensils, and food preparation areas clean by washing them with soap and water and allowing them to dry thoroughly.
- Thoroughly cook meats and seafood. Cooking to a temperature of 180°F (82°C) will kill disease-causing organisms. Use a meat thermometer when cooking roasts or whole turkeys in a Dutch oven to be sure food is cooked to a safe temperature.
- Keep raw food away from cooked food. Avoid cross-contamination by using separate plates for cooked food and raw food.
- Thoroughly wash raw vegetables (carrots, lettuce, tomatoes, etc.) and soak in vinegar or Grapefruit Seed Extract for 30 minutes to kill bacteria.
- Wash melons and similar fruits and vegetables to avoid transferring any dirt or contamination from the rind or skin to the inside of the fruit during cutting or peeling.

- Drink purified water and use purified water for washing hands and cleaning food preparation areas.
- Don't let cooked food sit at room temperature; to slow bacterial growth, promptly pack in shallow containers and cool at or below 4°C/40°F. If refrigeration is unavailable, cook only the amount of food you or your group can consume. Do not eat spoiled food, or any food that has an unpleasant smell or taste. When in doubt, throw it out.

Other

Disease	Type	Page
Hantavirus Pulmonary Syndrome	virus	231
Leptospirosis	bacteria	230
Schistosomiasis	parasite	230
Rabies	virus	228

Leptospirosis and schistosomiasis are transmitted by contact with contaminated water or mud via swimming, wading, etc. Rabies may be transmitted via aerosolized bat urine or feces. Hantavirus Pulmonary Syndrome is transmitted via aerosolized rodent urine and feces.

- Avoid walking barefoot in mud or swimming in water that may be contaminated by feces or urine.

Infectious Disease Index by Transmission Route

Transmission Route	Possible Disease	Type	Page
Body Fluids	Meningococcal Meningitis	bacteria	226
	Diphtheria	bacteria	227
	Hepatitis B	virus	228
	Bacterial Dysentery (Shigella)	bacteria	242
Animal Bite	Rabies	virus	228
	Tetanus	bacteria	229
Deep Wounds	Tetanus	bacteria	229
Swimming, or wading in or contact with contaminated water or mud	Leptospirosis	bacteria	230
	Schistosomiasis	parasite	230
Aerosolized Rodent Urine & Feces	Hantavirus Pulmonary Syndrome	virus	231
Flea Bite	Plague	bacteria	231
	Murine Typhus	bacteria	239

Transmission Route	Possible Disease	Type	Page
Mosquito Bite	Malaria	parasite	232
	Yellow Fever	virus	233
	Japanese Encephalitis	virus	233
	Dengue Fever	virus	234
	West Nile Encephalitis	virus	235
Tick Bite	Rocky Mountain Spotted Fever	bacteria	235
	Lyme Disease	bacteria	236
	Colorado Tick Fever	virus	237
	Q-Fever	bacteria	237
	Tularemia	bacteria	237
	STARI	unknown	238
	Heartland Virus	virus	239
	Relapsing Fever	bacteria	238
	Ehrlichiosis	bacteria	238
Assassin Bug Bite	Chagas Disease	parasite	239
Sand Fly Bite	Leishmaniasis	parasite	240
Chigger Bite	Scrub Typhus	bacteria	239
Louse Bite	Epidemic Typhus	bacteria	239
Ingested Contaminated Food Fecal/Oral Route	Cholera	bacteria	241
	Typhoid Fever	bacteria	243
	Hepatitis A	virus	243
	Bacterial Dysentery (Shigella)	bacteria	242
Ingested Contaminated Water or Ice Fecal/Oral Route	Cholera	bacteria	241
	Bacterial Dysentery (Shigella)	bacteria	242
	Hepatitis A	virus	243
	Typhoid Fever	bacteria	243
	Giardia	parasite	244

Meningococcal Meningitis

Pathophysiology

Meningococcal meningitis is an infection of the lining of the brain or spinal cord that can result from exposure to infectious bacteria. Close contact to an infected patient is required to spread the disease since primary transmission is by respiratory droplets; 5-10% of the people infected are asymptomatic carriers. The disease moves from the respiratory system into the blood and from there to the central nervous system. The bacteria may cause septic shock, meningitis, or pneumonia. Outbreaks of the disease have occurred in locations where relatively large numbers of people come into close contact, such as college dormitories, army bases, and highly populated regions of sub-Saharan Africa, India, Nepal, and China.

Prevention

• Vaccination: Meningococcal conjugate vaccine (MCV4) is the preferred vaccine for people aged 2-55. One dose is generally sufficient to confer immunity; those at high risk may require two. The vaccine is recommended for children, adolescents and those traveling to parts of the world where the disease is common. Avoid epidemic areas. Refer to the CDC website for updates.

- Persons in close contact with infected persons should receive prophylaxis: ciprofloxacin given by mouth as a single 500 mg dose OR ceftriaxone IM.

Assessment

- The patient has a history of exposure to the respiratory droplets of an infected person within the last ten days.
- S/Sx include a severe headache, nausea, vomiting, light sensitivity, fever, general weakness, and altered mental status; some will have a skin rash.
- Patients often present with a stiff neck and complain of extreme pain when their chin is flexed toward their chest.
- Definitive assessment requires a positive culture from the patient's cerebrospinal fluid.

Treatment

- Treatment of choice is 2 grams of ceftriaxone IM (adult dose) two times a day for 7-10 days. Note: ceftriaxone treats all forms of bacterial meningitis. Alternate treatment is a 7-10 day course of penicillin G; IV adult dose is 300,000 units/kg/day given in divided doses every two hours (maximum dose is 24,000,000 units per day). Some strains are resistant to penicillin.
- Immediately following the initial antibiotic course, rifampin is given to prevent relapse: adult dose is 600 mg twice a day for two days.
- Relapse requires retreatment; consider alternative drug therapy.
- Problems associated with the treatment of the disease often require the invasive procedures available only to intensive care units.

Diphtheria
Pathophysiology

Humans are natural hosts for the bacteria that cause Diphtheria. The bacteria release a toxin that can lead to kidney failure, platelet deficiency and bleeding, chronic heart disease, and demyelination of both central and peripheral nerves. While transmission can occur from direct contact with infected persons, it usually occurs from contact with people who have been previously infected or immunized

and have become asymptomatic carriers. The disease takes two forms. The more serious is associated with a respiratory tract infection and transmission occurs from contact with respiratory secretions. The disease may progress to include swelling of the pharynx and severe respiratory tract damage. In addition, the toxin directly injures the patient's heart and brain often causing congestive heart failure and paralysis. A second form associated with skin lesions is commonly seen in the tropics and is rarely fatal.

Prevention

- A vaccine is available and children are routinely immunized via a five-shot series (DTaP) that includes protection against pertussis and tetanus; DTaP may be given at the same time as other vaccines. DTaP is not for children 7 and older. Tdap vaccine is similar and a single dose is recommended for people aged 11-64. A booster shot is required every 10 years for persons at low risk and every 5 years for persons at high risk. Anyone working or playing in the outdoors is at high risk. Unimmunized persons who come into close contact with the respiratory form of the disease should receive the entire vaccine series and a 7-10 day oral course of erythromycin dosed at 1 gm per day.
- Those who are immunized but who have not had a booster within the past 5 years should receive a booster as soon as possible.

Assessment

- History of exposure to infected patients within the past week.
- Initial signs and symptoms are nonspecific and flu-like. Symptoms include a sore throat, low-grade fever, general muscle soreness, and fatigue.
- Definitive diagnosis is obtained through culturing.

Treatment

- An antitoxin is available but it is only effective on the free toxin and does not affect tissue-bound toxin. It is made from horse serum and associated with anaphylaxis. The antitoxin is given as a single IM dose 20,000-100,000 units depending on the duration and severity.
- Additional treatment includes antibiotic therapy to destroy the bacteria and respiratory support. Antibiotics of choice are procaine penicillin G (PPG) or erythromycin. Penicillin PPG is dosed

IM at 1.2 million units per day in two divided doses OR erythromycin dosed at 40-50 mg/kg/day until patient can swallow; then, oral penicillin VK is dosed at 125-250 mg four times a day or oral erythromycin is dosed at 250-500 mg four times a day for a total treatment of 14 days.

Hepatitis B
Pathophysiology

Hepatitis B is a viral disease transmitted through contact with the body fluids of infected persons (especially blood and semen); it is a serious disease but can be easily prevented. Some of the adults and most of the infants who survive the disease are carriers. In third world and developing countries, 20% of the total population may be chronic carriers. Although this virus replicates in the liver and destroys liver cells, it is unrelated to the Hepatitis A virus. The disease is usually self-limiting within 4-6 weeks with a complete recovery after six months. The majority of patients recover completely, many become asymptomatic chronic carriers, and some develop chronic persistent hepatitis or chronic active hepatitis; very few die. Those who develop chronic active hepatitis develop progressive signs and symptoms and eventually die from cirrhosis of their liver.

Prevention

• All persons should be vaccinated against Hepatitis B.
• Avoid contact with the patient's body fluids.
• A vaccine is available and typically given to children at birth with the series completed between 6-18 months. The vaccine is recommended for unvaccinated adults who may encounter blood during the course of their work, those with multiple sexual partners, and people traveling to areas where the disease is common. The vaccine requires three injections: the initial injection, the second at one month, and the third at six months.

Assessment

• History of exposure to body fluids of a potentially infected person within the last six months.
• The development of a rash, joint pain, arthritis, and fever is initially present in 20% of patients.
• Loss of appetite, nausea, vomiting, abdominal pain, and fever soon follow.
• Enlargement of the spleen and liver usually accompanies the later S/Sx.

• Jaundice usually appears a short time after the onset of gastrointestinal symptoms.
• Definitive assessment is possible with a positive blood test for the Hepatitis B antigen.

Treatment

• Because the infection is viral, treatment is supportive in nature and focused on relieving the patient's signs and symptoms.

Rabies
Pathophysiology

Rabies is a viral disease that affects the CNS and is found in the saliva of infected animals and transmitted by their bite. The disease can occur in all mammals. Common carriers are foxes, skunks, raccoons, bats, coyotes, cats, dogs, weasels, mongooses, wolves, and jackals. Rodents are unlikely carriers. In addition to bat bites and scratches infected with bat saliva, rabies may be transmitted by inhalation in heavily bat-infested caves where there is a high concentration of bat guano and urine. Once in the body, the virus travels to the central nervous system via the peripheral nerves at an estimated rate of 12-24 mm per day; once it reaches the spinal cord, it spreads much faster, approximately 200-400 mm per day. The average incubation period is 20-90 days, with 90% of cases showing S/Sx within one year. The virus establishes itself within the brain, multiplies, and then spreads throughout the entire body. The progression of the disease produces one of two distinctive forms, either furious or paralytic rabies. The signs and symptoms of furious rabies include hyperactivity, aggressive behavior, and seizures alternating with calm periods. Persons infected with furious rabies may develop hallucinations, pharyngeal spasms, and excessive salivation ("foaming at the mouth"). With paralytic rabies, the person becomes progressively uncoordinated and lethargic. Eventually all people infected with the rabies virus die. There is no effective treatment and attention is focused on prevention.

Prevention

• Pre-exposure vaccination is available and recommended for those traveling in endemic areas, countries with large dog populations, and those with a high risk of exposure. The vaccination is given in three doses over a 21-day period. Post exposure treatment is still required. Booster doses are given based on current antibody levels.

- Thorough post-exposure wound cleaning with soap and water and/or povidone-iodine may destroy the rabies virus and prevent infection.
- Post-exposure vaccine is given to all persons suspected of contracting the rabies virus including those who have already been vaccinated with the pre-exposure vaccination. The dose is given in the deltoid muscle to avoid absorption in local fatty tissue. Unimmunized persons should receive five 1.0 ml IM doses with the first dose on the day of exposure (day 0). Subsequent doses are given on days 3, 7, 14, and 28. Previously immunized persons should receive two 1.0 ml doses on days 0 and 3. Patients with severe head bites should receive a third dose on day 7.
- In addition to the post-exposure vaccine, post-exposure immune globulin (HRIG) is given to all previously unimmunized persons suspected of contracting the rabies virus. It must be given at a different site than the vaccine to prevent neutralization of both the vaccine and the immune globulin. HRIG is dosed at 20 International Units (IU)/kg. Half the dose is infused into the wound site and the remaining half is given by IM injection.

Assessment

- History of exposure to the saliva of a potentially infected animal or inhalation of aerosolized bat urine or feces. Because most bat bites are painless with little or no evidence of associated wounds, awakening in a room or tent where a bat is present is considered a positive exposure. The incubation period varies greatly in humans ranging from 9 days to 1 year and averaging 20-90 days in most cases.
- Assessment is focused on the type of bite and the behavior of the animal. Aggressive or unusual animal behavior increases the risk. If the animal is suspected of carrying rabies, post-exposure prophylaxis should begin immediately.

Treatment

- There is no effective treatment for the rabies virus. Attention is focused on prevention. All persons suspected of exposure to rabies should begin prophylactic treatment ASAP within 72 hours. With the onset of signs and symptoms, the disease is fatal.

Tetanus
Pathophysiology

Tetanus is caused by a toxin produced by an anaerobic bacteria. The toxin is usually introduced via deep lacerations, puncture wounds, or animal bites, although it may also attend even minor and inapparent wounds. The toxin travels via the blood and lymph to peripheral neural connections in the muscles and then on to the central nervous system. Once established in the CNS, it interferes with normal muscle innervation and causes uncontrolled muscle spasms. The muscle groups surrounding the jaw are often the first to be affected; hence, the colloquial term for tetanus is "lockjaw." All muscles eventually become affected including the smooth muscle of the heart and vessels. Death is usually caused by a prolonged spasm of the intercostal muscles and diaphragm, which leads to respiratory arrest. Once the toxin binds to neurons, it cannot be neutralized with antitoxin. Left untreated the disease has a 90% mortality rate among infants and 40% in adults. While treatment is possible, prevention is much easier. It is the only vaccine-preventable infectious disease that is not contagious.

Prevention

- A vaccine is available and children are routinely immunized in childhood via a five-shot series (DTaP) that includes protection against pertussis and diphtheria; DTaP may be given at the same time as other vaccines. DTaP is not for children 7 and older. Tdap vaccine is similar and a single dose is recommended for people aged 11-64. A booster shot is required every 10 years for persons at low risk and every 5 years for persons at high risk. Anyone working or playing in the outdoors is at high risk.
- ***Thorough wound cleaning is essential for tetanus prevention.***

Assessment

- All persons with deep lacerations, puncture wounds, and animal bites are at risk for tetanus.
- There is no test available to confirm a diagnosis of tetanus.

Treatment

- Field treatment is limited to thorough wound cleaning and prompt evacuation to a hospital or clinic.
- Unimmunized persons with tetanus prone-wounds should receive a shot containing tetanus immune

globulin (TIG) and begin the vaccination series within 24 hours of the incident.

- Those who are immunized but who have not had a booster within the past 5 years should receive a booster within 24 hours of the incident.

- Specific treatment for tetanus includes surgical removal of infected tissue, 3,000-6,000 International Units (IU) of the immune globulin IM 3, antibiotic therapy, and respiratory support. The antibiotic of choice is metronidazole delivered IV at 500 mg every six hours for 7-10 days.

Leptospirosis
Pathophysiology

Leptospirosis is caused by a group of bacteria (spirochetes) with over 200 identified strains. Cases range from asymptomatic or mild in areas where infections are endemic to severe depending upon the individual strain. Except for polar regions, leptospirosis is present worldwide and is considered a hazard to all people who are active in the outdoors. It is transmitted through the urine and feces of infected animals, usually via contaminated water. Carrier hosts include both domestic and wild animals. Common carriers are dogs, rats, swine, and cattle. Humans are usually infected by wading or swimming in water (or mud) contaminated by the urine of infected animals. Although the disease is more commonly found in catchment water, the bacteria may be present in clear streams. The spirochetes routinely enter through the victim's skin or mucous membranes. Abraded or cut skin increases the risk of transmission. Less common routes of transmission are ingestion or direct contact with an infected animal's urine, feces, or tissue. The infection has two phases which begin after an incubation period that usually ranges from 7-12 days but may be as long as four weeks. During the initial phase, the infecting spirochetes may be cultured from the patient's blood or cerebrospinal fluid. The second phase begins after a short remission of one or two days. During the second phase the organisms are no longer present in the patient's blood or CSF but may be isolated from their urine. Fatalities are possible and usually due to liver or kidney failure.

Prevention
- Avoid wading or swimming in water that may be contaminated by urine from livestock or wildlife.

- Vaccines are limited to individual strains of the bacteria and are rarely practical.

- Prophylaxis is possible in epidemic areas with a weekly dose of doxycycline given orally at 200 mg per dose.

Assessment
- The patient has a history of history of swimming or wading in potentially contaminated water within the last month. The incubation period is 2-20 days.

- The initial phase of the infection, is characterized by a sudden fever, chills, headache, muscle pain, especially in the calf and lumbar regions, and red, watery eyes. Additional signs and symptoms may include nausea, vomiting, abdominal pain, and a nonproductive cough.

- The second phase of the infection may immediately follow the first phase or may begin after a 1-2 day remission; it is characterized by a severe headache that is unresponsive to pain medications and may indicate developing meningitis. Nausea, vomiting, abdominal pain, and muscle pain may continue; some patients may develop a red skin rash. In severe cases, jaundice is present.

- Definitive diagnosis is through blood or CSF culture during the first 7-10 days or from culture of the patient's urine after the tenth day.

Treatment
- Oral antibiotic treatment is effective if begun during the first phase (week) of the disease.

- Doxycycline is the treatment of choice; it is administered orally at 100 mg twice a day for seven days. Doxycycline causes extreme sun hypersensitivity; sun block is usually ineffective in preventing sunburn. Alternative antibiotics include penicillins, cephalosporins, and erythromycin.

- Hospital care is necessary for more severe cases.

Schistosomiasis

Schistosomiasis is caused by parasitic flatworms that are transmitted by the larvae of infected fresh-water snails in tropical and sub-tropical areas worldwide. Serious infections result in Katayama fever and chronic schistosomiasis; infections are common in the Caribbean, eastern Mediterranean, South American, southeast Asian, and African countries. The larvae, called cercariae, burrow into the host's skin and travel to the heart, lungs, and through the systemic circulation and the portal veins or, depending on the species, the mesenteric veins of both the large and small intestines, where they develop into adult worms. The adult worms are typically not pathogenic and do not reproduce in the host's body, but they do lay eggs that are released in the host's feces. The parasitic load determines the severity of the disease and the patient's S/Sx. While most infections are benign or asymptomatic, serious infections can result in death.

Assessment

- The larvae produce an allergic dermatitis in many people. Previous exposure to the larvae is required to develop the rash. The rash appears in sensitized individuals from 4-60 minutes after the larvae penetrate the skin. Pustules may develop over the next 24-72 hours. The rash is extremely itchy and secondary bacterial infections are common when scratched.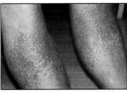

Katayama Fever

- Four to six weeks after the initial S/Sx, a heavy parasitic load may produce fever, lethargy, and muscle pain and less commonly cough, headache, weight loss, and rash. Because the S/Sx mimic most acute viral, bacterial, or malarial illnesses, the disease is often misdiagnosed unless schistosomiasis is suspected. A travel history that includes exposure to fresh water in an endemic area is an important clue in the patient's medical history.

Chronic Schistosomiasis

- While approximately 50% of the schistosoma eggs are excreted in the host's feces, the remainder become trapped in the host's tissues and over time cause local scarring and permanent organ damage. Onset of the disease is insidious and the S/Sx depend upon the number and location of trapped eggs (lungs, heart, intestines, etc.). While the initial inflammatory response is reversible with rapid treatment, the tissue and organ damage is not.

Treatment

- The dermatitis is treated with calamine lotion or oatmeal paste to sooth itching; it is self-limiting and typically resolves within two weeks.
- For serious infections of Katayama fever and chronic Schistosomiasis the drug of choice is praziquantel taken by mouth; the dose varies with the species.

Hantavirus Pulmonary Syndrome

Pathophysiology

Hantavirus pulmonary syndrome is a viral disease transmitted by inhalation of aerosolized rodent urine and feces. It is prevalent in the desert regions of the Southwestrn United States. Deer mice, pack rats, and chipmunks are the primary carriers. The incubation period varies from a few days to six weeks with a two week average. There is a 50% mortality rate.

Prevention

- Avoid disturbing rodent nests or burrows.
- Store food and water in rodent-proof containers.
- Do not use caves, cabins, or enclosed areas that have been infested by rodents.
- Do not camp in or near areas having a large rodent population.
- Maintain high standards for camp hygiene and water purification.
- The virus is susceptible to most disinfectants such as bleach. Spray contaminated areas thoroughly with water and disinfectant prior to cleaning.

Assessment

- The patient has a history of exposure to rodents within the last six weeks.
- The disease usually begins with general muscle soreness, fever, nausea, vomiting, and abdominal pain. The initial signs and symptoms are quickly followed by severe respiratory distress.

Treatment

- Because the infection is viral, treatment is supportive in nature and focused on intensive respiratory care.

Plague

(Bubonic & Pneumatic forms)

Pathophysiology

The Plague is a bacterial infection that is transmitted by the fleas of infected rodents, rabbits, or cats, or by the respiratory droplets of infected patients. Risk of contracting an infection is highest in rural mountain areas. The bacteria cannot penetrate unbroken skin and transmission may be prevented by washing after exposure. A serious infection may lead to meningitis and/or secondary pneumonia.

Prevention

- Avoid flea bites.
- Avoid close contact (face-to-face or within an enclosed space) with plague patients. The disease is transmitted through inhalation of respiratory droplets.
- Avoid areas with known outbreaks.
- The bacteria cannot penetrate intact skin and transmission may be prevented by washing after exposure.
- Preventive antibiotic therapy should be taken if risk of exposure is high. Prophylaxis may be obtained through oral tetracycline dosed at 15-30 mg per kg per day in four divided doses for one week following exposure.

Assessment

- The patient has a recent history of travel and flea bites in plague-epidemic areas or areas infested with rodents within the last week.
- Infection is characterized by a rapid onset of flu-like S/Sx, including fever, chills, headache, extreme exhaustion, and muscle soreness.
- Acute swelling of lymph nodes in the groin and occasionally the underarms and neck is characteristic of the Bubonic form.
- Coughing and respiratory distress are present in the pneumonic form.
- Definitive assessment is accomplished by culture and identification of the specific microorganism from the patient's blood, skin abscesses, cerebrospinal fluid (CSF), or sputum.

Treatment

- The drug of choice is Streptomycin IM given at 2-4 grams per day in two to four divided doses (adult dose) for 7-14 days; continue for 5-7 days once patient is afebrile. An alternate antibiotic is doxycycline.
- Place all patients thought to have plague and signs of pneumonia in strict respiratory isolation for 48-72 hours after starting antibiotic therapy.

Malaria
Pathophysiology

There are four different strains of Malaria. Each strain is a derivation of the same parasite: Plasmodium falciparum, P. vivax, P. ovale, and P. malariae. The infecting parasite is carried and transmitted by infected female Anopheles mosquitoes. Anopheles mosquitoes primarily feed between dusk and dawn. Malaria is common in Africa, Southeast Asia, Central and South America, the Indian subcontinent, and the Middle East. All wilderness travelers in these areas are at high risk for contracting malaria. Once infected, the parasite first matures in the host's liver and then within red blood cells, eventually destroying them. Once mature, the parasite acts like a "web" that "catches" red blood cells, causing micro clots. The clots may then migrate to the joints, lungs, kidneys, heart, spinal cord, and brain where they become lodged in small arteries and cut off perfusion; the clots may cause death in severe cases. Signs and symptoms follow an incubation period of 6-12 days. Improperly treated, infections of P. vivax, P. ovale, P. malariae can cause the disease to reoccur for years after the initial episode. Accurate diagnosis requires a blood test to identify the specific strain. Treatment varies depending upon the infecting strain. Some strains in some areas have become resistant to specific drugs; therefore, effective treatment hinges upon an accurate diagnosis, identifying resistant strains, and administering appropriate drug therapy.

Prevention

- No vaccine is available.
- Avoid mosquito bites. The Anopheles mosquito tends to feed in the early evening, throughout the night, and in the early morning; sleeping under protective netting is strongly advised. Travel during the transmission season, camping, and long-term trips are high-risk activities. Transmission typically does not occur at elevations higher than 6,000 feet.
- Prophylaxis is possible using antimalarial drugs (chloroquine, mefloquine, chloroquine phosphate). In some cases, doxycycline may be an effective chemoprophylaxis. Resistant strains are common in some regions. Outbreaks are unpredictable. The effectiveness of the prophylaxis depends upon the correct drug choice and dose. An overdose of antimalarial drugs can be fatal. Self medication is not advised. Visit the CDC website for current recommendations immediately prior to travel.
- Travelers can still get malaria despite the use of preventive measures.

Assessment

- The patient has a history of travel and mosquito bites within the past three weeks in countries where malaria is present.
- Travelers can still get malaria despite the use of prophylaxis.
- Flu-like symptoms follow the incubation period: headache, chills, fatigue, loss of appetite, muscle soreness, nausea, and vomiting.
- Early symptoms are soon followed by episodes of severe headache and joint pain, and high fever and sweating, followed by intense chills. Jaundice (yellow skin) may be present due to the destruction of both liver and red blood cells.
- The episodes commonly last 1-8 hours but may continue as long as 30 hours.
- Episodes are usually repeated every 2-3 days but may occur more frequently with a severe infection.

Treatment

- Because of the numerous drug-resistant strains, treatment for malaria is best done in a hospital setting. Self treatment is not recommended.
- Drugs used in the treatment of Malaria include chloroquine, quinine, mefloquine, halofantrine, primaquine, pyrimethamine-sulfadoxine (Fansidar), artemether, artesunate, or artemisinin. In some cases, Fansidar may be used as a field treatment until definitive care is reached. Artemether, artesunate, and artemisinin are derivatives of Chinese herbal remedies known to be clinically effective against malaria and without apparent significant toxicity. The drugs are currently available only in Southeast Asia.

Yellow Fever

Pathophysiology

Yellow fever is a viral disease transmitted by the infected Aedes aegypti mosquito; monkeys serve as animal reservoirs. Nicknamed "Jungle Fever," it is common in the tropical and forested areas of Africa, Central and South America, and some islands in the West Indies. After a 3-6 day incubation period, flu-like symptoms appear. Jaundice (yellow skin) occurs in most cases. In severe cases, as the virus continues to destroy red blood cells, the jaundice increases. The virus may also limit the patient's ability to clot and the patient may start bleeding more easily. Liver and kidney failure are possible; the disease is fatal in 50% of jaundiced patients.

Prevention

- A one-dose vaccine is available and is good for ten years; however, it requires a ten-day waiting period after administration before it is effective.
- The vaccine is a live virus vaccine and it is recommended for travelers to endemic areas. Infants, pregnant women, people allergic to eggs (the vaccine is prepared in embryonated eggs), and people with a suppressed immune system (HIV infection, AIDS, leukemia, lymphoma, etc.) should carefully weigh the risk of exposure to the risks associated with the vaccine.
- Cholera and yellow fever vaccines should be given three weeks apart.
- A certificate of vaccination is issued (yellow card) and remains valid for 10 years. It must be presented to meet entrance and exit requirements to some countries. A booster is required every 10 years.
- Avoid mosquito bites.

Assessment

- Yellow fever should be suspected in unvaccinated, symptomatic patients with a history of travel during the past week and mosquito bites in countries where yellow fever is present.
- Flu-like symptoms follow a 3-6 day incubation period: sudden fever, headache, muscle soreness, nausea, and vomiting.
- Jaundice is possible and the patient may easily bleed and vomit blood.
- Skin rashes are possible, but rare.

Treatment

- Because the infection is viral, treatment is supportive in nature and focused on relieving the patient's signs and symptoms.

Japanese Encephalitis

Pathophysiology

Japanese encephalitis is a mosquito-borne viral disease common in rural rice-growing and pig-farming regions in China, Korea, the Indian subcontinent, the Philippines, Southeast Asia, eastern Russia, and

Infectious Diseases 233

the Japanese archipelago. Pigs and aquatic birds are the primary reservoirs. The Culex mosquitoes that carry Japanese encephalitis represent a small portion of the entire mosquito population. The word, encephalitis, means swelling of the brain. The majority of persons infected do not develop any illness or exhibit only mild signs and symptoms. Infants and older people are at increased risk of developing serious signs and symptoms. Of those who develop encephalitis, only one third will recover without further incident, one third will survive with severe brain damage or paralysis, and one third of cases are fatal. AVPU and behavioral changes may occur as the disease progresses to infect the patient's brain.

Prevention

- A vaccine is available. A total of three doses is required; the second and third doses follow the initial dose on days 7 and 30. A waiting period of 10 days is necessary before the vaccine offers protection. A booster dose is required every two years. Monitor for anaphylaxis for 48 hours following each dose. The vaccine should not be given to people who are acutely ill, to those who have heart, kidney, or liver disorders; pregnant women, or people with a history of anaphylaxis.
- Avoid mosquito bites.

Assessment

- The patient has a history of travel and mosquito bites within the last 3 weeks in countries where Japanese Encephalitis is present.
- Initial S/Sx are flu-like with headache and fever.
- AVPU and behavioral changes accompanied by high fever, stiff neck, and jerky abnormal movements may occur as the disease progresses to infect the patient's brain.

Treatment

- Because the infection is viral, treatment is supportive in nature and focused on relieving the patient's signs and symptoms.

Dengue Fever

Pathophysiology

Dengue fever is a viral disease transmitted by infected Aedes aegypti and rarely Aedes albopictus mosquitoes. The Aedes mosquitoes feed during the day. Dengue fever is endemic to the semi-tropical and tropical regions of the Caribbean, Central and South America, Africa, Mexico, the Indian subcontinent, the Philippines, New Guinea, Southeast Asia, and northern Australia. Symptoms begin after a 3-to-14-day incubation period; the disease is self-limiting. Fatalities are rare with dengue fever. Dengue hemorrhagic fever, a different but related disease, has similar signs and symptoms, but is much more serious. Left untreated, dengue hemorrhagic fever has a mortality rate of 50%. The risk of contracting both diseases is high in endemic areas and low elsewhere; it is rarely found at elevations above 4,000 feet.

Prevention

- The mosquitoes that transmit dengue fever tend to feed during the daylight hours and bite below the waist; avoid mosquito bites.
- There is no vaccine available.
- Persons who have had previous bouts of dengue fever are more susceptible to dengue hemorrhagic fever.

Assessment

- The patient has a history of travel and mosquito bites within the past two weeks in countries where dengue fever is present.
- Dengue fever is commonly known as "bone-break" fever and is characterized by an acute fever and intense bone and joint pain. The febrile episodes usually last 3-5 days and no more than 7 days.
- Patients also complain of a severe headache, sore muscles, pain behind their eyes, and mild GI distress.
- A red, itchy rash usually appears on the patient's chest, back, abdomen, upper arms, and legs as the fever dissipates. The rash may begin on the chest and expand outward; it is rarely visible on dark-skinned races.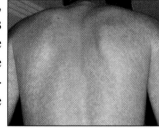
- Microscopic hemorrhages occur in the vascular beds causing minor bleeding from the nose and gums and pinpoint bruising throughout the body.
- Definitive assessment is by a blood test that detects the presence of the virus or antibodies.
- A simple field test using a blood pressure cuff can verify the presence of dengue hemorrhagic fever:

The cuff is inflated to a point halfway between the patient's systolic and diastolic pressures. The test is positive if pinpoint hemorrhages appear on the patient's skin distal to the cuff.

- A clinical pattern for volume shock after the febrile episodes have subsided indicates dengue hemorrhagic fever.

Treatment

- Because the infection is viral, treatment is supportive in nature and focused on relieving the patient's signs and symptoms; the disease is self-limiting.
- Aggressive fluid replacement and oxygen therapy significantly reduce fatalities in dengue hemorrhagic fever.
- Avoid aspirin, ibuprofen, and naproxen sodium; they impede the clotting process and exacerbate the bleeding. Give acetaminophen for pain and fever.
- The disease may last up to 10 days; complete recovery often requires 2-4 weeks.
- Relapses are rare, but possible.

West Nile Encephalitis

Pathophysiology

West Nile encephalitis is a worldwide viral disease with natural reservoirs in numerous species of wild birds; it is transmitted to humans via the Culex, Aedes, and Anopheles mosquitoes. Once in the blood, the virus crosses the blood-brain barrier and infects the brain. The incubation period is typically 1-6 days. Most people who are infected are asymptomatic or have a flu-like illness; few develop neurologic S/Sx.

Prevention

- Avoid mosquito bites.
- There is no vaccine available.

Assessment

- Most patients present with a low-grade fever and general malaise, including headache, sore muscles (especially backache), joint pain, vomiting, and diarrhea.
- Patients may exhibit changes in mental status, typically awake and confused, and decreased AVPU.
- A stiff neck indicates meningitis.
- 20% of patients present with a rash on the trunk of their bodies.

Treatment

- Because the infection is viral, treatment is supportive in nature and focused on relieving the patient's S/Sx.

Rocky Mountain Spotted Fever

Pathophysiology

Rocky Mountain spotted fever (RMSF) is caused by a tick-borne parasite active in the late spring and early summer. Many ticks carry the parasite, but dog ticks and wood ticks are the most common carriers. In order to transmit the disease, the ticks must have been actively feeding for a minimum of four hours. The disease is more common with feeding times greater than six hours. It is also possible to contract the disease during tick removal, if the person removing the tick comes into contact with tick tissue or fluids. Infections are prevalent in parts of North, Central, and South America. Signs and symptoms follow an incubation period of 2-14 days. In severe cases, the parasites multiply and progressively destroy the lining of the blood vessels; this destruction increases vascular permeability and leads to both organ dysfunction and volume shock. Left untreated, the mortality rate is 20-25%; mortality in those treated with the correct antibiotics is 5%; the mortality rate increases with age.

Prevention

- Avoid tick bites. Monitor patients with known tick bites for 14 days.

Assessment

- The patient has a history of a tick bite within the past two weeks. Definitive assessment is difficult without the history of a tick bite. In endemic areas during tick season, consider empirically treating the combination of rash and fever as RMSF.
- A sudden fever (103°-104° F) and chills immediately follow the incubation period and last for 2-3 weeks. They are accompanied by headache and muscle pain. Within 2-6 days of the onset of the fever, 50% of the patients develop a red-spotted rash on the extremities that spreads towards their core during the first three days; 90% develop the rash within 6 days. The rash emerges on the hands, wrists, and feet, then spreads to include the chest,

abdomen, and back. Other signs and symptoms include light sensitivity, joint pain, swollen hands and feet, ataxia, coughing, and abdominal pain with nausea, vomiting, and diarrhea.

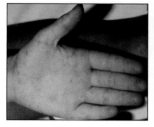 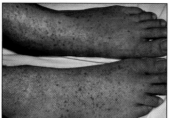

- RMSF is the only tick-borne disease that can directly cause congestive heart failure.

Treatment
- Prevent dehydration.
- The drug of choice is doxycycline, administered for 7 days. Adults typically receive a 200 mg loading dose twice a day for the first three days then 100 mg twice a day for the remainder of the course or until the patient is fever-free for three days. Doxycycline may cause severe photosensitivity; sun block is usually ineffective in preventing sunburn.

Lyme Disease
Pathophysiology

Lyme disease is a tick-borne bacteria commonly carried by the adult and nymphal forms of the deer tick. Signs and symptoms appear 3-32 days following an infected-tick bite. The organism can exist in human hosts for years without causing symptoms. The spirochete can penetrate human cells and live intracellularly and successfully avoid body defenses and antibiotics. The disease can progress through three stages. If the bacteria remain in the skin during the first stage and if they are treated with antibiotics within 3-6 weeks before antibodies are present, a complete recovery is likely. During the second stage, the disease begins to affect the heart, the central and peripheral nervous systems, the liver, the digestive system, and the musculoskeletal system. If still untreated or treatment is unsuccessful, the disease will progress to chronically infect the patient's nervous system, skin, eyes, and joints. Excessively late treatment may result in an incomplete recovery. Many patients complain of persistent fatigue, sleep disorders, depression, and cognitive difficulties.

Prevention

- Avoid tick bites. Monitor patients with known tick bites for five weeks.
- A single 200 mg dose of doxycycline may be used for prophylaxis in adults.

Assessment
- The patient has a history of a tick bite. Typically, ticks must be attached 24-48 hours to transmit the bacteria.
- The normal incubation period is typically 2-32 days; however, people can remain asymptomatic for years.
- Most infections occur during the late spring and early summer when ticks are most active.
- The first stage of the disease is usually heralded by a distinctive rash in 75% of the cases. The rash begins as a small red spot and grows outward forming an irregular circle; the rash may also appear in the form of hives. The classic bulls-eye pattern occurs in a small percentage of the population. The rash may be accompanied by non-specific flu-like signs and symptoms. Left untreated, the rash disappears after 1-4 weeks and the flu-like signs and symptoms appear or intensify.

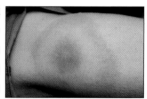
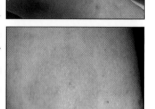

- The second stage of the disease leaves the patient with a feeling of extreme lethargy, loss of appetite, general malaise, low-grade fever, chills, swollen lymph glands, severe headaches, conjunctivitis, light sensitivity, and muscle and joint pain. Abdominal pain, nausea, and vomiting are possible. 60% of the patients in this stage develop arthritis.
- Definitive diagnosis is reached through the analysis of the patient's blood for the presence of Lyme-specific antibodies.
- Because early treatment is highly successful, assessment often consists of a positive history of a tick bite together with the presence of a rash.

Treatment
- Early treatment consists of an oral course of 100 mg of doxycycline (adult dose) twice a day for 2-3 weeks. Doxycycline causes severe sun hypersensi-

tivity; sun block is usually ineffective in preventing sunburn. Amoxicillin may be used in place of doxycycline. Amoxicillin is given orally at 500 mg four times a day for 2-3 weeks. Patients allergic to penicillin are also allergic to amoxicillin.

- Once the disease has become established internally, it must be treated more aggressively with an oral course of doxycycline at 200 mg twice a day for three days, followed by 100 mg twice a day for 25 days. Alternatively, erythromycin or ceftriaxone may be used.
- Intravenous antibiotics (usually high doses of ceftriaxone or penicillin) are required for difficult cases.

Colorado Tick Fever
Pathophysiology

Colorado tick fever is a viral infection transmitted by the wood tick and common to all areas of the mountain west. S/Sx of the disease follow an average incubation period of 3-5 days. The worst part of the infection is usually self-limiting within 5-7 days; however, the patient may continue to feel weak with general malaise for another 3-4 weeks.

Prevention
- Avoid tick bites. Monitor patients with known tick bites for five weeks.
- Infection usually confers lifelong immunity.

Assessment
- The patient has a history of a tick bite within the past week.
- Avoid tick bites. Monitor patients with known tick bites for five weeks.
- Signs and symptoms are flu-like. Fever (102°-104° F), severe headaches, muscle pain, and lethargy are common. In greater than 50% of the cases, the fever disappears for a few days and then returns. Light sensitivity, eye pain, nausea, vomiting, and abdominal pain occasionally occur. In a small number of cases, a mild skin rash may appear.
- Definitive diagnosis may be made by isolating the virus from the patient's blood.

Treatment
- Because the infection is viral, treatment is supportive in nature and focused on relieving the patient's signs and symptoms.

Q-fever
Pathophysiology

Q-fever is caused by tick-borne bacteria with a worldwide natural reservoir in mammals, birds, and ticks. In addition to tick bites, the disease can aerosolize and spread with the wind. The disease can be acute or chronic; mortality is 60% in patients with the chronic disease.

Prevention
- Avoid tick bites and endemic areas. Check the CDC website for updates.

Assessment
- The incubation period ranges from 2-6 weeks but averages 20 days.
- Other than an abrupt onset of high fever and chills, with or without a flu-like illness and joint pain, Q-fever has no classic clinical pattern. Chronic infections can involve the heart (endocarditis), lungs (pneumonia), liver (hepatitis) and/or brain (meningitis). GI problems and rashes are rare. S/Sx depend on the system involved.

Treatment
- Preferred treatment is an oral course of doxycycline (adult dose) with a 200 mg loading dose, followed by 100 mg twice a day for 3 days. Doxycycline causes severe sun hypersensitivity; sun block is usually ineffective in preventing sunburn.

Tularemia
Pathophysiology

Tularemia is caused by tick-borne bacteria with a natural reservoir in rodents, rabbits, hares, muskrats, and beavers. The disease is transmitted by ticks and occasionally by deer flies or by handling, skinning, and dressing an infected animal. The disease may present as a local papule that ulcerates, a distinct glandular infection, or GI distress after eating poorly cooked meat.

Prevention
- Avoid tick and deer fly bites.
- Handle potential mammal vectors carefully. Wear gloves and protective eye wear and wash yourself, your clothing, and other gear afterwards. Thoroughly cook all meat prior to consumption.

Assessment

- The incubation period is 3-5 days.
- The patient develops an abrupt onset of fever, chills, malaise, and fatigue.
- 80% of cases present with a small red papule that progresses into an ulcer within 2-3 days.
- Sore throat, abdominal pain, nausea, vomiting, diarrhea; frank gastrointestinal bleeding may occur if the mechanism is ingestion of poorly cooked meat (usually rabbit); pneumonia is possible.
- The glandular disease will present with swollen lymph glands, medically referred to as bubos.

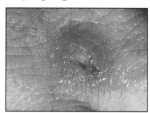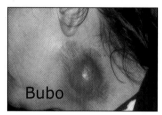

Bubo

Treatment

- Streptomycin is the drug of choice, and may ony be given in a hospital. The adult dose is 1/2-1 gram IM twice a day for 7-14 days or until the patient is afebrile for 5-7 days; do not exceed 2 grams per day.

Relapsing Fever
Pathophysiology

Relapsing fever is a bacterial infection that is spread by lice and ticks. Humans are the sole host of the disease spread by lice, while mammals and reptiles are the reservoir for the tick-spread disease. Lice-borne relapsing fever is uncommon; however, tick-borne relapsing fever tends to occur annually in mountainous regions at elevations above 8,000 feet.

Prevention

- Avoid tick bites and endemic areas. Check the CDC website for updates.

Assessment

- Average incubation time is 7 days.
- The patient experiences two or more episodes of high fever typically greater than 102° F (39° C), headaches, and muscle soreness. The initial febrile episode lasts an average of three days with an average of seven days between the initial episode and the first relapse. On average, patients with the tick-borne disease experience three relapses, while those with the lice-borne disease experience only one.

Patients tend to feel better between bouts; the febrile periods are characterized by a potentially lethal, although rare, period of unstable blood pressure.
- Chills, joint pain, nausea and vomiting, abdominal pain, mental status changes, nonproductive cough, diarrhea, dizziness, neck pain, photophobia, rash, and painful urination are possible.

Treatment

- Louse-borne relapsing fever is treated with a single dose of 100 mg of doxycycline by mouth. Tick-borne relapsing fever is treated with 100 mg of doxycycline by mouth every 12 hours for 7-10 days. Doxycycline causes severe sun hypersensitivity; sun block is usually ineffective in preventing sunburn.

Ehrlichiosis
Pathophysiology

Ehrlichiosis is a bacterial infection of white blood cells and is transmitted by ticks; mammals are the natural reservoir. The majority of cases are characterized by mild flu-like S/Sx that go unreported; however, serious infections resemble Rocky Mountain spotted fever and may be fatal.

Prevention

- Avoid tick bites.

Assessment

- The incubation period for ehrlichiosis is 5-14 days.
- Severe headache, muscle pain, and fever are the primary S/Sx. Shaking chills, nausea, and vomiting are common. Abdominal pain and rash are rare.

Treatment

- The preferred treatment is 100-200 mg of doxycycline by mouth every 12 hours for 7-10 days.

STARI

Southern Tick-Associated Rash Illness (STARI) is transmitted by the lone star tick (Ambylomma americanum). The microorganism that causes STARI is unknown.

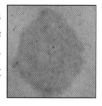

Assessment

- The saliva from lone star ticks can be irritating. Redness and discomfort at the site of a bite does not necessarily indicate an infection. An expanding rash roughly 3 inches in diameter, appears within seven days. The rash is similar to that of lyme disease, however, lone star ticks do not cause or carry lyme disease.

• Fatigue, headache, fever, and muscle pains.

Treatment

• Treatment with Doxycycline has been successful.

Heartland Virus

The heartland virus is related to a virus recently discovered in China and spread by the lone star tick. Consider this virus for tick-bitten persons who do not get better following treatment using antibiotics. Treatment is supportive only.

Typhus
Pathophysiology

Typhus refers to a group of infectious bacterial diseases that cause an acute febrile illness. There are three types: epidemic typhus, scrub typhus, and murine typhus; of the three types, epidemic typhus is the most severe. Epidemic typhus is transmitted by lice; humans are the primary reservoir, although flying squirrels are linked to infections within the United States. Epidemic typhus occurs in parts of North America, Central and South America, Africa, northern China, and certain regions of the Himalayas. Scrub typhus is transmitted by chiggers, which are the larval form of mites; mites are the primary reservoir while rodents and humans are secondary hosts. The disease is limited to eastern and southeastern Asia, India, northern Australia, Japan, and the adjacent islands. Murine typhus is transmitted by fleas; rats, mice, opossums, and cats are the primary reservoirs. Murine typhus occurs in most parts of the world, particularly in subtropical and temperate coastal regions. The transmitting organism—louse, chigger, or flea—defecates on the patient's skin while feeding; infection occurs when the victim scratches the bite site, providing an entrance for the excrement and bacteria, which subsequently travel to the blood. The rickettsial bacteria that cause typhus are extremely small and are able to "hide" within cells; reinfection is possible months to years after an apparent cure.

Prevention

• Avoid chigger, flea and louse bites.

Assessment

• Incubation period is 10-12 days.

• The disease is characterized by abrupt onset of

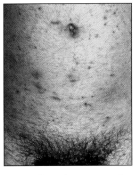

high fever (102°-105° F; 39°-41° C), headache, and rash are common symptoms in rickettsial infections. The rash occurs on days 4-7 and usually presents on the armpits and trunk before spreading to the extremities. Less common symptoms include nonproductive cough, swollen lymph glands, and deafness or tinnitus.

• An obvious bite site and subsequent scab are common with scrub typhus.

Treatment

• The duration of most clinical S/Sx in untreated typhus is approximately 2 weeks. Several months may pass before complete recovery from fatigue and malaise.

• The preferred treatment is 100-200 mg of doxycycline by mouth every 12 hours for 7-10 days or until the patient is afebrile for 2-3 days.

• 0.5-1 gram IV chloramphenicol every 6 hours—not to exceed 4 grams per day—is recommended for doxycycline-resistant strains.

• A second course of antibiotic therapy is usually curative in cases of recurring typhus.

Chagas
Pathophysiology

Chagas is a parasitic disease transmitted through the fecal matter of the blood-sucking species of the assassin bug (Trypanosoma cruzi), also known as the kissing bug because they tend to target the eyes and lips. Mammals are the natural reservoir. When the infected insects feed, they deposit parasite-laden feces. The parasites are then transmitted via contact with breaks in the skin, mucosal surfaces, or the eyes. The disease can also be transmitted when mammalian hosts ingest infected insects or by blood transfusions. Chagas disease occurs in three phases: an acute phase, an asymptomatic phase, and a chronic phase. S/Sx in the acute and chronic phases can range from mild to severe; many people don't experience S/Sx until the chronic stage.

Prevention

• Avoid assassin bug bites. Avoid sleeping in primitive living quarters, as they are often infested.

Assessment
Acute phase

- The incubation period of the disease is 7-14 days; many victims are asymptomatic. If S/Sx occur, they may include redness and swelling at the site of infection—which is not necessarily the bite site—and dermatitis and swelling around the eyes and eyelids if the victim has rubbed their eyes. Additional S/Sx include malaise, intermittent fever, fatigue, sore muscles, headache, loss of appetite, nausea, diarrhea, vomiting, swollen lymph glands, increased pulse, and inflammation and enlargement of the liver and/or spleen.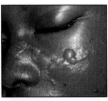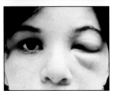

- Left untreated, S/Sx tend to spontaneously resolve within 3-8 weeks and are followed by the asymptomatic phase of the disease.

Chronic phase

- The chronic phase of chagas disease may occur 10 to 30 years after the initial infection with 10-30% of patients developing clinical S/Sx. Lesions appear on various organs of the body, including the heart, esophagus, colon, or peripheral nervous system; the damage done to organs during this phase is irreversible.

- S/Sx of an enlarged heart include arrhythmias and congestive heart failure, swelling of hands and feet, increased pulse & respirations, and respiratory distress (due to developing pulmonary edema).

- S/Sx of an enlarged esophagus include weight loss, difficulty swallowing and accompanying substernal discomfort, swollen salivary glands, inflammation of the walls of the alveoli because of the regurgitation and aspiration of stomach acids typically during sleep.

- S/Sx of an enlarged colon include abdominal pain, distention, and constipation.

Treatment

- Benznidazole or nifurtimox are used to treat patients in the acute phase; both may be available locally or from the CDC. The adult dose of nifurtimox is 8-10 mg/kg/day for 90-120 days; the adult dose of benznidazole is 2.5 mg/kg/day by mouth

twice a day for 60 days. Efficacy of either drug is assessed by monitoring disappearance of T. cruzi-specific antibodies; this may take several years in some patients. A cure is possible if the disease is diagnosed and treated early in the acute phase; once in the chronic phase, the parasite is untreatable.

Leishmaniasis
Pathophysiology

Leishmaniasis is a worldwide protozoal disease transmitted by sand flies; mammals are the primary reservoir. Infections present with a range of S/Sx from skin ulcers to a systemic infection involving the liver, spleen, and bone marrow. Infections may heal spontaneously or may progress to chronic disease, often resulting in death from secondary infection. Presentation and severity of the disease depends upon the patient's immune response, the virulence of the infection species, and the parasite burden. Four varieties of the disease are possible: cutaneous, mucocutaneous, visceral, and viscerotropic leishmaniasis.

Prevention

- Avoid sand fly bites.

Assessment
Cutaneous leishmaniasis

- The incubation period of the disease is weeks to months. The initial bite may evolve into a non-tender, firm, red papule that is several centimeters in size and that later becomes a small, painless ulcer with a crusty scab with a raised rim; secondary bacterial infections are possible and prolong healing. Healing often occurs spontaneously within 2-12 months with a loss of skin pigmentation.

- With a poor immune response, the lesion may spread, resulting in large non-ulcerating plaques that may ultimately cover the patient's entire body.

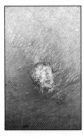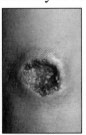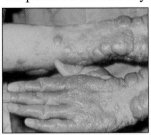

- Even with apparent healing, the disease may resurface after months or years following the initial infection and with new ulcers forming on the patient's cheek.

Mucocutaneous leishmaniasis

- This form of the disease develops from a persistent cutaneous lesion that eventually heals. Several years later, the patient develops a runny nose, nose bleeds, and nasal congestion, as the respiratory mucosa become inflamed. Severe infections cause nasal deformities referred to as "parrot's beak" or "camel's nose"; prolonged infection often results in death from respiratory compromise.

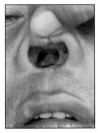 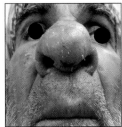 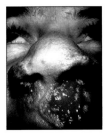

Visceral leishmaniasis

- The most fatal form of the disease, known as Black Fever, causes systemic infection of the liver, spleen, and bone marrow; incubation time varies. S/Sx include enlarged liver and spleen, excess production of IgG, and low red blood cell, low white blood cell, and low platelets counts resulting in a grossly distended abdomen.

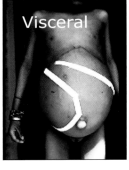

Viscerotropic leishmaniasis

- This form of the disease causes an inflammation of the GI tract one month to two years after exposure. S/Sx include malaise, fatigue, intermittent fever, cough, diarrhea, abdominal pain, and pain when swallowing. Nose bleeds and petechiae are common.

Treatment

- Sodium stibogluconate is the drug of choice for the treatment of cutaneous, mucocutaneous, and visceral leishmaniasis in the United States. The adult dose is 20 mg/kg/day IV. The length of course varies depending on the diagnosis: 10-20 days for cutaneous leishmaniasis; 28 days for mucocutaneous leishmaniasis; and 28-40 days for visceral leishmaniasis. Cure rate is greater than 90%.

- Miltefosine is the drug of choice for visceral leishmaniasis in India. The adult dose is 100 mg/day by mouth for 28 days. It may also be used to treat cutaneous leishmaniasis caused by L viannia braziliensis: 2.25-2.5 mg/kg/day by mouth for 3-4 weeks.

Cholera
Pathophysiology

Cholera is a bacterial infection caused by fecal-oral transmission and the ingestion of contaminated food or water; it may remain active for weeks in some foods. Cholera is wildly prevalent throughout the world; 50% of the reported cases occur in the western hemisphere. Cholera may also be transmitted in "hand-to-mouth" person-to-person contacts. The cholera bacteria may also live in coastal rivers and waters, contaminating shellfish. In most cases, the cholera bacteria are destroyed by normal stomach acids. Infection occurs when the bacteria are able to establish themselves in the small intestine and multiply. The incubation period is 1-5 days. The bacteria produce a toxin that prevents fluid absorption and causes an influx of fluids into the gut from the rest of the body; the result is profuse, watery diarrhea. Most infections occur either without symptoms or extremely mild symptoms. A severe cholera infection occurs in one fifth of the cases, causing extreme and painless diarrhea. Once diarrhea begins, death from dehydration can occur within hours. There is a 50% fatality rate associated with untreated cases.

Prevention

- Treat suspected food and water.

- The use of antacids, histamine receptor blockers, and proton pump inhibitors increases the risk of cholera infection and predisposes patients to more severe disease as a result of reduced gastric acidity.

- A vaccine is available but provides only 25-50% protection. Cholera and yellow fever vaccines should be given three weeks apart.

Assessment

- The patient has a history of ingestion of potentially contaminated food or water or contact with an infected person within the past 5 days. Incubation is typically 24-48 hours.

- Cholera causes fluid accumulation, distention, and diarrhea. The diarrhea may initially be brown in color but quickly becomes a watery gray with a fishy odor. Severe fluid loss occurs within the first 24 hours. Vomiting may also occur and is usually the result of dehydration.

- Fever is present in 25% of the cases.
- Definitive diagnosis is made via a stool culture.

Treatment

- ***Death from dehydration can occur within hours.***
- ***Begin immediate and aggressive fluid and electrolyte replacement until the patient's urine is clear.*** If the patient is not producing clear urine, aggressively continue fluid replacement. Fluid replacement should continue as long as diarrhea is present. In 90% of the mild-to-moderate cases, oral rehydration is successful. The World Health Organization (WHO) recommends the following oral fluid replacement formula: 20 grams per liter glucose (table sugar), 3.5 grams NaCl (table salt), 1.5 gram KCl (potassium chloride/salt substitute), 2.5 grams $NaHCO_3$ (baking soda).
- Intravenous therapy may be necessary in severe cases. Use WHO diarrhea solution and replace 30 ml/kg of fluid IV within the first 30 minutes; then switch to oral replacement.
- With fluid treatment, the disease is self-limiting.
- An oral course of antibiotics shortens the duration of the disease. Some areas report drug-resistant strains. Tetracycline is generally the antibiotic of choice. The adult dose is 500 mg four times a day for three days. Tetracycline causes severe sun hypersensitivity; sun block is usually ineffective in preventing sunburn. Trimethoprim-sulfamethoxazole (TMP/SMX) may be substituted for tetracycline at 320 mg TMP/1600 mg SMX two times a day for three days. Patients allergic to sulfa medications should not take TMP/SMX. Alternate antibiotics include azithromycin, doxycycline, ciprofloxacin, and erythromycin.

Bacterial Dysentery (Shigella)

Pathophysiology

Bacterial dysentery is caused by Shigella bacteria. Shigella bacteria are extremely hardy. They can survive freezing and are easily transmitted by the fecal-oral route through ingestion of contaminated food or water, including ice. Person-to-person spread ("hand-to-mouth") is common especially among groups in close physical contact. Expeditions with questionable sanitary conditions are at high risk of contracting the disease. Shigella is responsible for many cases of traveler's diarrhea. The incubation period is 1-3 days. Shigella produces local toxins that affect the patient's intestinal tissue. Mild cases are common and indistinguishable from other illnesses that cause headache, fever, abdominal cramps, watery diarrhea, muscle soreness, and general exhaustion. If the bacteria become established in the large intestine, they may invade local tissue causing a severe infection and ulcers. This classic form of infection is characterized by a fever, severe abdominal cramps, and bloody diarrhea. Mild infections tend to resolve within 7 days, but severe cases may last up to a few weeks. One quarter of untreated severe cases result in death.

Prevention

- Treat all suspect food and water.
- Maintain appropriate sanitary procedures.
- Avoid contact with the fecal matter of infected persons.

Assessment

- The patient has a history of ingestion of potentially contaminated food or water or close contact with an infected person within the past week.
- Initial signs and symptoms include headache, fever, abdominal cramps, watery diarrhea, muscle soreness, and general exhaustion.
- After 1-3 days, dysentery may develop. The signs and symptoms of dysentery are fever and bloody diarrhea. The urgency and frequency of diarrhea increases as the volume decreases; 20-30 watery yellow, green, or brown bowel movements containing mucus and blood are possible per day. Most patients report that each bowel movement requires effort and strain. Vomiting is present in 50% of the cases.
- Definitive diagnosis is made via a stool culture. Since antibiotic resistance is common with Shigella, bacteria cultured from the patient's stool are subjected to laboratory trials to determine which antibiotics would be most effective.

Treatment

- In cases involving severe fluid loss, treatment is focused on fluid and electrolyte replacement. The disease is self-limiting and fluid replacement is highly effective in preventing fatalities.
- Vomiting and diarrhea should not be controlled using medications.
- An oral course of antibiotics decreases the severity and duration of the disease. Administer ciprofloxa-

cin; the adult dose is 500 mg two times a day for 3-5 days. TMP/SMX and azithromycin are alternatives.

Hepatitis A

Pathophysiology

Hepatitis A is a viral infection transmitted through a fecal-oral route by contaminated food and water or "hand-to-mouth" contact with an infected person. It is the most common serious viral infection among travelers worldwide. It is prevalent in countries with poor sanitation. The incubation period is 2-7 weeks. The virus replicates in the liver destroying liver cells in the process. In most cases, the cells regenerate without complications after the disease has run its course. Signs and symptoms include loss of appetite, nausea, vomiting, abdominal pain, and fever. Jaundice usually follows within a few days or weeks. The disease is usually self-limiting within three weeks of the appearance of jaundice; however, it may take months for a full recovery.

Prevention

- Treat suspect food and water.
- A two-dose vaccine given six months apart is recommended for all children and adolescents living in communities where the disease is common and for travelers to third world countries. The vaccine may be given concurrently with other vaccines.
- An immune globulin shot will help prevent infection and is recommended for persons with potential intermittent or short-term exposure (3-6 months). The immune globulin interferes with normal antibody development and should be given 2-4 weeks after other vaccines and immediately prior to potential exposure since its protection disappears after 3-6 months. The shot may also be given within two weeks after exposure.
- Infection confers lifelong immunity.

Assessment

- The patient has a history of ingestion of potentially contaminated food or water or "hand-to-mouth" contact with an infected person within the past 7 weeks.
- S/Sx of the disease include loss of appetite, nausea, vomiting, abdominal pain, and fever.
- Enlargement of the spleen and liver usually accompanies the initial signs and symptoms.

- Jaundice follows within a few days or weeks.
- A few patients may initially present with a rash and joint pain.
- Definitive assessment is possible through a blood antibody count.

Treatment

- Because the infection is viral, treatment is supportive in nature and focused on relieving the patient's signs and symptoms.
- Do not attempt to restrict vomiting and diarrhea unless they interfere with necessary fluid and electrolyte replacement.
- A liver-friendly diet consisting of bland, low-fat foods is recommended.

Typhoid Fever

Pathophysiology

Typhoid fever is a bacterial disease transmitted through a fecal-oral route by contaminated food or water or direct "hand-to-mouth" contact with an infected person. The disease is common in third world and developing countries with poor sanitation. In a majority of the cases, most of the bacteria are destroyed by stomach acids while the remaining pass through the gut without transmitting the disease. If the bacteria become established in the digestive tract, they multiply, invade local tissues, and multiply again. The typical incubation period is 7-21 days, but may extend to three months. From the digestive tract, the disease moves into the blood, causing a systemic infection that may last 2-3 weeks. Left untreated, typhoid fever may resolve itself within 3-4 weeks; however, life-threatening complications cause a 12-32% fatality rate.

Prevention

- Treat all suspected food and water.
- A vaccine is available and recommended for travelers where typhoid fever is common; the vaccine is NOT 100% effective. An oral live vaccine is available in four doses taken over eight days, one capsule every other day. A oral booster is required every five years. An older, inactivated vaccine, given by a single-dose injection, is less effective and requires a booster shot every two years.
- The use of antacids, histamine receptor blockers, and proton pump inhibitors increases the risk of

typhoid infection and predisposes patients to more severe disease as a result of reduced gastric acidity.

Assessment

- The patient has a history of ingestion of potentially contaminated food or water or "hand-to-mouth" contact with an infected person within the past three weeks. The incubation period is typically 7-14 days.

- The systemic signs of the disease are usually preceded by gastrointestinal distress, abdominal pain, and constipation. Diarrhea may occur, but is less common.

- A slowly increasing fever follows the GI distress and indicates a systemic infection. The fever tends to rise during the day and drop by the next morning, gradually increasing with time. Left untreated, the fever will remain constant for 2-3 weeks.

- Symptoms include head-ache, loss of appetite, muscle soreness, and general exhaustion. A skin rash develops in 25% of the patients on the trunk of their body.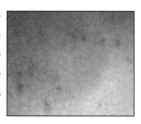

- Enlargement of the spleen and liver is common.

- Definitive diagnosis is through a blood or bone-marrow culture.

Treatment

- The bacteria causing typhoid fever have developed widespread antibiotic resistance that varies according to location. Generally, uncomplicated cases can be successfully treated by an oral dose of 500 mg of Levofloxacin every day for 7-14 days; complicated cases require IV antibiotic therapy. The fever will usually subside after 3-4 days of the correct antibiotic treatment.

- Relapse can occur after two weeks and requires retreatment; consider an alternative antibiotic.

- Do not attempt to restrict diarrhea unless it interferes with necessary fluid and electrolyte replacement.

Giardia

Pathophysiology

Giardia lamblia is a flagellate protozoan that is transmitted in cyst form in contaminated water. The adult organism is a filter feeder and restricts itself to clear running brooks and streams. Except during runoff, it is not usually found in large rivers or lakes; although, the mouths of streams where they join rivers or lakes should remain suspect throughout the year. The protozoan may remain dormant in its cyst form for long periods of time and it is the cysts that are transmitted in the feces of most animals, including humans. Fecal-oral "hand-to-mouth" contamination is the primary method of transmission especially among groups. The incubation period ranges from 7-20 days. Once the cysts are ingested, they emerge in a form that damages the lining of the small intestine, restricting food absorption. Most patients present with mild S/Sx while a small percentage experience an acute infection. The disease is usually self-correcting and often requires weeks or months for a complete recovery.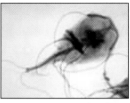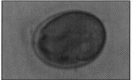

Prevention

- Treat all suspect water.
- Maintain high standards for personal and group hygiene.

Assessment

- The patient has a history of ingestion of potentially contaminated water or poor expedition hygiene within the past three weeks.

- Most patients present with mild signs and symptoms that include flatulence, loose and foul-smelling stools, nausea, and mild abdominal cramps.

- A small percentage of patients experience an acute infection with severe abdominal cramps; explosive, foul-smelling diarrhea; sulphurous burps; fever; nausea; and vomiting. An acute infection may result in severe dehydration. Fever and vomiting are usually limited to the first few days of the acute form, while general malaise, loose stools, and mild GI distress may continue for weeks to months.

Treatment

- Giardia is eventually self-correcting (weeks to months) and treatment is usually symptomatic. Fast relief may be obtained by administering tinidazole or metronidazole as described below:

- Tinidazole is taken by mouth in a single 2 gram dose.

- Metronidazole (Flagyl®) may be given at 250 mg twice a day for 5 days.
- A patient taking either medication should supplement their diet with acidophilus capsules and/or yogurt containing live cultures to prevent yeast infections.
- Patients who present with the symptoms of lactose intolerance (cramping, bloating, diarrhea), may benefit from adopting a lactose-free diet for several months.
- Do not attempt to restrict vomiting and diarrhea, unless they interfere with necessary fluid and electrolyte replacement.

SECTION X

Basic Pharmacology

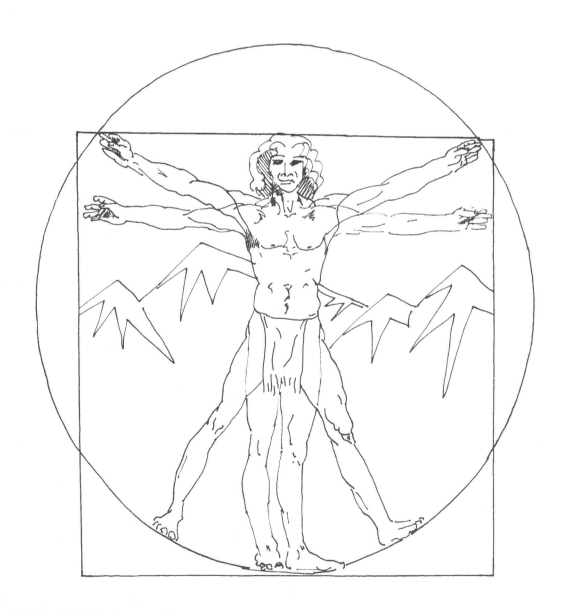

Basic Pharmacology

Introduction

Pharmacology is the study of drugs. Drugs are defined as chemical substances that have an effect on living organisms; medicines are drugs used to prevent or treat disease. The administrative route, health and age of the patient, and the chemical structure and dose of the drug all play a role in how fast it will act. A drug is considered effective if it elicits the desired therapeutic response with minimal side effects.

ALL drugs elicit more than one response and the use of multiple drugs at the same time may lead to desirable or dangerous drug interactions. Fortunately, due to effective drug control laws, the desired therapeutic response usually occurs and the side effects of most FDA-approved drugs are predictable, minimal and can be reduced by adjusting the dose of the drug. That being said, a few patients experience side effects strong enough to warrant discontinuing the drug treatment regime. Unlike most side effects, systemic allergic reactions are unpredictable and while most result in hives some cause respiratory distress, vascular collapse, and death. Interactions between multiple drugs taken concurrently may result in either an increase or decrease in the effectiveness of one or both drugs due to changes in each drug's absorption, distribution, metabolism, or excretion (ADME) characteristics. The majority of drug interactions are known and can be prevented by checking the appropriate database. Patients taking any form of a drug should be monitored for side effects, systemic allergic reactions, and drug interactions (if taking more than one drug).

Drug Classifications

Drugs fall into two distinct categories: those that require a physician's prescription to obtain (Rx) and those that can be purchased over-the-counter (OTC); both are regulated by the United States Food and Drug Administration (FDA).

Within these categories, drugs are further classified by the body system they affect, how they are used, or how they elicit their response. Drugs may be referred to by their chemical names, official names, brand names, or by their generic names. Because it describes the drug's exact molecular structure, the chemical name is complex and really only useful to chemists. Upon approval, the FDA gives each drug an official name. Trademark or brand names are proprietary and assigned and registered by the drug's manufacturer. In order to distinguish them from generic names, official drug names and brand names are capitalized when in print. The generic name is non-proprietary, simpler, and not capitalized when in print.

How Drugs Work—A Conceptual Overview

Most drugs act by forming chemical bonds with specific receptor sites within the body to stimulate or inhibit a response. While drugs alter the body's physiological activity along existing chemical pathways, they DO NOT create new pathways or responses. The success of a drug's response depends on two factors: its molecular fit and the number of receptor sites it bonds to. The better the fit and the greater the number of receptor sites occupied, the stronger the response. Chemical agonists fit and bond well into receptor sites and therefore elicit a strong response. Partial chemical agonists bond, but only fit well enough to elicit a partial response. Chemical antagonists also bond to receptor sites but do NOT fit well enough to elicit a response; their main role is to occupy the site and prevent agonists from bonding. If a receptor site is occupied, other drugs cannot bond to it.

In order for drugs to elicit a response, they must first be dissolved in the patient's blood or plasma and then transported to their respective receptor sites. Once dissolved, they go through four distinct stages: absorption, distribution, metabolism, and excretion (ADME).

Absorption is the process by which a drug is transported from its administration site into general circulation. The rate of absorption depends on the patient's hydration status, the administration route, the blood flow through the tissue at the administration site, and the solubility of the drug. Once absorbed, most drugs bind to and are carried by plasma proteins in the blood and lymph for distribution. When bound, the large size of the resulting drug/protein complex prevents the drug from crossing the vascular membranes into the tissue. A drug MUST cross into tissue to bathe receptor sites, become metabolized by the liver, or be excreted by the kidneys.

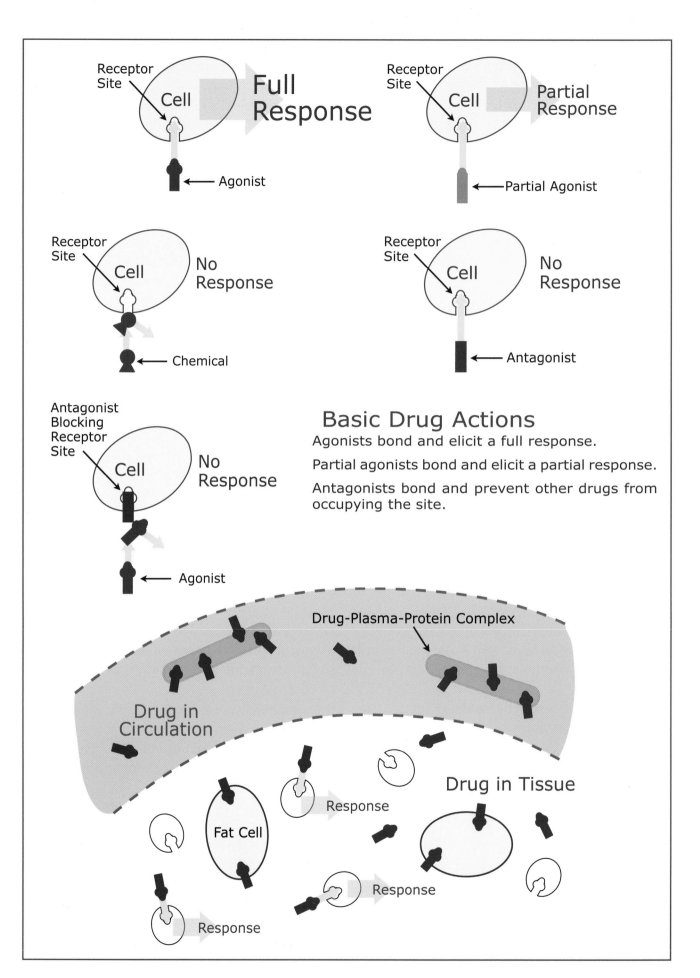

Receptor Site

Cell

Full Response

← Agonist

Receptor Site

Cell

Partial Response

← Partial Agonist

Receptor Site

Cell

No Response

← Chemical

Receptor Site

Cell

No Response

← Antagonist

Antagonist Blocking Receptor Site

Cell

No Response

← Agonist

Basic Drug Actions

Agonists bond and elicit a full response.

Partial agonists bond and elicit a partial response.

Antagonists bond and prevent other drugs from occupying the site.

Drug-Plasma-Protein Complex

Drug in Circulation

Drug in Tissue

Fat Cell

Response

Response

Response

Furthermore, once in the extracellular space, fat-soluble drugs are likely to bind to fat cells rendering them temporarily inactive. As serum drug levels change due to a drug response, metabolism, or excretion, molecules of the bound drug are released from the drug/protein complex and/or fat cells to maintain the equilibrium between the free and the bound drug. It is only the unbound drug in solution that is pharmacologically active. The amount of the drug that reaches the receptor sites determines the strength of its response. Serum levels of the drug MUST remain within a specific range in order to render the desired therapeutic effect.

Enzymes produced by the liver are the body's primary method of breaking down drugs and preparing them for removal (metabolism). Once inactivated, drug metabolites—and in some cases the active drug—are excreted from the body primarily through the urinary system and kidneys. Other less utilized removal methods are via the gastrointestinal tract (bile), lungs (exhalation), and skin (perspiration). Age, disease, smoking, and dehydration may decrease liver and renal function, thereby slowing both drug metabolism and excretion.

Drug Administration
in a Wilderness Environment

Drugs are administered by one of three routes: through the digestive system via ingestion, directly into the body's fluid reservoir via injection, and through body membranes via the lungs, mucous membranes, or skin. Choosing and administering a drug in a wilderness context by non-physicians should be done only in specific circumstances and according to protocols established by the expedition's or organization's physician advisor. Hydration, even in healthy people, is always a concern in a wilderness environment and becomes even more so when administering drugs. Dehydration causes poor absorption, distribution, metabolism, and excretion (ADME) and inhibits the desired therapeutic response; ***make sure that your patient is well hydrated before administering any drugs.***

Because oral drugs are effective, easy to carry, and simple to administer, they tend to make up the majority of the drugs carried in an expedition first aid kit. Before an oral medication can reach general circulation, it must survive the acids and enzymes of the digestive system, be successfully transported across the stomach or intestinal lining, and survive the initial pass through the liver. Throughout the process, hydration is extremely important; even in a well-hydrated patient, oral medications should be given with at least eight ounces of water.

Absorption through the skin and mucous membranes are also common drug administration routes used in a wilderness setting because, like oral drugs, they are effective, easy to carry, and simple to administer. Ear and eye drops are used to treat local infections. Rectal suppositories are used to treat constipation and nausea. Vaginal suppositories or creams are used to treat vaginitis. Topical skin ointments are used to treat local allergic reactions, promote healing in partial-thickness wounds, and treat a variety of cutaneous fungal infections. Sublingual or buccal glucose tablets are used to treat hypoglycemia in the insulin-dependent diabetic, and sublingual tablets are used to treat angina.

Absorption via inhalation is influenced by the depth of the patient's respirations. Absorption in the lungs is more effective when a spacer is used to disperse the medication prior to inhalation. The patient must take a deep breath and hold the drug in their lungs for a few seconds before exhaling in order for it to work. In a wilderness setting, the inhalation route tends to be reserved for participants suffering from asthma.

While all types of injections bypass the digestive system and frequently offer the fastest absorption and distribution routes, they should NOT be the first choice for an expedition first aid kit because they are expensive, difficult to carry, and require advanced training to use. Subcutaneous (SC) and intramuscular (IM) injections of epinephrine are commonly given, primarily by auto-injectors, to treat systemic allergic reactions. Because there are more blood vessels in muscles than in subcutaneous tissue, absorption is faster via IM injection. Give IM injections in the belly of the muscle where blood flow is the greatest and there are no large arteries or veins; the most common site used in the field is the anterior thigh.

Infusions are similar to injections in that they are an invasive procedure requiring a needle; however, during infusions, the needle or a catheter remains in place for hours or occasionally days. Intravenous (IV) infusions provide the most direct route to the blood and are commonly used in the acute pre-hospital setting where large amounts of fluid are required. Subcutaneous (SC) infusions are easier to start, maintain, have significantly fewer problems and potential problems than other infusion methods, and may be of value in the marine environment when used to treat dehydration secondary to sea sickness (hypodermoclysis). Intraosseous (IO) or bone infusions are similar to IVs in that they require specialized equipment and training, but are easier to use in hazardous environments. Infusion solutions and kits are rarely carried in the backcountry because of their relatively high weight, low need, storage problems, difficulty of administration in challenging environments, and the high level of training needed to administer them correctly even under the best of circumstances. As a result, infusions tend to be reserved for inbound rescue teams and remote field clinics that have the capacity to carry or store the necessary equipment and that are staffed with field paramedics, nurses, or physicians.

When choosing a drug, make sure that you:

• have authorization,
• adhere to your organization's protocols,
• review the patient's history for prior systemic allergic reactions to the drug,
• confirm that there is no possibility of dangerous drug interactions if multiple drugs are to be administered.
• review and advise the patient of the possible side effects.

Prior to administration, assess and document the patient's response to any prior medications and make sure they are hydrated. Make sure that you have the:

• right patient,
• right drug,
• right administration route,
• right dose, and
• right time.

After administering the drug, document all of the above information in the patient's SOAP note and/or a separate drug log.

Herbs

Medicinal herbs have been successfully used to treat ailments for thousands of years. Their gathering, preparation, and use have been documented in the writings and folklore of numerous cultures worldwide. Their use has been refined by generations and provides a built-in safety factor unavailable in modern drugs. Although herbs may be evaluated according to their pharmacological actions and chemical compounds, the constituents of the entire plant are greater than the sum of its parts. Some plant components are synergistic and enhance the herb's action far beyond the synthesized "active" compound, while other constituents buffer chemicals that would, without their presence, cause harmful side effects. In addition to their direct therapeutic effect, many medicinal herbs provide necessary trace elements and vitamins required for effective healing. Pharmaceutically, both herbs and drugs are chemicals that work within the body in a similar manner. That said, the line between therapeutic and toxic doses tends to be much broader with herbs than with drugs, thus increasing the safety factor of herbs when used by lay people. Herbs may be gathered and stored for use as the dried herb, dried powders, essential oils, tinctures, ointments, liniments, capsules, lozenges, and syrups. Teas may be made from fresh or dried herbs, tinctures, and tonics.

• *Essential oils* extracted from a plant are used as inhalants and when diluted, for massage; they should not be taken internally.
• *Fresh herbs* steeped in alcohol or cider vinegar produce concentrated tinctures. *Tinctures* are taken internally or used to make teas, compresses, or ointments. Be aware that some herbs, such as comfrey, should not be taken internally. A single tincture made from multiple herbs is referred to as a *tonic*. Unless you are a trained herbalist or have done your research, take care in mixing herbs. Different herbs taken together, much like different drugs, can be either synergistic and amplify their effects, nullify one another, or produce an unexpected and potentially dangerous side effect.
• *Infusions* are teas made from the flowers and leaves of fresh or dried herbs. To make an infusion, pour boiling water over the herb, cover, and allow it to steep for 10-15 minutes before straining. Infusions reserve the volatile oils present in the herb.
• *Decoctions* are teas made by boiling the hard, woody parts of an herb. The roots, woody stems,

bark, or nuts are first chopped (or ground) and then boiled for 10-15 minutes before straining.

- **Compresses** are made by soaking a clean cloth in an infusion or decoction. **Poultices** are similar to compresses but are made by wrapping the herb in gauze before applying to the skin. Both compresses and poultices are applied hot to the injured area and changed once they become cool. The active components are absorbed through the skin.
- **Ointments** are made by combining the fresh herb or tincture with a base of wax, fat, or oil that is then applied to the skin.
- **Liniments** are an oil-based herbal extract and used externally.

- **Capsules** are gelatin containers filled with powdered herbs or oils.
- **Lozenges** are powdered herbs or oil combined with gum or dried sugar.
- **Syrups** are tinctures added to sugar.

Herbs may be carried and stored in chopped or powdered form for later use in infusions, decoctions, compresses, or poultices. Since they do not keep well, water-based infusions and decoctions should be used immediately. Essential oils, ointments, liniments, and tinctures are prepared prior to use and for specific purposes; they are easily carried and last for years.

Antifungal Drugs

Drug	Rt	Contraindications	Notes
Clotrimazole	Topical	Hx of hypersensitivity. Caution in pregnancy.	Discontinue if irritation or sensitivity appears. Avoid contact with eyes.
Econazole	Topical		Discontinue if irritation or sensitivity appears. Avoid contact with eyes.
Itraconazole	Oral		Use with caution. Numerous drug interactions are possible. Discontinue if neuropathy appears.
Ketoconazole	Oral Topical		Discontinue if irritation or sensitivity appears. When using topical preparation, avoid contact with eyes.
Miconazole	Topical		Discontinue if irritation or sensitivity appears. Avoid contact with eyes.
Naftifine	Topical		Discontinue if irritation or sensitivity appears. Avoid contact with eyes.
Sertaconazole nitrate	Topical		Discontinue if rash, itching, dry skin, or local tenderness appear. Avoid contact with eyes.
Terbinafine	Oral Topical		Concurrent use with oral cyclosporine, phenobarbital and/or rifampin may decrease therapeutic levels. When using topical preparation, avoid contact with eyes.

Antiviral Drugs

Drug	Rt	Contraindications	Side Effects	Notes
Acyclovir	Oral Topical	Hx of hypersensitivity. Kidney disease. Pregnancy, children.	CNS: headache, dizziness, fatigue. GI: nausea, vomiting, diarrhea. GU: kidney failure. Skin: rash.	Most effective when started with the onset of S/Sx. Avoid contact with eyes.
Valacyclovir	Oral Topical	Hx of hypersensitivity. Kidney disease. Pregnancy, children.	CNS: fever, weakness, fainting. Circ: easy bruising or petechiae, bloody diarrhea, vomiting. Jaundice.	Most effective when started with the onset of S/Sx. Avoid contact with eyes.
Famciclovir	Oral	Hx of hypersensitivity. Kidney disease.	CNS: headache, dizziness, fatigue, confusion. GI: nausea, vomiting, diarrhea, abdominal pain. Skin: rash.	Most effective when started with the onset of S/Sx. Avoid contact with eyes.

Antibiotic Drugs

Drug	Rt	Contraindications	Side Effects	Notes
Amoxicillin	Oral	Hx of hypersensitivity to penicillins. Pregnancy.	GI: diarrhea, nausea, vomiting. GU: vaginal yeast infections.	
Azithromycin	Oral	Hx of hypersensitivity. Pregnancy, nursing mothers, children.	**Anaphylaxis.** GI: diarrhea, nausea, vomiting, abdominal pain.	May decrease effectiveness of birth control pills.
Ceftriaxone	IM	Hx of hypersensitivity to cephalosporins. Pregnancy.	GI: diarrhea, abdominal cramps. GU: vaginal yeast infections.	
Ciprofloxacin	Oral	Hx of hypersensitivity to quinolines. Pregnancy, nursing mothers, children.	CNS: headaches, vertigo, malaise, seizures. GI: nausea, vomiting, diarrhea, abdominal cramps.	
Clarithromycin	Oral	Hx of hypersensitivity. Caution in patients with liver, kidney & heart disease.	CNS: dizziness, headaches. GI: diarrhea, nausea, vomiting, abdominal pain. Facial swelling.	May decrease effectiveness of birth control pills.
Clindamycin	Oral	Hx of hypersensitivity. Pregnancy. Caution with Hx of GI Px.	GI: diarrhea, nausea, vomiting, abdominal pain. Skin: rashes.	Stop drug if severe diarrhea develops. Do NOT take concurrently with diarrhea drugs.
Doxycycline	Oral	Hx of hypersensitivity to tetracyclines. Pregnancy, nursing mothers, children.	GI: nausea, vomiting, diarrhea, abdominal cramps. Skin: phototoxic reaction.	Avoid sun during therapy & 5 days after course is complete; sun blocks are ineffective.
Erythromycin	Oral	Hx of hypersensitivity. Pregnancy. Patients with impaired liver function.	CNS: vertigo, tinnitus. GI: nausea, vomiting diarrhea, abdominal cramps. GU: vaginal yeast infection.	Not for prolonged use due to potential for developing resistant organisms.
Levofloxacin	Oral	Hx of hypersensitivity to quinolines. Pregnancy, nursing mothers, children. Caution in patients with liver, kidney & heart disease.	Irreversible peripheral neuropathy, central nervous system toxicity, cardiovascular toxicity, tendon & articular toxicity, & hepatic toxicity.	Do not take concurrently with NSAIDs.
Penicillin G	Oral IV	Hx of hypersensitivity to penicillins or cephalosporins. Pregnancy.	**Anaphylaxis.** CNS: fever, malaise. Skin: rash.	Take oral meds 1 hour before or 2 hours after meals.
Penicillin VK	Oral	Hx of hypersensitivity to penicillins or cephalosporins. Pregnancy.	**Anaphylaxis.** GI: nausea, vomiting, diarrhea.	
Streptomycin	IM	Hx of hypersensitivity to aminoglycosides. Pregnancy, children.	**Anaphylaxis** CNS: headache, weakness, vertigo, tinnitus.	
Tetracycline	Oral	Hx of hypersensitivity to tetracyclines. Pregnancy, nursing mothers, children.	GI: nausea, vomiting, diarrhea, abdominal cramps. Skin: phototoxic reaction.	Avoid sun during therapy & 5 days after course is complete; sun blocks are ineffective.
Trimethoprin sulfamethoxazole	Oral	Hx of hypersensitivity to sulfa drugs. Pregnancy.	GI: nausea, vomiting, diarrhea. Skin: rashes, photosensitivity, jaundice.	Discontinue if skin rash or jaundice appear.

Angina Medication

Drug	Rt	Contraindications	Side Effects	Notes
Nitroglycerin	Sublingual	Hx of hypersensitivity to nitrates. Pregnancy, nursing mothers, children. Head trauma, increased ICP, hypotension.	CNS: headache, vertigo. Circ: postural hypotension, palpitations, collapse. Skin: flushing, cold sweat.	Tingling or burning sensation under tongue is normal. Once pain is relieved with tablet, patient can spit out remainder.

Antimalarial Drugs

Drug	Rt	Contraindications	Side Effects	Notes
Artemether	IM	Hx of hypersensitivity. Caution in pregnancy.	CNS: potential neurotoxicity.	For use in severe cases with quinine resistant strains and in combination with other antimalarials.
Artemisinin	Oral	Hx of hypersensitivity.		
Artesunate	IM IV	Hx of hypersensitivity.	CNS: potential neurotoxicity.	
Chloroquine	Oral	Hx of hypersensitivity. Caution in pregnancy.	CNS: dizziness, headache. GI: nausea, diarrhea, abdominal pain.	Avoid prolonged use.
Halofantrine	Oral	Hx of hypersensitivity. Patients on cardiac drugs. Pregnancy.		Do not use concurrently or after mefloquine.
Mefloquine	Oral	Hx of hypersensitivity. Caution in pregnancy, children. Patients on cardiac drugs. Patients with psychiatric and seizure disorders.	CNS: dizziness, insomnia. GI: nausea, diarrhea, abdominal pain.	Do not use concurrently with halofantrine or chloroquine.
Pyrimethamine-sulfadoxine	Oral	Hx of sulfonamide intolerance. Caution in pregnancy.		Taken with chloroquine. Tx is temporary; seek medical evaluation ASAP.
Primaquine	Oral	Hx of hypersensitivity. Caution in pregnancy.	Circ: hypotension, arrhythmias. GI: abdominal cramps.	
Quinine	Oral IV	Hx of hypersensitivity. Pregnancy.	CNS: tinnitus, vertigo, confusion. GI: nausea, vomiting, diarrhea.	Avoid tetracyclines. Do not use if patient has taken mefloquine during the past 2 weeks.

Pain Medications

Drug	Rt	Contraindications	Side Effects	Notes
OTC & Rx Nonsteroidal Anti-inflammatory Drugs (NSAIDs)				
Acetaminophen	Oral	Hx of hypersensitivity. Alcoholism.	Liver toxicity at high doses.	Avoid alcohol. No anti-inflammatory properties. Do NOT take with food. May be crushed & dissolved.
Aspirin	Oral	Hx of Hypersensitivity to NSAIDs. Infections in children (Reye's syndrome).	***Anaphylaxis.*** CNS: tinnitus, hearing loss. GI: nausea, vomiting, heartburn, bleeding.	Take with food. Do NOT crush or dissolve.
Ibuprofen	Oral	Hx of Hypersensitivity to NSAIDs. Hx of GI ulcers.	***Anaphylaxis.*** GI: nausea, heartburn, bleeding.	Do NOT exceed 2400 mg in 24 hours.
Naproxen Sodium	Oral	Hx of Hypersensitivity to NSAIDs. Hx of GI ulcers.	***Anaphylaxis.*** CNS: headache, drowsiness, dizziness. GI: nausea, heartburn, bleeding.	Take with food.
Rx Opioids				
Acetaminophen & Codeine Acetaminophen & Oxycodone	Oral	Hx of Hypersensitivity to acetaminophen or opioids. Pregnancy. Liver or kidney disease. Caution with breathing disorders. Mental illness. Hx of drug or alcohol addiction.	CNS: headache, dizzy, drowsy blurred vision. GI: nausea, vomiting, constipation. Dependence.	Avoid alcohol. For short-term use ONLY. Do NOT operate machinery.

AMS Drugs

Drug	Rt	Contraindications	Side Effects	Notes
Acetazolamide	Oral	Hx of hypersensitivity to sulfa drugs. Pregnancy. Caution with diabetics.	CNS: malaise, depression, fatigue, muscle weakness. GI: nausea vomiting, diarrhea, thirst, dry mouth.	Take with food to minimize GI Px. Increase fluid. Requires potassium supplement.
Dexamethasone	Oral IM	Hx of hypersensitivity. Systemic fungal infections, acute infections, concurrent with live virus vaccine.	CNS: euphoria, insomnia, increased ICP, vertigo. Circ: CHF, hypertension, edema. Endocrine: menstrual irregularities, hyperglycemia,. GI: hiccups, nausea, abdominal distension, ulcers, oral yeast infections. Musc: weakness, tendon rupture, pathogenic fractures. Skin: impaired wound healing.	Requires potassium supplement.
Nifedipine	Oral Sublingual	Hx of hypersensitivity. Caution in pregnancy.	Circ: hypotension.	Avoid concurrent use with any drug that lowers BP.
Sildenafil Citrate (Viagra)	Oral	Hx of hypersensitivity.	CNS: headaches. Circ: flushing, rhinitis, prolonged painful erection. GI: indigestion. Back pain, muscle soreness.	Avoid alcohol and concurrent use of nitrates.
Tadalafil (Cialis)	Oral	Hx of hypersensitivity.	CNS: headaches. Circ: flushing, rhinitis, prolonged painful erection. GI: indigestion. Back pain, muscle soreness.	Avoid alcohol and concurrent use of nitrates.
Salmeterol	MDI DPI	Documented hypersensitivity. Caution in pregnancy. Cardiac: angina, tachycardia.	Mild tachycardia.	

Allergy Medications

Drug	Rt	Contraindications	Side Effects	Notes
Antihistamine				
Diphenhydramine	Oral	Hx of Hypersensitivity to antihistamines. Pregnancy, nursing mothers, children under 12. Asthma. Caution in patients with cardiovascular disease and diabetes.	CNS: drowsiness, dizziness, headache, impaired coordination, insomnia, tinnitus. Circ: tachycardia, collapse. GI: vomiting, diarrhea, constipation. Resp: wheezing, thickened secretions.	Take with food. Avoid alcohol and other CNS depressants. Avoid activities that require alertness. Increase fluid intake.
Emergency Bronchodilator				
Epinephrine	Oral	Hx of hypersensitivity. Caution in pregnancy. Cardiac arrhythmias.	Circ: tachycardia, hypertension, MI. CNS: anxiety, severe headache, dizziness, stroke. GI: nausea, vomiting. Skin: sweating, pale.	May increase blood glucose levels; diabetic patients may have control Px.

Emergency Hypoglycemia Medication

Drug	Rt	Contraindications	Side Effects	Notes
Glucagon	IM	Hx of hypersensitivity. Pregnancy.	GI: nausea, vomiting.	After patient becomes alert (5-20 min), follow with complete meal. Headache, nausea & weakness may persist for hours after recovery.

Ointments, Creams, & Suppositories

Drug	Use	Rt	Contraindications	Side Effects	Notes
Clortimazole	Vaginal yeast infections	Vaginal	Pregnancy, nursing mothers, children.	Local: mild burning. GI: lower abdominal cramps, bloating. GU: UTI.	Avoid intercourse during Tx. Supplement with acidophilus capsules or yogurt with live cultures.
Metronidazole	Vaginal bacterial infections	Vaginal	Pregnancy, nursing mothers. Patients with yeast infections.	CNS: vertigo, headache, depressions, fatigue. GI: nausea, vomiting, diarrhea, abdominal pain. GU: UTI, pelvic pressure, yeast infection vagina & vulva dryness. Dark brown urine.	Avoid alcohol and intercourse during Tx. Discontinue if seizures or peripheral numbness develop. Supplement with acidophilus capsules or yogurt with live cultures.
Miconazole	Vaginal yeast infections	Vaginal	Hx of hypersensitivity. Pregnancy, nursing mothers, children.	Circ: tachycardia, arrhythmias. GU: mild burning, itching, pelvic cramps. GI: nausea, vomiting, diarrhea.	Identify organism prior to Tx. Avoid intercourse during Tx. Supplement with acidophilus capsules or yogurt with live cultures.
Gentamicin	Eye infections	Topical	Hx of hypersensitivity to aminoglycoside antibiotics.	Photosensitivity, burning, stinging, redness.	Avoid contact use during Tx. Avoid prolonged sun exposure.
Neomycin-polymyxin B-gramicidin ophthalmic	Eye infections	Topical	Hx of hypersensitivity to neomycin, polymyxin, or gramicidin. Caution in pregnancy, nursing mothers.	**Anaphylaxis.** Local allergic reaction: redness, itching, swelling.	Do NOT let tip of container touch patient's eye. Do NOT use with multiple patients; may spread infection.
Promethazine	Nausea	Oral Rectal	Hx of hypersensitivity to phenothiazines.	CNS: sleep, drowsiness. Resp: depression. GI: nausea, vomiting, constipation. Skin: photosensitivity.	Avoid prolonged sun exposure.
Silver Sulfadiazine	Burns	Topical	Hx of hypersensitivity to sulfa drugs.	Local: pain, burning, itching, rash.	Normal color of cream is white; do NOT use if dark.
Diazepam	Continuous Seizures	Rectal	Hx of hypersensitivity. Narrow-angle glaucoma. Caution in pregnancy & with CNS depressants.	CNS: occasionally patients may have psychotic reactions or suicidal ideation after use.	Monitor for respiratory depression & changes in blood pressure/cardiac output.

Antiparasitic Drugs

Drug	Rt	Contraindications	Side Effects	Notes
Metronidazole	Oral	Hx of hypersensitivity. Pregnancy, nursing mothers. Patients with preexisting yeast infections.	CNS: vertigo, headache, depression, fatigue. GI: nausea, vomiting, diarrhea, abdominal cramps, constipation. GU: UTI, pelvic pressure, dryness of vagina & vulva, yeast infection.	Avoid alcohol. Pts urine may be dark or reddish brown. Discontinue if seizures or peripheral numbness develop. Supplement with acidophilus capsules and/or yogurt with live cultures.
Praziquantel	Oral	Heart, liver or kidney disease.	**Anaphylaxis.** CNS: fever, vertigo, headache, fatigue. GI: nausea, vomiting. Skin: rash.	Do not use to Tx parasitic eye infections. Do not take concurrently with rifampin.
Quinacrine hydrochloride	Oral	Pregnancy.	CNS: vertigo, headache, irritability, insomnia. GI: nausea, vomiting, diarrhea, abdominal pain. Jaundice.	Skin discoloration disappears about 2 weeks after Tx.
Tinidazole	Oral	Pregnancy, nursing mothers. Patients with preexisting yeast infections.	GI: nausea, vomiting, diarrhea, abdominal cramps, constipation. GU: UTI, pelvic pressure, dryness of vagina & vulva, yeast infection.	Supplement with acidophilus capsules and/or yogurt with live cultures.

Common Asthma Medications

Drug	Rt	Contraindications	Side Effects	Notes
Short-acting Bronchodilators				
Albuterol Levalbuterol Pirbuterol	MDI	Hx of hypersensitivity. Pregnancy, nursing mothers. Caution with cardiovascular disease & diabetes.	CNS: anxiety, headache, hallucinations. Circ: hypotension, hypertension. Eye: blurred vision. GI: nausea, vomiting. Musc: cramps.	Avoid OTC cold medications or drugs that mimic sympathetic actions.
Inhaled Corticosteroids				
Fluticasone Triamcinolone Beclomethasone	MDI DPI	Hx of hypersensitivity. Caution in pregnancy. Infections.		Often used with inhaled long-acting bronchodilators. Do NOT use for acute treatment. Rinse mouth after use.
Long-acting Bronchodilators				
Formoterol Salmeterol	MDI DPI	Hx of hypersensitivity. Pregnancy, nursing mothers. Caution with cardiovascular disease.	While decreasing the number of acute attacks, both drugs may increase severity of attacks that do occur and increase the chance of asthma-related deaths.	Use with inhaled or oral corticosteroids. Do NOT use for acute treatment.
Oral Corticosteroids				
Prednisone	PO	Hx of hypersensitivity. Caution in Pregnancy. Infections. Liver or GI Px. Ulcers.	CNS: Headache, insomnia, psychosis. Circ: CHF. GI: nausea, vomiting, ulcers. Musc: weakness. Hyperglycemia.	Avoid aspirin during Tx. Taper gradually if course is greater than a week.
Mast Cell Stabilizers				
Cromolyn sodium	MDI	Hx of hypersensitivity. Kidney/liver Px.		
Nedocromil	DPI	Hx of hypersensitivity.	CNS: headache. GI: upset stomach.	
Emergency Bronchodilator				
Epinephrine	IM	Hx of hypersensitivity. Caution in Pregnancy. Cardiac arrhythmias.	Circ: tachycardia, hypertension, MI. CNS: anxiety, severe headache, dizziness, stroke. GI: nausea, vomiting. Skin: sweating, pale.	May increase blood glucose levels; diabetic patients may have control Px.

Herbs

Common Name	Latin Name	Parts Used	Route	Action
Agrimony	Agrimonia eupatoria	aerial parts	tea	Increase clotting up to 50%. Tones mucous membranes. Slows profuse menstruation. Mouthwash, gargle, eye wash, wound irrigation.
Aloe	Aloe vera	fresh juice & gel	poultice ointment	Burns, cuts, wounds. Encourages skin regeneration.
Angelica	Angelica archangelica	roots, stems, seeds	tea	Colds. UTI. Sweat inducing expectorant. Antimicrobial. Antiseptic. Antispasmodic. Relieves abdominal cramps. Diuretic.
Arnica	Arnica montana	dried flowers, extract	poultice compress ointment	Bruises & sprains. Increases resistance to bacterial infection. Stimulates local circulation. ***Do NOT take internally.***
Astragalus	Astragalus membranaceus	root	tea	Strengthens the immune system. Use with ginseng.
Bayberry	Myrica cerifera	dried root bark	tea	Colds & fevers. Inflammation & infection of digestive tract. Antibacterial. Stimulating astringent.

Herbs continued

Common Name	Latin Name	Parts Used	Route	Action
Black Cherry	Prunus serotina	bark collected in fall	tea	Cough suppressant.
Black Cohosh	Cimicifuga racemosa	dried root, rhizome	tea	Dilates blood vessels & lowers BP. Antispasmodic. Anti-inflammatory. Reduces menstrual cramps. Relieves asthma.
Boldo	Peumus boldus	leaves	tea	UTI. Diuretic & urinary antiseptic.
Boneset	Eupatorium perfoliatum	aerial parts	tea	Colds & flu. Stimulates circulation & promotes sweating. Weak anti-inflammatory.
Catnip	Nepeta cataria	dried aerial parts	tea	Colds, flu, infectious diseases. Promotes sweating. GI sedative that counters flatulence & diarrhea. Relieves menstrual cramps.
Chamomile	Chamomilla	dried flowers	tea	Sedative. Induces sleep. Relaxes smooth muscle of the intestine & uterus. Wound irrigation (relieves pain & promotes healing). Eye wash. Antimicrobial. Antifungal. Antispasmodic. Antihistamine.
Clove	Eugenia aromatica	dried buds	oil	Relieves toothache pain.
Comfrey	Symphytum officinale	fresh or dried roots & leaves	poultice compress salve	Fractures, bruises, burns. **Do NOT use internally.**
Couch Grass	Agropyron repens	rhizome	tea	UTI. Soothing diuretic & antibacterial.
Echinacea	Echinacea	dried root, rhizome	tea	Strengthens immune system. Wound irrigation. Antibacterial & antiviral. Increases general tissue repair.
Eucalyptus	Eucalyptus	oil of leaves	oil	Strong antiseptic. Inhalation therapy for colds & flu. Chest rub. **Do NOT use internally.**
Eyebright	Euphrasia officinalis	aerial parts	tea compress	Nasal congestion. Eye infections. Mouthwash.
Evening Primrose	Oenothera lamarkiana, Oenothera biennis	extracted oil	oil	PMS. Heart disease. Reduces blood clotting & BP. Relieves menstrual cramps. GI sedative. Antiarthritis.
Five Finger Grass	Potentilla erecta	root	tea ointment	GI infections & diarrhea. Cuts & wounds. Eye wash.
Garlic	Allium sativum	cloves	crushed raw poultice	Lowers blood cholesterol & fats. Reduces BP and blood clotting. Antifungal. Antibacterial. Lowers blood sugar levels.
Ginger	Zingiber officinale	rhizome	tea raw	Nausea, sea & motion sickness, poor circulation, colds. Stimulates heart & circulation. Lowers cholesterol. Anti-inflammatory. Expectorant.
Oriental Ginseng	Panax ginseng	dried root	tea	Strengthens immune system. Especially useful for people weakened by disease.
Globe Artichoke	Cynara scolymus	flower heads, leaves, root	tea	Lowers blood cholesterol & triglyceride levels. Diuretic.
Goldenseal	Hydrastis canadensis	rhizome, roots	tea	Antibacterial & antiviral. Heals inflamed mucous membranes. Skin wash for infections. Gargle for sore throat & gums. Eye wash.
Gravel Root	Eupatorium purpureum	rhizome, roots	tea	UTI, PID, menstrual cramping. Diuretic.
Hawthorn	Crataegus oxyacanthea, Crataegus monogyna	rhizome, roots	tea	Dilates coronary & peripheral arteries. Slows pulse & reduces high BP. Relieves S/Sx of Raynauds disease.
Hops	Humulus lupulus, Humulus americana	dried female strobiles	tea	Relaxes the smooth muscle of the digestive tract. Antibacterial. Anti-inflammatory.

Herbs continued

Common Name	Latin Name	Parts Used	Route	Action
Horse Chestnut	Aesculus hippocastanum	fruit, bark	tea ointment	Strengthens veins. Externally for Hemorrhoids. **Nuts are poisonous.**
Hyssop	Hyssopus officinalis	flowering herb	tea compress	Use internally in small doses. Expectorant. Externally for bruises, burns & cold sores.
Jewelweed	Inpatiens pallida	stems, leaves	raw juice ointment	Juice from crushed stems & leaves prevents or relieves poison ivy.
Licorice	Glycyrrhiza glabra	roots, runners	tea	Colds & lung infections. Wound irrigation.
Lily of the Valley	Convallaria majalis	leaves	tea	Increases strength of heart contractions. Lowers high BP. Encourages arterial vasodilation. Diuretic.
Lung Wort	Pulmonaria officinalis	dried flowering plant	tea	Soothing expectorant.
Mullein	Verbascum thapsus	leaves, flowers	tea	Soothing expectorant. GI sedative. Diuretic. Wound irrigation.
Osha	Ligusticum porteri	root	tea	Colds & lung infections. Wound irrigation.
Parsley	Petroselinum crispum	leaves, roots, seeds	tea	UTI. Strong diuretic.
Peppermint	Mentha piperita	flowering herb	tea	Antispasmotic effect on smooth muscle of the digestive tract. Anti-inflammatory. Antibacterial & antiparasitic.
Pleurisy Root	Asciepias tuberosa	root	tea	Sweat-inducing expectorant. Respiratory sedative.
Northern & Southern Prickly Ash	Zanthoxylum	bark, berries	tea	Stimulates circulatory system. Promotes peripheral circulation, sweating & reduces fevers. Chew bark for toothache.
Prickly Pear	Opuntia	inner flesh, flowers	raw juice poultice tea	Externally for bruises & burns. Take juice internally for anti-inflammatory diuretic. Reduces pain associated with UTI. Adult onset diabetes. Tea from flowers strengthens capillary beds & submucosa.
Rue	Ruta graveolens	aerial parts	ointment	Strains & sprains. Chilblains. Strengthens blood vessels.
Sage	Salvia officinalis, Salvia lyrata, Salvia urticifolia	leaves	tea	Antibacterial & antiseptic. Stops sweating. Strengthens the nervous system. Relieves congested sinuses & eustachian tubes. Steam can be inhaled. Mix with apple cider vinegar & gargle for sore throat.
Slippery Elm	Ulmus fulva	inner bark	tea poultice	Diarrhea. Lubricates & relieves GI irritation. Wounds.
Skunk Cabbage	Symplocarpus foetidus	root	tea	Antispasmodic & expectorant with sedative properties.
Thyme	Thymus vulgaris, Thymus serpyllum, Thymus pulegioides	flowering aerial parts	tea	Sore throats, colds, cough. Antibacterial & antifungal. Antispasmodic. Sweat-inducing expectorant. Gargle. Relieves flatulence.
Witch Hazel	Hamamelis virginiana	leaves, bark	tea compress	Bruises. Stops mild bleeding. Eye wash.
White & Black Willow	Salix	bark	tea	Fevers, arthritis. Antipyretic. Antireheumatic. Analgesic. **Do NOT give to persons allergic to aspirin.**
Yarrow	Achellea millefolium, Achellea lanulosa	aerial parts, especially flowering heads	tea	Sweat inducing. Reduces fever. Expels toxins. Anti-inflammatory. Lowers BP.

SECTION XI

First Aid Kits

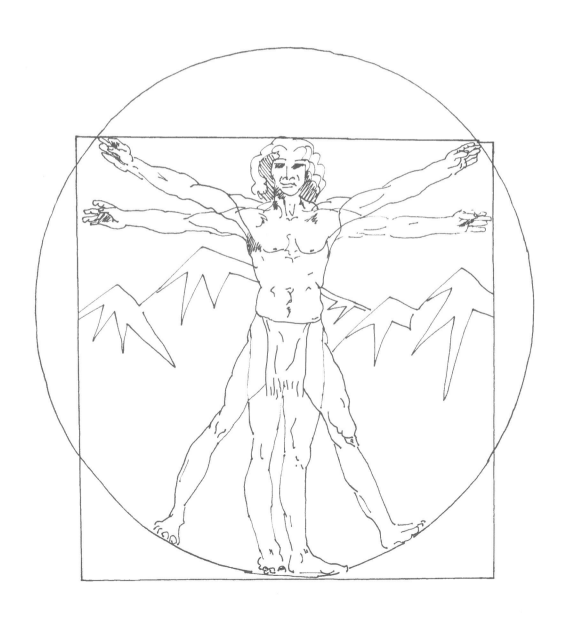

First Aid Kits
Introduction

Whether you are traveling alone, taking part in an expedition, or responding as a member of a search and rescue (SAR) team, you will need a first aid kit. What you should carry and how you should package it depends on many things. *There is no generic first aid kit.* Here are a few basic concepts that you will need to know in order to begin building a first aid kit that will meet your needs.

Size and Weight

The type of activity or expedition will dictate the amount of weight and space available for your kit. For example, a sailboat can carry more than a raft and a raft can carry more than a climber, etc. The farther you are from "help," generally the larger your first aid kit needs to be; consider resupplying your kit one or more times on a longer expedition. The level of training of the medical "officer" will also limit the amount of invasive equipment or prescription drugs that you can carry. Have each expedition or team member complete a thorough medical form well in advance of the trip. You may need to add special equipment or medications to your kit depending upon the needs of the expedition members. Pay attention to any allergies. If your experience in wilderness medicine is limited, consider carrying the Wilderness Medicine Training Center's waterproof field manual, *the Wilderness Medicine Handbook.* In addition consider carrying their weatherproof *Patient SOAP Notes* to thoroughly document your assessment and treatment. Remember to bring a pen and/or pencil.

Expedition and SAR Team Kits

First aid kits used by expeditions are conceptually very different from those used by Search and Rescue teams. Expeditions hope that they will NOT use their first aid kits and adhere to the principles of improvisation: They limit specialized items, focus on multipurpose equipment, and adapt expedition gear for medical uses. As your ability to improvise increases, the size of your expedition first aid kit decreases. SAR teams know they WILL use their equipment and often carry specialized gear with them rather than scavenging their gear for improvisation.

Packaging

Packaging is extremely important. Well thought-out and organized packaging protects valuable and irreplaceable equipment. It permits fast and easy access to emergency gear without "vomiting" kit contents everywhere. Critical concepts to organization and packaging are:

- Use different colored pockets, compartments, and/or packs for organizing related items so they can be found quickly and easily; avoid using plastic bags as pack or compartment substitutes. Clearly label each compartment or pack. First aid kits may be organized according to use: For example, materials used to treat basic life support problems (or emergencies) are packed in one pack, items used to treat minor traumatic problems in another pack, and medications in a third pack. In many expeditions, each member carries their own personal care kit that includes items for treating minor blisters, cuts, and scrapes. The kit also includes any personal prescription and over-the-counter medications, and personal-care items, such as sunscreen, tampons, etc. In addition to helping ensure the expedition first aid kit is complete when it is needed, having each individual carry a personal care kit with commonly used first aid items reduces the overall weight and size of the expedition first aid kit by focusing its contents on minor and major trauma, environmental emergencies, and expedition-based medical problems.

- Laminate a contents list for each pack and include the intended use for each item.

- Protect soft goods from moisture by placing them in individual mini self-sealing bags (Ziplock®) or vacuum sealed in heavy-duty plastic (Seal-a-Meal®).

- Tubes break. Repackage ointments in wide-mouth Nalgene® bottles.

- Liquids leak. Package liquids in narrow-mouth Nalgene® bottles.

- Use a weatherproof logbook for ALL medications so that you know who is using them and why. The log should include space for the patient's name, drug name, administration route, dose, time, and reason/diagnosis.

Training

Train expedition members to use your kit. Until they are trained, only you know why you assembled the kit as you did. Without specific training, most people will not know how to use the equipment you have so thoughtfully assembled. Restrict access to compartments or packs that members are not trained to use.

An effective first aid kit is built from a comprehensive possible problem list. A checklist for many possible problems and first aid supplies follows; use it as a guide. In remote areas, consider a resupply.

Within the United States a physician consultation and prescription is required for all prescription drugs.

Basic Life Support and Major Trauma

Possible Problem	First Aid Supplies
Respiratory Distress and Arrest	~ Simple face mask or face shield (or commit to mouth-to-mouth rescue breathing) ~ Pulse oximeter
Cardiac Arrest	~ AED (only if Advanced Life Support and transport are available)
Severe Bleeding	~ Trauma scissors ~ Trauma gloves ~ Trauma dressings (maxi-pads, diapers) ~ Elastic wrap or self-adhering bandage(s) for pressure bandages
Vomiting	~ 60 cc suction syringe and tube
Unstable Spine	~ Safety pin for spine assessment ~ SAM splint (for improvised C-collar) ~ Improvise a backboard or litter from expedition equipment
Urgent Evacuation	~ Detailed Emergency Action Plan ~ Cell phone, radio or satellite phone

Minor Trauma

Possible Problem	First Aid Supplies
Stable and Unstable Extremity Injuries	~ Improvise splint from expedition equipment ~ SAM splint and self-adhering bandage (vet wrap) ~ Pain and anti-inflammatory drugs and herbs
Friction Blisters	~ Tincture of Benzoin ~ Cloth or flexible medical tape ~ 2nd Skin® for treating blisters ~ ENGO® for blister prevention and treatment
Superficial and Partial-thickness Wounds	~ Aloe Vera gel and Vitamin E gel for superficial wounds ~ White/light petroleum jelly for partial-thickness wounds
Full-thickness Wounds	~ Irrigation syringe ~ Scalpel and blades and/or surgical scissors ~ Forceps or tweezers ~ Exam gloves ~ Povidone-iodine solution ~ Steri-strips®, super glue or skin adhesive, suture kit or wound staples ~ Local analgesic for infiltrating wound prior to cleaning ~ Topical and oral herbs and antibiotics (Rx) ~ Micro-thin film dressing (Tegaderm®) ~ Roller gauze for cleaning, packing and dressing ~ Self-adhering bandage for holding dressing in place

Environmental Problems

Possible Problem	First Aid Supplies
Hypothermia	~ Hypothermia thermometer ~ Space bag for inner vapor barrier of hypothermia package ~ Improvise hypothermia package and heat packs from hydropacks, water bottles, etc. and other expedition equipment
Heat Illnesses	~ Mist bottle for cooling in arid climates ~ Extended-range digital thermometer ~ Oral rehydration solution/salts
Sun Exposure	~ Sun block ~ Aloe Vera gel and Vitamin E gel for superficial wounds
Allergic Reactions	~ Epinephrine (Rx) for anaphylaxis ~ OTC oral antihistamine (Benadryl®)
Poison Ivy, Oak and Sumac	~ Pre-exposure lotion ~ Post-exposure soap (Tecnu Oak and Ivy Cleanser®, Goop®) ~ Post-exposure treatment (Tecnu Extreme Gel®)
Acute Mountain Sickness	~ Herbs: Ginkgo biloba ~ AMS (Rx) drugs ~ Portable hyperbaric chamber
Sea and Motion Sickness	~ Scopolamine tablets or patch (Rx) ~ Herb: Ginger root ~ Wrist bands (acupressure) ~ OTC and Rx antihistamines ~ Hypodermoclysis (HDC) infusion set for dehydration (Rx)

Medical Problems

Possible Problem	First Aid Supplies
Disease	~ Disease-specific Rx drugs ~ Disease-specific herbs
Angina and Heart Attack	~ Chewable baby aspirin ~ Nitroglycerin (Rx) ~ AED (if ALS and rapid evacuation are possible)
Diabetes	~ OTC Glucose tablets and paste ~ Glucagon kit (Rx) ~ Urine test strips for ketones
Asthma	~ Asthma medication (Rx oral, inhalers) ~ Epinephrine (Rx)
Pain	~ NSAIDs (Ibuprofen or Naproxen preferred) ~ Rx codeine-based pain meds
Nosebleed Broken Nose	~ Vasoconstricting nasal spray or drops ~ Gauze, small tampons, or commercial nasal tampons ~ Petroleum jelly, saline gel, or aloe vera gel for moisturizing dry nasal passages

Medical Problems continued

Possible Problem	First Aid Supplies
Nausea/Vomiting	~ Ondansetron ODT (Rx, preferred) or promethazine suppositories (Rx); preload Tx with promethazine suppositories with OTC diphenhydramine
Diarrhea	~ OTC Loperamide
Constipation	~ OTC stool softener, lubricating agent, osmotic agent, intestinal stimulant, or bulking agent
Acid Stomach	~ OTC antacid, proton pump inhibitor
Foreign Body Corneal Abrasion Corneal Ulcer Chemicals Photokeratitis Conjunctivitis	~ Synthetic wetting solution (artificial tears) ~ Cotton-tipped applicators to invert eyelids ~ Fluorescein strips/solution and cobalt blue light for assessment ~ Ophthalmic anesthetic to control pain during assessment ~ Sterile saline and/or irrigation syringe for flushing eye ~ Ophthalmic antibiotic ointment/solution for bacterial eye infections ~ Ophthalmic NSAID solution to control pain during healing ~ Rx pain meds to control severe pain during evacuation
External Ear Infection Middle/Inner Ear Infection Ruptured Ear Drum	~ Otoscope (for assessment) ~ Vinegar or GSE to treat external ear infections ~ Rx antibiotic drops to treat external ear infections ~ Rx antibiotics to treat middle or inner ear infections ~ Mineral oil, alcohol, and irrigation syringe for removing ear wax ~ Ear plugs to prevent or treat external ear infections and ruptured ear drums in a wet environment
Broken Teeth Avulsed Teeth Lost Fillings and Crowns Infected Teeth and Gums	~ Cavit® is a dental putty/cement without oil of clove ~ Dentemp® is a dental putty/cement with oil of clove ~ Oil of clove topical analgesic ~ Cavity varnish to seal and protect tooth repairs (paint on) ~ NSAIDS and Rx analgesics for pain ~ Dental mirror and probe/forceps to see/work in patient's mouth
Vaginitis	~ Supplemental bacteria (yogurt, acidophilus capsules, etc.) for women taking antibiotics to help prevent yeast infections ~ OTC vaginal suppositories or creams for yeast infections ~ Rx vaginal suppositories or creams for bacterial infections ~ Rx oral antimicrobials for protozoal infections
Urinary Tract Infection	~ Urine test strips for nitrites ~ Over-the-counter Phenazopyridine (AZO®, Uristat®) relieves S/Sx but is not a cure; use for two days maximum during evacuation. ~ Rx antibiotics
Tinea Fungal Infections	~ OTC creams, lotions, and powders ~ Rx oral antifungal meds, creams, and lotions
Ectopic Pregnancy	~ Early pregnancy test (EPT)
Seizures/Epilepsy	~ Rectal Diazepam for stopping continuous seizures

If size, weight, and space restrictions, and medical training permit, consider carrying: a blood pressure cuff and stethoscope, advanced airways, oxygen, BVM, Foley catheter kit, and chest tube set.

SECTION XII

Medical Abbreviations & Symbols

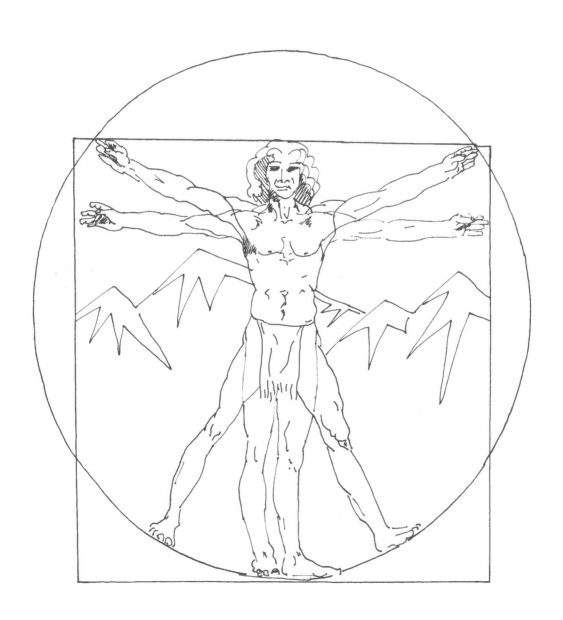

Abbreviations

A

AED	Automated External Defibrillator
ALS	Advanced Life Support
AMS	Acute Mountain Sickness
ASR	Autonomic Stress Response
AVPU	Alert, Voice-responsive, Pain-responsive, Unresponsive

B

bid	twice a day
BLS	Basic Life Support
BP	Blood Pressure
BSI	Body Substance Isolation

C

c̄	with
c/o	complaining of
cc	cubic centimeter
CC	Chief Complaint
CCR	Cardiocerebral Resuscitation
CHF	Congestive Heart Failure
CNS	Central Nervous System
CPR	Cardiopulmonary Resuscitation
CSF	Cerebral Spinal Fluid
CSM	Circulation, Sensation, Motor
CVA	Stroke

D

Dx	diagnosis
DDx	differential diagnosis
DKA	diabetic ketoacidosis
DPI	Dry Powder Inhaler

E

ET	Endotracheal Tube

F

Fx	Fracture

G

g	gram
GI	Gastrointestinal
GSE	Grapefruit Seed Extract
gtts	drops
GU	Genitourinary

H

HACE	Hige Altitude Cerebral Edema
HAPE	High Altitude Pulmonary Edema
Hx	History

I

IM	Intramuscular
ICP	Intracranial Pressure
IO	Interosseous
IV	Intravenous

K

kg	kilogram

L

lb	pound
L	liter
LOC	Loss of Consciousness

M

MDI	Multi Dose Inhaler
MDR	Mammalian Diving Reflex
mg	milligram
MI	Myocardial Infarction
MOI	Mechanism of Injury/Illness

N

N/V	Nausea/Vomiting

O

OTC	Over the Counter

P

PAC	Portable Altitude Chamber
PEA	Pulseless Electrical Activity
PAS	Patient Assessment System
PFA	Pain Free Activity
PE	Pulmonary Embolism
PI	Povidone Iodine
PO	By mouth
PPV	Positive Pressure Ventilations
PR	By rectal administration
PRN	as necessary
Pt	Patient
Px	Problem

Q

q	every
qd	every day
qid	four times a day
qod	every other day

R

RICE	Rest, Ice, Compression, Elevation
RO	Rule Out
ROM	Range of Motion
Rt	Route
Rx	Prescription

S

s̄	without
S/Sx	Signs/Symptoms
SOB	Short of Breath
SPF	Sun Protection Factor
STD	Sexually Transmitted Disease
SQ	Subcutaneous

T

TBSA	Total Body Surface Area
tid	three times a day
TIP	Traction into Position
tsp	teaspoon
tbls, tbsp	tablespoon
Tx	Treatment

V

VF	Ventricular Fibrillation
VT	Ventricular Tachycardia

Y

y/o	year old

Symbols

2°	secondary; due to
+	positive; good
−	negative; poor
Δ	change
↑	increasing
↓	decreasing
♂	male
♀	female
±	with or without

SECTION XIII

Wilderness Medicine Training Center's
Patient SOAP Note

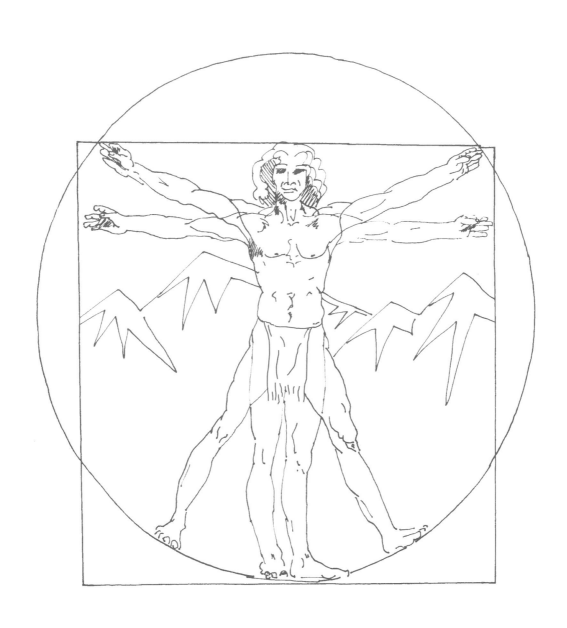

Patient SOAP Note

The following two pages show a Patient SOAP Note from the Wilderness Medicine Training Center. This SOAP note is designed to be printed on 8.5 by 11 inch legal paper and may be folded into thirds so it takes up less space in your first aid kit. The front side contains space for the patient's contact information, Basic Life Support assessment and treatment, SAMPLE History, Physical Exam, Vital Signs, and the results of the focused spine assessment if the MOI is trauma.

Patient SOAP Note

Lead rescuer's name

Patient information

Name

Age	Weight		Male	Female
Address			Phone	
			Date	
			Time	
Contact Person				
			Phone	

Describe MOI ☐ Trauma ☐ Environmental ☐ Medical

If Trauma, tell a brief story that addresses speed, dispersal of KE, & location of impact.

Describe weather conditions

Temp _____ ☐ Sun ☐ Partly Cloudy ☐ Overcast ☐ Wind ☐ Rain ☐ Snow

Patient found
☐ Right Side ☐ Left Side
☐ Front ☐ Back
☐ Sitting ☐ Standing ☐ Walking

Initial PX
☐ No Respirations ☐ No Pulse ☐ Vomiting
☐ Unstable Spine ☐ Severe Bleeding
☐ Blocked Airway ☐ V P U on arrival

Initial treatment

☐ Direct Pressure ☐ Pressure Dressing ☐ Tourniquet
☐ Chest Compressions ☐ Rescue Breathing ☐ Abdominal Thrust ☐ Suction
☐ C-Collar ☐ Stabilize Spine ☐ Remove Wet Clothes ☐ Hypothermia Package
☐ Cool Pt ☐ Glucose ☐ Med ☐ Shelter ☐ Evac 1 2

Subjective Information = What the patient tells you

Symptoms = Describe onset, cause, and severity (1-10) of chief complaints.

Time

Allergies = Local or systemic, cause, severity and treatment.

Medications = prescription, over-the-counter, herbal, homeopathic, & recreational.

DRUG	REASON	DOSE	CURRENT
			Yes / No
			Yes / No

Notes

Past relevant medical history = Relate to MOI

Last food & fluids = Intake & Output

H₂O	Calories	Electrolytes
Urine Color	Urine Output	Stool

Events = Patient's description of what happened.   Memory Loss Yes / No

---

Objective Information = What you see

Physical exam = Look for discoloration, swelling, abnormal fluid loss, & deformity. Feel for tenderness, crepitus, & instability. Check ROM & CSM.

Time

Vital Signs = Get a baseline, then record changes. Record normal VS if known.

Time	Pulse	Resp	O₂ Sat	BP	Skin	Temp	AVPU
Normal							

Focused spine assessment

Time	Yes	No		Yes	No	
	☐	☐	Reliable Patient	☐	☐	Squeeze 1st & Ring Finger
☐ Pass	☐	☐	Spine Pain	☐	☐	Press Down on Hand or Fingers
☐ Fail	☐	☐	Spine Tenderness	☐	☐	Press Up on Foot or Big Toe
	☐	☐	Shooting Pain	☐	☐	Press Down on Foot or Big Toe
	☐	☐	Distinguish between Pinprick & Light Touch on hands and feet			

wildmedcenter.com

The back side of the note contains a Possible Problem List, a Current Problem List, and an Anticipated Problem list together with your treatment and evacuation plans, rescuer and witness contact information, and a call log. You can purchase a paper Patient SOAP Note tablet and/or individual weatherproof Patient SOAP Notes from the Wilderness Medicine Training Center's website store at http://wildmedcenter.com/store.html. You may also download a pdf file of the SOAP note at no charge for your personal use.

Additional Information

RESCUER 1 Name _____ Age ____
Male ____ Female ____
E-mail _____
Address _____ Phone ____ Cell ____ Organization ____

RESCUER 2 Name _____ Age ____
Male ____ Female ____
E-mail _____
Address _____ Phone ____ Cell ____ Organization ____

WITNESS 1 Name _____ Age ____
Male ____ Female ____
E-mail _____
Address _____ Phone ____ Cell ____ Relationship ____

WITNESS 2 Name _____ Age ____
Male ____ Female ____
E-mail _____
Address _____ Phone ____ Cell ____ Relationship ____

WITNESS 3 Name _____ Age ____
Male ____ Female ____
E-mail _____
Address _____ Phone ____ Cell ____ Relationship ____

EMERGENCY CALL LOG

Time	Number	Person/Organization

Plan = What you are going to do

FIELD TREATMENT
Time

MONITOR

EVACUATION PLAN

Time	Level		Type		
	1 2 3 4	☐ None ☐ Self ☐ Assist	☐ Carry ☐ Litter ☐ Vehicle		
	1 2 3 4	☐ None ☐ Self ☐ Assist	☐ Carry ☐ Litter ☐ Vehicle		
	1 2 3 4	☐ None ☐ Self ☐ Assist	☐ Carry ☐ Litter ☐ Vehicle		

Assessment = What you think is wrong

POSSIBLE PX	TIME	CURRENT PX	ANTICIPATED PX
Traumatic Px			
Unstable Spine			
Concussion / ↑ ICP			
Trunk Injury			
Respiratory Distress			
Volume Shock			
Unstable Extremity Injury			
Stable Extremity Injury			
Wounds			
Environmental Px			
Dehydration / Low Sodium			
Cold / Hypothermia			
Heat Exhaustion / Stroke			
Frostbite / Burns			
Local / Systemic Toxin			
Local / Systemic Allergy			
Near Drowning			
Acute Mountain Sickness			
Lightning			
SCUBA / Free Diving			
Medical Px			
Circulatory System Px			
Respiratory System Px			
Nervous System Px			
Endocrine System Px			
Gastrointestinal System Px			
Genitourinary System Px			
Ear Px			
Eye Px			
Tooth & Gum Px			
Skin Px			
Infectious Disease			

RED FLAGS FOR URGENT MEDICAL PROBLEMS

ADDITIONAL PATIENT NOTES

Patient SOAP Note 269

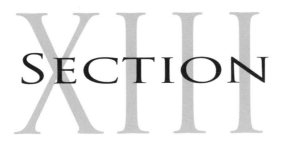

Section XIII

Problem & Treatment Index

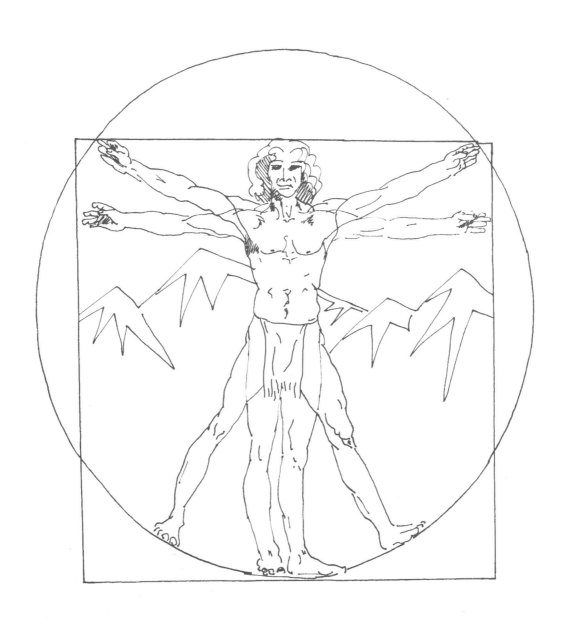